Comprehensive
PAEDIATRIC NURSING

Comprehensive

PAEDIATRIC NURSING

By

Rajalakshmi Murugan

Assistant Professor and Head
Department of Paediatric Nursing, Centralized
School of Nursing Faculty of Medicine,
Addis Ababa University, Ethiopia

Reviewed by

Dr Amha Mekasha

Associate Professor
Paediatric and Child Health Department, and
Head of Medical Education in Ethiopia Unit,
Addis Ababa University, Ethiopia

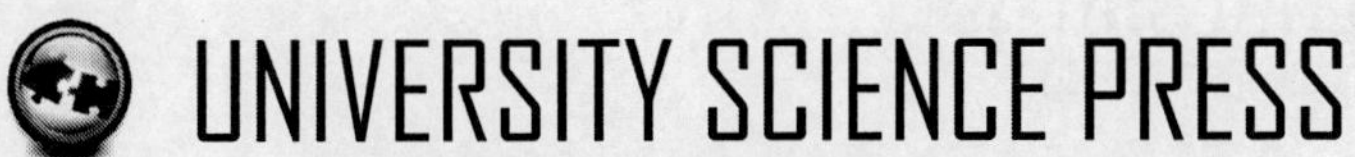

UNIVERSITY SCIENCE PRESS

(An Imprint of Laxmi Publications Pvt. Ltd.)

An ISO 9001:2008 Company

BENGALURU • CHENNAI • COCHIN • GUWAHATI • HYDERABAD
JALANDHAR • KOLKATA • LUCKNOW • MUMBAI • RANCHI • NEW DELHI
BOSTON (USA) • ACCRA (GHANA) • NAIROBI (KENYA)

Comprehensive **PADIATRIC NURSING**

Printed and bound in India
Typeset at Sukuvisa Enterprises, Delhi
First Edition : 2012, Reprint 2013, Second Edition : 2017
ISBN 978-93-81159-30-9

Branches

	Branch	Phone	
✆	Bengaluru	080-26 75 69 30	
✆	Chennai	044-24 34 47 26,	24 35 95 07
✆	Cochin	0484-237 70 04,	405 13 03
✆	Guwahati	0361-254 36 69,	251 38 81
✆	Hyderabad	040-27 55 53 83,	27 55 53 93
✆	Jalandhar	0181-222 12 72	
✆	Kolkata	033-22 27 43 84	
✆	Lucknow	0522-220 99 16	
✆	Mumbai	022-24 91 54 15,	24 92 78 69
✆	Ranchi	0651-220 44 64	

PUBLISHED IN INDIA BY

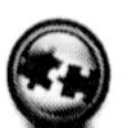

UNIVERSITY SCIENCE PRESS
(An Imprint of Laxmi Publications Pvt. Ltd.)

An ISO 9001:2008 Company
113, GOLDEN HOUSE, DARYAGANJ,
NEW DELHI - 110002, INDIA
Telephone : 91-11-4353 2500, 4353 2501
Fax : 91-11-2325 2572, 4353 2528
www.laxmipublications.com info@laxmipublications.com

C—
Printed at: Repro Knowledgecast Limited, Thane

To my beloved Parents
and
All children in Ethiopia, who could have benefited
from treatment of different diseases and
appropriate nursing care

FOREWORD

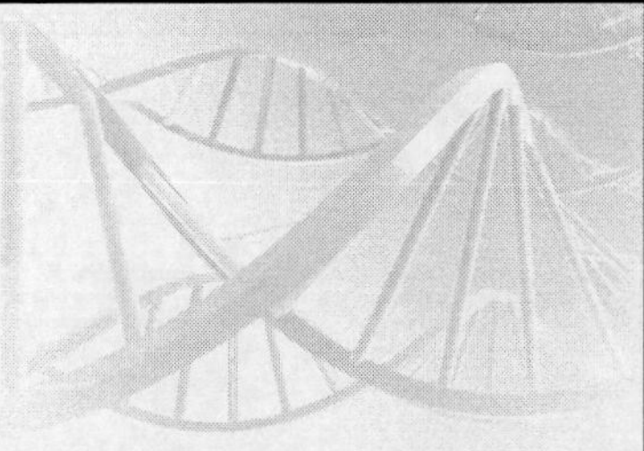

As the number of children in the world, younger than age 15 increases annually, now representing more than 30% of the total population. It becomes apparent that clinical nursing and midwifery students need to know about well-child health care, acute and chronic diseases states in paediatric population and appropriate nursing intervention. Recognizing development stages, acquiring skills and teaching families are critical in the care of children and require different skill sets than caring for adults. Nurses and midwives with strong grasp of these important concepts are in a good position to help the families deal with everyday situation, resulting in positive outcomes for their children. Unfortunately, the clinical experience in the care of children are commonly limited in nursing programmes because most ill children are cared for in the home and hospital stays are short. Therefore, to be well prepared to care for these patients and their families and to have adequate knowledge and competence on paediatric practice.

This edition has a wide range of coverage and includes the relevant issues of all paediatric diseases and care. The book also has evidence based neonatal and children interventions, including instructional and community based care aspects.

Mrs Rajalakshmi has worked hard to structure the text especially according to our context, so this book is educationally sound and very relevant in the field of neonatal and child health nursing. It is my sincere belief that this book will contribute to reduce the neonatal and child mortality and morbidity in this country, besides it helps to overcome the shortage of paediatric nursing textbook. I appreciate her efforts to our nursing profession especially for child health, surely all nursing and midwifery students will get benefit from this book.

Mr Asrat Demisse

Director, Centralized School of Nursing

Faculty of Medicine, Addis Ababa University

Ethiopia

PREFACE TO THE SECOND EDITION

This fully revised book, now in its Second Edition, continues to provide a compact state of the art resource for clinicians in simple, lucid and user-friendly manner for easy understanding.

I have received numerous emails, and letters from readers commenting on the book and suggesting how it could be improved. With the aid of all this information, I have completely revised. In this Edition, new topics such as paediatric formulas, calculation of drugs, degrees of malnutrition as for IPA/WHO, calculation of weight according to age, and to find out the degree of malnutrition, identification of dehydration, current immunization schedule, and breast feeding and calculation of artificial feeding have been included at appropriate places. Some sections are also updated to enrich the contents.

Let me thank everyone who has provided me with suggestions and corrections for improving the First Edition. I am extraordinarily grateful to them all.

Author

PREFACE TO THE FIRST EDITION

It gives me immense pleasure and satisfaction in introducing *Comprehensive Paediatric Nursing* to the Ethiopian society. Today nurses are challenged to make quick yet critical and update clinical practice about variety of patient's/client's problems occurring within the context of a complex and rapidly health care system. Our nursing profession is increasingly in the development of scientific knowledge related to its practice. I have been teaching paediatric nursing in Ethiopia for the last 8 years. There is no adequate books and those available are costly and of the standard of developed countries. Keeping in view the problems and needs of Ethiopian nursing students and nurses, I conceived the idea of writing a book on paediatric nursing since there is a lacunae of such books in Ethiopia by the local authors.

This edition of the *Comprehensive Paediatric Nursing* provides a compact state of the art resource for clinicians in simple, lucid and user-friendly language for easy understanding. It has been designed to ensure that specific information can easily be identified and applied in clinical setting. This book provides special information on Care of Children with HIV/AIDS and Integrated Management of Neonatal Childhood Illness (IMNCI).

The text of the book has been divided into 14 chapters. Chapter 1 focuses on growth and development and includes concepts, principles, theories, assessing and measuring of growth and development from newborn to adolescent period. Chapter 2 provides an essential component of the physical assessment like purpose, approaches and detailed physical examination. Chapter 3 provides a summary of twenty neonatal common health problems and interventions. Each illness/disorders includes concise description of the problems, schematic presentation of pathophysiology, clinical sign and symptoms, investigations, treatment and nursing management. Chapter 4 deals with the care of newborn with congenital anomalies. It includes anomalies of each organ system in detail. Chapter 5 provides the details of altered respiratory conditions. It includes etiology, pathophysiology, clinical manifestations, treatment and nursing management. Chapter 6 details the alteration in cardiovascular functions and their management. Chapter 7 describes the details of altered gastrointestinal functions and their nursing management. Chapter 8 deals with the alterations in genitourinary functions and their nursing care. Chapter 9 provides the information about neurological disorders and the role of nursing care in their management. Chapter 10 deals with the management and care of altered musculoskeletal conditions. Chapter 11 provides the details of altered haematological conditions, their management and nursing care. Chapter 12 is specially devoted to the causes, pathophysiology, complications, clinical manifestations, investigations, medical management and nursing care of common oncological conditions and Chapter 13 deals with altered endocrine conditions, finally Chapter 14 describes care of children with HIV/AIDS.

I hope the *Comprehensive Paediatric Nursing* will fill the gap for a book on paediatric nursing in the Ethiopian context as well as for developing countries. This book will provide enough knowledge related to paediatric nursing and enable the students to apply it in clinical practice and it will be definitely useful for faculty who is teaching paediatric nursing.

The suggestions for improvement would be gratefully accepted and will be incorporated in next revised edition.

Author

ACKNOWLEDGEMENTS

I take this opportunity to express my deepest sense of gratitude to *Mr Asrat Demisse, Director of School of Nursing, Addis Ababa University* and the *President, Ethiopian Nurses Association* for his inspiration for writing this book, great encouragement and cordial support.

I am deeply appreciative of *Dr Amha Mekasha, Associate Professor of Paediatrics and Child Health, Medical Faculty, Addis Ababa University* for his valuable guidance and wholehearted efforts in editing the book.

I am greatly indebted to all my professional colleagues and friends in the institution who have initiated and encouraged me to write this textbook.

Finally not least but most, my acknowledgement goes to my sons and husband Mr Murugan for their enthusiastic encouragement and continuous effort to complete this book.

I also take this opportunity to express my heartfelt thanks to management, consultant and the staff of Laxmi Publications Pvt. Ltd. for giving proper shape to bring out and efforts to publish the first Indian book in the field of nursing in Ethiopia.

Author

CONTENTS

LIST OF PLATES

LIST OF FIGURES

LIST OF TABLES

Introduction To Paediatric Nursing

PRINCIPLES OF PAEDIATRIC NURSING

Patient Population

- Children from birth to adolescence.
- Care spans the continuum from well-child care to illness and death.

Intervention Goals and Considerations

- All interventions are family-centered: The child and family are treated as a unit.
- Interventions are geared towards helping the child and family unit attain, maintain, or regain optimal health.
- Health interventions are guided primarily by the children's level of development and secondarily by chronological age.

ROLE OF THE NURSE IN PAEDIATRIC OR CHILD HEALTH

Clinical Practice

Paediatric nursing focuses on protecting children from illness and injury, assisting them to attain optimal levels of health, regardless of health problems, and rehabilitation. The scope of nursing practice encompasses, "the diagnosis and treatment of human responses to actual or potential health problem." The nursing roles in caring for children and their families include direct care, patient education, advocacy and case management.

Direct Nursing Care

The primary role of paediatric nurse is to provide direct nursing care to children and their families. The nursing process provides the framework for delivery of direct paediatric nursing care. The nurse assesses the child, identifies the nursing diagnosis that describes the responses of the child and family to the illness or injury, and implements and evaluates nursing care. This care is designed to meet the child's physical and emotional needs. It is tailored to the child's developmental stage, giving the child additional responsibility for self-care with increasing age.

Nurses play an important role in minimizing the psychological and physical distress experienced by children and their families. Providing support to children and their families is one component of direct nursing care. This often involves listening to the concerns of children and parents, being present during stressful or emotional experiences, and implement strategies to help children and family members. Nurses can help families by suggesting ways to support their children in the hospital, and in the home.

Patient Education

In paediatric nursing, patient education is especially challenging, because nurses must be prepared to work with children at various levels of understanding and to change the behaviour of family members.

As patient educators, nurses help children adapt to the hospital setting and prepare them for procedures. Most hospitals encourage parent to stay with the child and to provide advanced care. Taking an active role prepares the parent to assume total responsibility for care after the child leaves the hospital.

Counselling is another form of patient education. Counselling may involve provision of information such as injury-prevention strategies and anticipatory guidance to promote development. Advance practicing nurse or other experienced nurse is often responsible for counselling. That is directed towards helping them or family in solving a problem.

Patient's Advocacy

Advocacy acting to safeguard and advance the interests of another is directed at enabling the child and family to adjust to the changes in the child's health in their own way. To be an effective advocate, the nurse must be aware of the child's and the family's needs, the family's resources, and the health care services available in the hospital and the community. The nurse can then assist the family and the child to make informed choices about these services and to act in the child's best interests.

Nurse, acting as an advocate also ensures that the policies and resources of health care agencies meet the psychosocial needs of child and its family. The nurse must also protect the child and its family by taking appropriate actions against any incidents of incompetent, unethical, or illegal practice by any member of the health care team.

Case Management

What happens when a child has significant health problems? Can you handle it all?

When a child has a significant health problem or handicapping condition, health care professionals (physician, nurse, social worker, physical and occupational therapist, and other specialist) create an interdisciplinary plan to meet the child's medical, nursing, developmental, educational, and psychosocial needs. Because nurse spends large amounts of time providing nursing care for the child and family, she often knows more than other health care professionals about the family's wishes and resources. As a member of the interdisciplinary care plan team, the nurse serves as an advocate to ensure that the care plan considers the family's wishes and contains appropriate services. The nurse often becomes the child's case manager, coordinating the implementation of the interdisciplinary care plan. Sometimes, the parent or a social worker becomes the case manager.

Case management is a process of coordinating the delivery of health care services in a manner that focuses on both quality and cost outcomes. This is often a collaborative practice with other health care providers that promotes continuity of care, an interdisciplinary process of facilitating a patient's transition between and among settings based on changing needs and available resources. The nurse as case manager has control over the use of health care resources that are considered appropriate for the patient's condition and links the child and family to these services. The goal is to help the child and family to have the best health care outcome and decrease fragmentation of care, while controlling the cost of health care services. Case management may be used for the care of the patient when hospitalized as well as for long-term care of chronic conditions.

Discharge planning is a form of case management. Good discharge planning promotes a smooth, rapid, and safe transition into the community and improves the results of treatment begun in the hospital. To be a discharge planner, the nurse needs to know about community medical resources, home care agencies qualified to care for children, educational interventions, and services reimbursed by the child's health plan or other financial resources.

NURSING PROCESS IN PAEDIATRIC CARE

Can you describe how the five steps of the nursing process relate to children? Paediatric nurse uses the nursing process to identify and solve problems and to plan patient care. The systematic framework for practice that the nursing process provides is the same for paediatric patients as for other patients.

- Assessment involves collecting patient and family data and performing physical examinations during community-based health services, at admission, periodically during the child's hospitalization, and when home care services are provided. The nurse analyzes and synthesizes data to make a judgment about the patient's problems.
- Nursing diagnoses describe the health promotion and health patterns that nurse can manage. Once health patterns have been identified, specific nursing actions can be planned.
- Nursing care plans are based on goals that will improve the child's or family's dysfunctional health patterns. Specific expected outcomes should be realistic. The family and the nurse (and the child, when old enough) should agree with care plan goals.

  Standard care plans for specific diagnosis are often used in the paediatric unit of the hospital and by home health agencies. The nurse is responsible for individualizing standard care plans based on data collected from the child's assessment and from evaluation of the child's response to care. Individualized nursing action plans provide directions for nursing care.
- Implementation is the carrying out of interventions outlined in the nursing care plan. Interventions may be modified if the child's response is undesirable.
- Evaluation is the use of specific objective and subjective measures (often called outcome measures or criteria) to assess the child's and family's progress in reaching the goals defined in the nursing care plan. Following the evaluation of their progress towards the goals, the nursing care plan may be modified. For example, as the child's

condition improves and goals are attained, new goals and nursing action plans must be defined. Data from ongoing assessments are collected to guide the revision of the care plan.

Clinical practice guidelines and critical pathways are comprehensive interdisciplinary care plans for specific conditions, which describe the sequence and timing of interventions that should result in expected patient outcomes. The care plans are increasingly evidence-based, using a synthesis of research, group consensus, and past medical decisions to identify the most effective practices for a patient's condition.

Family-Centered Care

Efforts to address and meet the emotional, social, and developmental needs of children and families seeking health care in all settings is a concept known as family-centered care. The importance of the family in helping the child recover from an illness or injury is recognized. Families are often considered as partners in care, learning about children's health care problems. The key elements of family-centered care are as follows:

Key Elements of Family-Centered Care

- Incorporating into policy and practice the recognition that the family is the constant in a child's life, while the service systems and support personnel within those systems fluctuate.
- Facilitating family/professional collaboration at all levels of hospital, home, and community care:
  - Care of an individual child
  - Programme development, implementation, evaluation, and evolution
  - Policy formation.
- Exchanging complete and unbiased information between family members and professionals in a supportive manner at all times.
- Incorporating into policy and practice the recognition and honouring of cultural diversity, strengths, and individuality within and across all families, including ethnic, racial, spiritual, social, economic, educational, and geographic diversity.
- Recognizing and respecting different methods of coping and implementing comprehensive policies and programmes that provide developmental, educational, emotional, environmental, and financial supports to meet the diverse needs of families.
- Encouraging and facilitating family-to-family support and networking.
- Ensuring that home, hospital, and community service and support systems for children needing specialized health and developmental care and their families are flexible, accessible, and comprehensive in responding to diverse family-identified needs.
- Appreciating families and children as children, and recognizing that they possess a wide range of strengths, concerns, emotions, and aspirations beyond their need for specialized health and developmental services and support.

Chapter 1 GROWTH AND DEVELOPMENT

The concepts of growth and development are fundamental to the practice of paediatric nursing. Throughout the periods of child development, major milestones are accomplished. For each of these development periods, important aspects of care involving such topics as nutrition, language, safety and discipline must be addressed.

CONCEPTS OF GROWTH AND DEVELOPMENT

Definition

Growth: Growth implies an increase in size, such as height and weight. Height is measured in centimetre or inches. Weight is measured in kilogram or pound.

Development: Development refers to the acquisition of skills and abilities or milestones the baby achieves according to age and grasping knowledge and its practice.

Principles of Growth and Development

1. Growth and development are continuous processes from conception until death.
2. Growth and development proceed in an orderly sequence.
3. Different children pass through predictable development stages at different rates.
4. All body systems do not develop at the same rate (developmental pace).
5. Physical development is in cephalocaudal direction (head to tail).
6. Physical development proceeds from proximal to distal body parts.
7. Development proceeds from gross to refined skills.
8. There is an optimum time for initiation of development experiences or learning.

Factors Influencing or Affecting the Growth and Development

- Cultural and socioeconomic status:
  - Cultural environment determines a child's language and greatly influences his actions.
  - Socioeconomic status may affect the child's access to medical care, housing and nutrition —all of which can impact growth and development.
- Hereditary factors:
  - Family characteristics,
  - Genetic factors.
- Race and nationality
- Illness or injury
- Exercise
- Sex
- Prenatal factors:
  - Drugs
  - Infections
  - Nutrition
  - Radiations
  - Maternal illness.

Growth and development occur in following ways:

1. Physically (in body)
2. Mentally (mind/intellect)
3. Emotionally (personality formation)
4. Socially (contact with others/interaction).

Theories of Growth and Development

Cognitive Theory (Jean Piaget)

- Mental activity occurs in successive stages during childhood.
- By successfully encountering new experiences, the child adapts and progresses to the next stage.
- The child incorporates new ideas, skills and knowledge into familiar pattern of thought and

action. When faced with a problem that's new or too complex to fit into existing pattern of thought, the child accommodates, drawing on past experiences that are closest to his current problem to solve it.

- Development occurs in four stages. The child cannot progress to more advanced stages if he has not accomplished the one preceding it.
  - *Sensorimotor stage* (*birth to age 2*): During this stage, the child progresses from reflex activity through simple repetitive behaviours to imitative behaviours.
  - *Preoperational stage* (*ages 2–7*): This stage is marked by egocentricity (the child cannot comprehend a point of view different than his own), it is a time of magical thinking and increases the ability to use symbols and language.
  - *Concrete operational stage* (*ages 7–11*): The child's thinking processes become more logical and coherent; he/she can use inductive reasoning to solve the problems but still cannot think abstractly; he/she is less self-centered.
  - *Formal operational thinking stage* (*ages 12–15*): This stage is characterized by adaptability and flexibility; the adolescent can think abstractly, from logical conclusions from his observations and establish and test hypothesis.

Psychosocial Theory (Erik Erikson)

- Major personality changes occur throughout an individual's life cycle.
- Passage from one stage to another depends on the use of skills acquired in the preceding stage; however, new situations may provide opportunities for learning to cope with deficits experienced in earlier stages.

There are five childhood stages:

- *Trust vs. mistrust* (*birth to age 1*): The child develops trust on the primary caregiver who meets his/her needs.
- *Autonomy vs. shame and doubt* (*ages 1–3*): The child learns to control his body functions and becomes increasingly independent, preferring to do things himself.
- *Initiative vs. guilt* (*ages 3–6*): The child learns about the world through play and develops a conscience.
- *Industry vs. inferiority* (*ages 6–12*): The child enjoys working on projects and with others and tends to follow rules; competition with others is keen, and forming social relationships takes on great importance.
- *Identity versus role confusion* (*ages 12–18*): Changes in his body are taking place rapidly, and the child is preoccupied with how he looks and how others view him. While trying to meet the expectations of his peers, he's also trying to establish his own identity.

Psychosexual Theory (Sigmund Freud)

- The human mind (personality) consists of three major entities:
  - The Id (seeks immediate gratification)
  - The Ego (orients the individual to reality)
  - The super-ego (is responsible for the existence of a conscience and individual's ideas)
- Each stage must be mastered before the child moves to the next stage:
  - *Oral stage* (*birth to age 1*): The child seeks pleasure through sucking, biting and other oral activities.
  - *Anal stage* (*ages 1–3*): The child undergoes toilet training and learns to control his excreta.
  - *Phallic stage* (*ages 3–6*): The child is interested in his genitalia and various sensations and discovers the difference between the boy and girl.
  - *Latency period* (*ages 6–12*): The child expands on traits developed in earlier stages and concentrates on playing and learning.
  - *Genitalia stage* (*age 12 and older*): The production of sex hormones becomes intense and the reproductive system reaches maturation.

Moral Development (Lawrence Kohlberg)

- This theory addresses the way children develop a sense of right and wrong. They develop stages of thought as well as to moral behaviour.
- There are three sequential levels of cognitive development:
  - *Preconventional levels of morality* (*ages 2–7*): The child attempts to follow rules set by those in authority; he tries to adjust his behaviour according to good, bad, right, and wrong.
  - *Conventional levels of morality* (*age 7–7*): The child seeks conformity and loyalty; he attempts to justify, support, and maintain the social order and follows fixed rules.

- *Post conventional autonomous levels of morality (age 12 and older)*: The adolescent strives to construct a personal and functional value system independent of authority figure and his peers.

Spiritual Development

- Spiritual beliefs are closely related to the moral and ethical portion of children self concept and as such must be considered as part of the child's basic need assessment.

Fowler Theory

He identified seven stages in the development of faith, five of which are parallel and closely associated with congnitive and psychosocial development in childhood.

Stage 0: *Undifferentiated*—This stage of development encompasses the period of infancy, in which there is no concept of right or wrong, no beliefs, and no convictions to guide behaviour. However, the development occurs through relationships with the primary caregiver.

Stage 1: *Intuitive-projective*—Toddlerhood is primarily a time of imitating the behaviour of others. The children imitate religious gestures and behaviours of others without comprehending the meaning or significance of the activities. In preschool age they assimilate some of the values and beliefs of their parent's attitudes towards their religion

Stage 2: *Mythical-literal*—Through the school age years spiritual development parallels cognitive development and is closely related to the children experience and social interaction. Most children have a strong interest in religion during school age. They accept that good behaviour is rewarded and bad behaviour is punished. They relevance for many thoughts and matters and are able to articulate their faith. They may even begin to question its validity.

Stage 3: *Synthetic-convention*—As children approach adolescence they become increasingly aware of spiritual disappointment. They recognize that prayers are not always answered. They begin to reason, to question some of the established parental religion standards and to drop or modify some religious practices.

Stage 4: *Individuating-reflexive*—Adolescence become more sceptical and begin to compare the religious standards of their parents with the standards of others. They attempt to determine which to adopt and incorporate into their own set of values. They also begin to compare religious standard with the scientific viewpoint. Adolescents are uncertain about many religious ideas but will not achieve profound insight until late adolescence or early adulthood.

Language Development

Children learn the complex symbol system of language with astonishing speed. Infants use abstract signifiers (word) to refer to objects and activities before they can talk. However, at all stages of language development, children's comprehension and vocabulary is greater than their expressed vocabulary, and the acquisition of vocabulary and language keeps pace with cognitive advancement.

Children are born with the mechanism and capacity to develop speech and language skills, using intact physical functions of:

- The respiratory system.
- Speech control centers in the cerebral cortex.
- Articulation and resonance structure of the mouth and nasal cavities.

In addition, acquisition of language requires

- An intact and discriminating auditory apparatus
- Intelligence
- A need to be communicable
- Stimulation.

Stages in Development of Language

Prelinguistic stage: The period before a child utters its first meaningful word; develops in step like fashion over first 10–12 months from crying through cooing to babbling.

Holophrastic stage: The period when children's speech consists of one-word utterance, some of which are thought to be holophrases (single word utterances that represent the meaning of an entire sentence) begins at appropriately 1 year of age.

Telegraphic stage: The period when children's speech consists solely of content word, omitting the less meaningful part of speech (such as articles, prepositions and auxiliary verbs) begins at approximately 18 to 24 months of age.

Preschool period: The period when children begin to produce some very lengthy sentences and speech increases in complexity (age 3 months to 5 years).

Middle childhood period: The period when children refine their language skills and increase linguistic competence (ages 6 to 14 years). They use bigger words. Produce longer and more complex utterances, and learn suitable exceptions to grammatical rules. They begin to understand even the most complex syntactic structures of their native language.

Theories of Growth and Development

The child development theories discussed in this chart should not be compared directly because they measure different aspects of development. Erik Erickson's psychosocial-based theory is the most commonly accepted model for child development although it cannot be empirically possible or reliable.

Table 1.1: Theories of Growth and Development

Age-Group	Psychosocial Theory	Cognitive Theory	Psychosexual Theory	Moral Development
Infancy period (birth to age 1)	Trust vs. mistrust	Sensorimotor (birth to age 2)	Oral	Not applicable
Toddler period (age 1 to 3)	Autonomy vs. shame and doubt	Sensorimotor to preoperational	Anal	Preconventional
Preschool period (age 3 to 6)	Initiative vs. guilt	Preoperational (age 2 to 7)	Phallic	Preconventional
School age (age 6 to 12)	Industry vs. inferiority	Concrete operational (age 7 to 11)	Latency	Conventional
Adolescence (age 12 to 19)	Identity vs. role confusion	Formal operational thought (age 12 to 15)	Genitalia	Postconventional

ASSESSING AND MEASURING OF GROWTH AND DEVELOPMENT

- **Chronological age**
  - Years or months since birth date
- **Mental age**
  - Level of cognitive function
  - This determination is based on atleast two types of intelligence test administered over 6 months; with the child in optimal health.
- **Bone age**
  - Radiographic studies of the tarsal's and carpal's indicate the degree of ossification.
  - This measure is used for the child who's shorter or taller than chronological age suggests.
- **Adjusted or corrected age**
  - Chronological age minus the number of weeks born prematurely.
  - Used upto age 2.
- **Developmental assessment**
  - Determines whether the child has achieved certain expected goals during a development stage.
  - If an expected goal is not achieved, the acquisition of subsequent skills may be delayed.
  - Denver Developmental Screening Test (Denver II).
    - The test is designed for a child upto age 6.
    - It measures gross motor, fine motor, language, and personal – social development; it does not measure intelligence.
    - Other standardized screening tests in use include
      - Parents Evaluation of Developmental Status (PEDS) for children age 0 to 8; has 10 items and is accompanied by a decision path way.
      - Ages and Stages Questionnaire (ASQ) for children age 0 to 5; measures development of communication, gross motor, fine

motor, problem-solving, and personal (social) skills.

INFANT (BIRTH THROUGH AGE 1)

Neonatal Period (Birth to 28 days)

- Head and chest circumferences are relatively equal; head circumference may be upto 2 cm (3/4″) greater than the chest circumference (HC- 33–35 cm, CC- 31–33 cm).
- Head length is one-fourth of total body length.
- Brain growth depends upon the myelinisation.
- All behaviour is under reflex control; extremities are flexed.
- Hearing and touch are well developed; a hearing screening is recommended for all neonates.
- Vision is poor; the neonate fixates momentarily on light.
- The neonate is stimulated by being held or rocked, listening to music and watching a black and white object.
- When lying prone, the neonate can lift its head.
- Normal pulse rate ranges from 110/beat to 160 beat/minute (Count the apical pulse for one minute).
- Normal respiratory rate ranges from 32 to 60 breath/minute.
  - Respiration is irregular
  - The neonate is an obligate nose breather.
- Average blood pressure is 82/46 mm Hg (use the correct size of cuff, one and one-half times the diameter of the extremity or no less than one-half and no greater than two-thirds the length of the part of the extremity being used to measure the BP).
- Temperature regulation is altered because of poorly developed sweating and shivering mechanism.
  - Limit exposure time during bath.
  - When the neonate is wet or cold, cover the head and body (dry with towel when wet).
  - Mortality is higher in the neonatal period than in any other growth stage.

Ages 1 to 4 Months

- The posterior fontanel closes (usually within two months).
- The infant begins to hold up its head.
- At ages 4 to 8 weeks, reflexes reach their peak, especially the sucking reflex, which affords nutrition, survival and psychological pleasure.
- At the age 3 months, the most primitive reflexes begin to disappear except for the protective and postural reflexes (blinking, parachute, cough, swallow and gag reflexes) which remain for life.
- The infant observes the people's faces and watches mobiles (an appropriate toy for an infant younger than age 3 months).
- The infant develops binocular vision; the eyes can follow an object 180 degree and any intermittent strabismus should be resolved by age of 4 months.
- The infant begins to put its hand to its mouth.
- The infant reaches out voluntarily but uncoordinatedly.
- The infant cries to express needs.
- The infant's instinctual smile appears at age 2 months and social smile at age 3 months.
  - The social smile is the infant's first social response.
  - The social smile initiates social relationships, indicates memory traces and signals the beginning of thought processes.
- At age 4 months, the infant laughs in response to its environment.
- The infant recognizes his parents voice.
- The infant sits in an infant seat.
- The infant explores its feet.

Ages 5 to 6 Months

- Birth weight doubles.
- The infant can sleep through the night with one or two naps a day.
- The infant begins teething (lower central incisors appear first); this may result in increased drooling and irritability.
- The infant rolls over from its stomach to its back.
- When lying prone, the infant uses its arms to push its chest up and to push its body toward its feet (crawl).
- The infant voluntarily grasps and releases objects.

- The infant sits with support.
- The infant cries when its parents leave; this is a normal sign of attachment.
- The infant discerns one face from another and exhibits stranger anxiety (is wary of strangers and clings to or clutches its parents).
- The infant begins to exhibit comforting habits—sucks his thumb, rubs his ear, holds a blanket or stuffed toy, rocks.
  - All these habits symbolize parents and security.
  - Thumb sucking in infancy does not result in malocclusion of permanent teeth.

Ages 7 to 9 Months

- The infant sits alone without assistance.
- The infant creeps on its hand and knees with its belly off of the floor.
- The infant stands and stays up by grasping for support.
- The infant develops a pincer grasp, places everything in its mouth, and is, therefore, at high risk aspirating the objects.
- The infant self-feeds crackers; the infant who is physically and emotionally ready can begin to be weaned to a cup.
- The infant verbalizes all vowels and most consonants but speaks no intelligible words.
- The infant begins to imitate the expressions of others.
- The infant likes to look in to the mirror.
- The infant develops objects permanence and searches for objects outside its perceptual field.
- The infant understands the word "no."

Ages 10 to 12 Months

- Birth weight triples and birth length increases about 50%.
- The infant cruises (takes side steps while holding on) at age 10 months, walks with support at age 11 months, and stands alone and takes its first steps at age 12 months.
- The infant says "mama" and "dada" and also responds to its name at the age of 10 months, it can say about five words but understands many more at age 12 months.
- The infant claps its hands, waves bye-bye and enjoys rhythm games.
- The infant enjoys books and toys to build with.
- The infant explores everything by feeling, pushing, turning, pulling, biting, smiling, and testing for a sound.

Care Needs During Neonatal Period

- Maintain a neonate airway
- Maintain a stable body temperature
- Prevent infection or injury
- Administration of vitamin K
- Provide optimum nutrition
- Elimination needs
- Exhibit attachment behaviour
- Immunization

Maintain a Patient Airway

- Suction: Clean the mouth and nasopharynx with bulb syringe or mechanical suction to prevent aspiration of fluid.
- Position: The infant should be kept on right side after feeding to prevent aspiration.
- Position the infant on back during sleep.
- Administration of oxygen if needed during first hour after delivery and also if infant is on respiratory distress.
- Take vital signs according to the institutional policy.
- Observe for signs of respiratory distress and report any of the following immediately.
  - Tachypnea
  - Grunting, stridor
  - Abnormal birth sound
  - Flaring of nostril
  - Severe chest indrawing
  - Cyanosis or pallor

Maintain a Stable Body Temperature

- Wrap the infant comfortably in a warm blanket.
- Place the infant under the radiant warmer or near to mother.
- Place the infant on a padded, covered surface.
- Frequently monitor the infant temperature.
- Maintain the room temperature between 24° C to 25.5° C.
- Infant temperature is stable—give bath, prevent chilling of infant during bath.

- Head should be covered to prevent heat loss, infant should be dressed and covered with blanket.
- Observe the sign of hypothermia or hyperthermia.

Prevent Infection or Injury

- Wash the hands before and after caring for each infant.
- Protect the infant from potential source of infection, e.g. a person with respiratory infection, skin infection, improperly prepared food source and other unclean items.
- Check the eyes every day for the evidence of inflammation or discharge.
- Apply appropriate eye prophylaxis if prescribed.
- Wear the hand gloves when in contact with body fluids.
- Keep the umbilical stump clean and dry.
- Assess the cord daily for odour, colour, and drainage.
- Apply antibacterial agent or alcohol to cord as per order.
- Place the diaper below the umbilical stump.
- Clean the perineal area to prevent foecal contamination.
- Infant should be properly identified for placement with correct mother.
- Ensure that the infant identification band is properly and securely placed.
- Never leave the infant alone in crib or room.
- Keep pointed or sharp objects away from infant.
- Keep infant fingernails short and trimmed, avoid jewellery that can scratch infant.
- Employ appropriate methods of handing and transporting infant.

Administration of Vitamin K

- Administration of vitamin K injection (1 mg IM) in anterior mid thigh.

Provide Optimum Nutrition

- Assess strength of suck and coordination with swallowing to identify the problem affecting feeding.
- Prepare the mother for breast feeding specially for demand feeding to her infant.
- Assist and support breast feeding mothers during initial feeding.
- Educate the mother about exclusive breast feeding upto six months to the infant, water or other supplements are not necessary for the infant.
- Educate the mother regarding good position and attachment.
- Behaviour such as restlessness, crying and moving the head can indicate hunger.
- Place the infant on right side to prevent aspiration, left side position compresses the stomach and causes regurgitation and aspirations.

Elimination Needs

- Newborn babies cannot control defecation and urination.
- Meconium is the first foecal material passed by the newborn, normally up to 24 hours after birth.
- The stool is black tarry colour, odourless and sticky in nature.
- The new born passes stool frequently, often after each feeding because intestine is immature.
- Educate the parents about infant feeding and sleeping behaviour; if it is changed it should be informed.
- Guide the parents placing the diapering and cleanliness of the perineal area.
- Urine output varies according to fluid intake but usually it is 15 to 60 ml/day after birth.
- Educate the mother to change the diaper frequently after baby void urine, to prevent infection.
- Check for diaper rashes.

Exhibit Attachment Behaviour

- Encourage the mother to see and hold infant; place newborn close to face of parent to establish visual contact.
- Rubbing the infant with finger tip.
- Keep the baby near to mother (rooming in) in same room.
- Encourage the parent to talk to newborn by responding verbally to the cries, cough and sneezes.
- Responding early to the newborn's needs.
- Explain the siblings to participate in newborn care.
- Encourage the parents to participate in newborn care.

Immunization

- After birth zero oral polio vaccine and BCG vaccine to be given.

Care Needs During Infant Period

- Nutrition
- Sleep
- Prevention of infection
- Immunization
- Prevention of accident
- Provide love and affection

Nutrition

- Breast feeding is most desirable and is the complete diet for first six months of the year (exclusive breast feeding).
- Formula feeding—Iron-fortified commercial formula is a complete food for the first half of the year in children, mothers died with HIV/AIDS condition and HIV mothers CD_4 count is decreased.
- After 6 months solid foods to be started (weaning).
- First foods are strained, pureed, or finely mashed.
- Finger foods such as teething crackers, cooked fruit or vegetables can be introduced by 6 to 7 months.
- As the quality of solid increases the amount of formula should be limited to approximately 900 ml daily and fruit juice to less than 360 ml daily.
- Calorie requirement for 0–6 month infant—weight in kg × 117, 6–12 months infant—weight in kg × 108.
- Protein requirement for 0–6 month infant—weight in kg × 2.2 gm, 6–12 months infant—weight in kg × 2 gm.

Sleep

- Concerns regarding sleep are common during infant stage.
- Normally infant should sleep 15 to 18 hours per day.
- Identify if the infant has any sleep disturbance from the parents.
- When a sleeping problem is presented, a careful assessment is essential.

Prevention of Infection

- Encourage the mother to give daily bath and change the clothes daily.
- Protect the child from infected persons.
- Protect child from cold.
- Wash the hands before and after caring for each infant.
- Protect the infant from potential source of infection *e.g.*, persons with respiratory infection, skin infection, improper prepared food source and other unclean items.

Immunization

One of the most dramatic advances in paediatrics has been the decline of infectious diseases during the twenty-first century because of the widespread use of immunization for preventable diseases. The recommended primary schedule begins during infancy period. The immunization for tuberculosis (BCG), oral polio, diphtheria, tetanus, pertussis, hepatitis B (Pentaviollent), haemophilus influenza type b (Hib), measels is included under health promotion during infancy.

Prevention of Accident

- Injuries are a major cause of death during infant period, especially for children aged 6 to 12 months.
- Encourage the parents to have vigilance. Awareness and supervision are essential as a child gains increased locomotors and manipulative skills.
- Children are more prone to get aspiration of foreign objects, suffocation/drowning, falls, burns etc., so do not leave the child alone.
- Educate the mother to keep all plastic bags stored out of infant reach.
- Always raise crib rails.
- Never leave alone on a raised, unguarded surface.
- Never leave infant alone in bath.

Provide Love and Affection

- Encourage parents to give love and affection by providing or satisfying the need of the child.

TODDLER (AGES 1 TO 3)

Introduction (Physical Development)

- This is a period of slow growth, with a weight gain of 1.8 to 2.7 kg per year.
- Growth is measured in height rather than length after 2 years. Between age 1 and 2 years, the average growth of the height is 10 to 12 cm and between ages 2 to 3 years it is 6–8 cm per year.
- Normal pulse rate is 100 beats/minute.
- Normal respiratory rate is 26 breaths/minute.
- Normal blood pressure is 99/64 mm Hg.
- Vision still is not mature, visual activity is fairly well established by 1 year, and however it is continually refined until the age 6 years.
- The senses of hearing, taste, smell, and touch become increasingly developed and associated with one another.
- Posture of toddlers has a pronounced lumbar lordosis and a protruding abdomen. The abdominal muscles develop gradually as the toddler grows and the abdomen flattens.
- The anterior fontanel closes between ages 12 and 18 months.
- The head circumference of the toddler increases in an average about 2.5 cm. The brain is 70% of its adult size by the time the infant is 2 years old.

Psychosocial Development

- The toddler is egocentric.
- The toddler follows wherever his parents go.
- Starts playing peek-a-boo to develop trust.
- Progresses to playing hide-and-seek to reinforce the idea that his parents will return.
- Separation anxiety arises.
- The toddler sees bedtime as desertion.
- The toddler develops a fear of the dark.
- Separation anxiety demonstrates closeness between the toddler and his parents; the toddler screams and cries when his parents leave and then may sulk and engage in comfort measures.
- The parents who are leaving should say so and promise to return.
  - The parent should leave a personal item with the toddler.
  - Prepare the parents for the toddler's reaction, and explain that this process promotes trust.
- Transitional objects (blankets, bottles, comforting habits) represent the toddler's parents and security; as long as they do not impede daily functioning and social interactions, they are not detrimental to mental health.
- If the toddler is a head-banger or rocks in bed, ensure his safety but ignore the behaviour.
- The toddler may engage in solitary play and have little interaction with others, this progresses to parallel play (the toddler plays alongside not with other children).
- To promote the development of autonomy, allow the toddler to perform tasks independently.

Cognitive Development

- The toddler understands object permanence.
- The toddler engages in ritualistic behaviour to master skills and decrease anxiety.
- The toddler exhibits magical thinking (believes that thoughts affect events).
- The toddler uses symbols (understands that gestures, such as waving bye-bye, have meaning).
- Memory and learning are enhanced by experiences.
- The toddler shows curiosity about everything but cannot lead to aspiration or ingestion of dangerous items.
- The toddler begins imitative play and role play to express his feelings.
- The toddler lacks the concept of sharing and does not know the value of items
- The toddler points to mentioned body part and recognizes himself in the mirror.

Motor Skills Development

- The toddler explores the environment and is usually active.
- The toddler uses his arms to balance.
- The toddler plants his feet wide apart and walks by age 15 months, if it does not happen, seek further evaluation.
- Feet are flat with no arches.
- Provide push-pull toys to encourage walking.

- The toddler climbs stairs at age 21 months, runs and jumps by age 2, and rides tricycle by age 3.
- The toddler has some difficulty coordinating the swallowing reflex and speaking.

Dentition

- First molar erupt (a child has 20 deciduous teeth by age 3 years).
- Introduce the toddler to a tooth brush but not yet to the tooth paste, because he swishes and swallows.
- As necessary, continue the fluoride use until age 12.
- Prevent tooth decay by giving the toddler a cup containing water.

Language Development

- Language aids the toddler's expression of feelings, experiences and memory and provides a new way to manipulate the world.
- By the age of two, the toddler uses 400 words as well as two-to-three-word phrases and comprehends many more.
- Speech is egocentric.
- The toddler becomes frustrated to communicate, which may result in temper tantrums; allow more time for the toddler to ask questions and share feelings.
- At age of 3, the toddler is a chatter box, using about 11,000 words a day.
- The toddlers speak four to five words sentences and may be 75% intelligible by age 3; if not, seek further evaluation and assess his hearing capacity.
- The amount the toddler speaks is influenced by the amount spoken in his home.
- The toddler's ability to understand speech is more important than his ability to vocalize.

Toilet Training

- Training depends on the toddler's emotional read -iness.
- Training also depends on the toddler's physical readiness.
- Toilet sitting should begin when the toddler demonstrates readiness and shows interest.
- With increased stress (such as new baby in the family, a divorce, a vacation) the toddler may regress; the toilet training may have to be delayed or retaught.
- Introduce underpants as a badge of success and maturity.
- If the toddler is not trained by age 5, seek further evaluation.

Personality Traits of the Toddler

- Negativism
- Ritualistic behaviour
- Temper tantrum
- Regression
- Sibling rivalry
- Slowness in carrying out parents request

Negativism

One of the most different aspects of rearing children in this age-group is their persistent "no" response to every request.

Management

- Parents approach is to be positive suggestion rather than commanding. Avoid an emotional climate of negativism, blame and punishment.

Ritualistic Behaviour

- Stylized expression in nursery rhymes and children's games. In many cultures ritualistic behaviour is characterized by repetitive elements and by adherence to rules, impressed by the child on his own behaviour and on the behaviour of others.

Temper Tantrums

Toddlers typically respond to frustrated efforts at independence by controlled outbursts of anger known as temper tantrums. These outbursts may include crying, throwing objects, striking out at others, breath holding and head banging.

How to Handle Temper Tantrums

Ignore the behaviour so that the tantrum accomplishes nothing, avoid giving in or responding in kind.

- Separate the child from the immediate situation.
- Calmly restrain the child on the floor away from other people, furniture or objects that may cause injury to the child or may be damaged.
- Provide distraction and comfort when the tantrum is waning.

Regression

- The retreat from one's present pattern of functioning to past levels of behaviour is referred to as regression.
- It usually occurs in instances of discomfort or stress when one attempts to conserve psychic energy by reverting to patterns of behaviour that were successful in earlier stages of development.
- Regression is common in toddlers because almost any additional stress hinders their ability to master present developmental tasks, any threat to their autonomy such as illness, separation or adjustment to a siblings, demand for the bottle, hospitalization, etc.
- At first such regression appears acceptance and comfortable for children.
- When regression does occur, the parent's best approach is to ignore it while praising existing pattern of appropriate behaviour. It is advisable not to attempt new areas of learning when an additional crisis is present or expected, such as beginning toilet training shortly before a sibling is born or attempting new areas of learning during a brief period of hospitalization.

Sibling Rivalry

The natural jealousy and resentment of children to a new child in the family is referred to as sibling rivalry, the arrival of a new infant represents a crisis for even the best prepared toddlers. It is not the infant that toddlers hate or resent.

How to Handle the Sibling Rivalry?

- Preparation of children for the birth of a sibling is quite individual.
- Preparing children too soon for the birth may lessen their interest by the time the event occurs.
- A good time to start talking about the new baby is when toddlers become aware of the pregnancy.
- Parents can minimize the visitors by alerting visitors to the toddlers needs, having some gifts on hand for the toddler, because visitors may initiate problems by talking about praising new baby, they may insult the toddler.

How to identify sibling rivalry or how children exhibit jealousy?

- Toddler will hit the infant.
- Push the child off the mother's lap or pull the breast or bottle from the infant's mouth.
- Verbally express their wish that the infant should go back.
- Toddler throw the infant dresses bottles spoiling their underpants.
- They divert the attention towards themselves aggressively acting out toward others.
- For this reason, infants must be protected by parental supervision during the interaction between the siblings.

Slowness in Carrying Out Parents Request

- The period of the development of a sense of autonomy is a time of expanding social contacts. Toddlers are curious and ask many questions. Children at this age are often creative, although the productive activity may not be perfect. Because of playful mood the toddlers show the slowness in carrying out a request.

Care Needs for the Toddlers

- Physical care
- Nutrition
- Prevention of accident
- Toilet training

Physical Care

- Encourage the mother to give daily bath and change the clothes.
- Provide attention on dental health—Regular teeth examination is essential, teach the parents correct methods of dental hygiene and provide nutritional counselling, especially related to preventing dental carries.
- Encourage hand washing with soap before and after food.

Nutrition

- During the toddler period the growth rate is slow, so slight adjustment is needed in the caloric requirement which is 102 kcal/kg of body weight.
- Protein requirements are 1.2 g/kg for toddlers but still higher at succeeding ages to meet the demands of muscle tissue growth and high activity level.
- Fluid requirement is 115 ml/kg.
- The requirement for most vitamins and minerals increases during toddler period.

- Encourage the children to drink milk, the chief source of calcium and phosphorus, it should average 2 to 3 cups a day.
- It may be necessary to withhold the bottle feedings, as well as other between meal foods and fluids other than water, until the child eats solid foods. It usually results in conflicts and does little to establish healthy eating habits.

Prevention of Accident

- The toddlers are very naughty and greatly curious too, so they may be prone to get the accidents in motor vehicles, drowning, burns, poisoning, falls, bodily damage.
- Supervise the child while playing outside.
- Teach the child to obey traffic regulations (safety rules).
- Supervise the child closely when they are near any source of water, keep bathroom door and lid on toilet closed.
- Teach swimming and water safety.
- Place the electric appliances, such as coffee maker, frying pan, etc. at safe places.
- Cover the electrical outlet devices.
- Do not keep the stove on the floor.
- Do not allow the child to go near firewood while preparing the food.
- Place all potentially toxic agents (including plants) in a locked cabinet or out of reach.
- Never remove labels from containers of toxic substances.
- Keep screens in windows, nailed securely and use guardrails.
- Supervise at playgrounds.
- Avoid large, round chunks of meat.
- Avoid fruits with pits, fish with bones, dried beans, hard candy, chewing gum, nuts, popcorn, grapes.
- Avoid giving sharp or pointed objects such as knives, scissors or toothpicks—especially while walking or running.
- Teach the child never to go with a stranger.
- Use safety gates at the top and bottom of stairs.

Toilet Training

- Begin training when the toddler demonstrates readiness.
- Provide a pleasant mood.
- Use a potty seat or potty chair.
- Be aware that the child is curious about excretion products.
- Do not refer to bowel movement as being "dirty" or "yucky."
- Teach hand washing.
- Teach wiping from front to back or wash the anus.

PRESCHOOL CHILD (AGES 3 TO 5)

Introduction

- Slow growth continues during this period, birth length doubles by age 4.
- Average pulse rate ranges from 90 to 100 beats/minute.
- Average respiratory rate is 20 to 25 breaths/minute.
- Normal blood pressure ranges from 85/60 to 90/70 mm Hg.
- Attendance at day care center or nursery school increases the child's contact with peers and they are prone to get infection.

Psychosocial Development

- Language is egocentric and used to boast, brag and shock others.
- The child identifies with the same sex parent or primary care giver; the child enjoys role playing, role modelling, and playing with dolls.
- The child shows anxiety about healthcare treatment and life events (use doll play to help the child prepare for or adjust to treatments).
- The child shows fear concerning body integrity.
    - Anticipate the child's fear of animal noises, new experiences and the dark.
- Egocentricity decreases and awareness of others' needs increases.
    - The child begins to share and take turns but continues to have difficulty with these concepts.
    - The child attempts to please others.
- The child begins to function socially.
    - Child learns rules.
    - Nursery school enhances the child's social development.

- The child may create an imaginary playmate to help deal with fear and loneliness.

Cognitive Development

- The child uses four to five sentences but he has a difficulty with pronouns.
- The child has limited perspective and focuses on one idea at a time.
- The child becomes aware of racial and sex difference.
- The child develops a body image.
- The child begins to have a concept of time.
- The child begins to have a concept of numbers, letters, colours.

Motor Skills

- The child dresses without help (but they tie the shoes at the age of 5).
- The child builds the tower of blocks, copies circles and lines, he uses scissors, and throws the ball over the head.
- The child alternates the feet on steps and hops on one foot, skips at the age of 5.
- The child develops hand dominance.
- The child enjoys with the sand, plays with water, blocks, crayons, clay and fingerprints.

Special Problems of Preschool Children

- Sucking of Thumbs
- Food likes and dislikes
- Enuresis
- Encopresis
- Selfishness or possessiveness
- Bad language
- Destructiveness or Aggression
- Hurting others

Sucking of Thumbs

It is the common habit of small children that they suck their thumbs. Generally at three months age babies commence thumb sucking and keep doing it for some time. The natural cause of this habit can be the breast-feeding of the baby.

Management of Thumb Sucking

- When the parents initially notice the tendency of thumb sucking in the child, they should try to find the reason, give it more milk if its hunger is not satiated, and if it gets hungry between the feeding schedules, give it some fruit juice or biscuits.
- Another method of checking this habit in children is to provide them with good and soft toys with a view to divert their mind from thumb sucking.
- The other alternative tool for avoiding thumb sucking is to give the child rubber-soothers to suck.

Food Likes and Dislikes

Preschool children still have food habits that are typical of toddlers, such as food feeds and strong taste preferences.

- Preschool children may enter another period of finicky eating, which is generally characteristic of the more rebellious and rowdy behaviour. The children are more agreeable to trying new foods, especially if they are encouraged to experiment with new taste or different dish. The meal times can become battlegrounds if parents expect perfect table manners. The amount and variety of foods consumed by young children varies greatly from day to day.

How to Approach

- Advice the parents to keep a weekly record of everything the child eats.
- Prepare the food according to likes of child.
- Provide small and frequent meals.

Enuresis or Nocturnal Enuresis

It is the medical term for bed-wetting. All over the world kids wet the bed. Bed-wetting is actually quite common among the children. Due to it children may feel very alone, and they can't talk to others about it. They may avoid certain social situations, like overnight camp and slumber parties. Other people may call them a "baby", or blame them for being wet, even though they cannot help it. Bed-wetting can cause real problems like loss of self-esteem and other psychological distress for the child and the family. It is very common in boys than girls.

Causes

There are two types of enuresis with different kinds of causes

- Primary nocturnal enuresis: It means the child has never had night time control, they have always wet at least two times a month. It can be caused by differences in bladder muscles, having a small bladder, secretion of more urine and sleeping too deeply to wake up when the bladder is full.

- Secondary nocturnal enuresis: The child may not wet the bed during night at least for 6 months, then started wetting again. The cause for these changes in the child is lifestyle, new stress like a divorce, a new baby sibling or death in the family and also medical problems like urinary tract infection, constipation.

Treatment

Usually there is no cause that can be directly treated. Some parents don't like to treat the child because medicine has side effects. Some medications may be utilized to relax the muscles of the bladder and to increase the volume that bladder can store. Newer agents decrease the production of urine at night. Medication like

- Tofranil (Imipramine) causes the relaxation of bladder muscles during sleep which in turn prevent the contraction of bladder during sleep
- DDAVP (Desmopressin) is similar to the hormone vasopressin, it signals the kidney to make less urine secretion at night.
- Detrol (tolterodine) is an anti-spasmodic and helps stop wetting caused by bladder spasms.

Motivation to the child is the key to the success of any treatment modality. Rewarding success and increasing the child responsibility work well. Modern alarms are safe and inexpensive.

Remember the nurse should educate the parents related to the point on treatment:

- Don't punish your child for wetting the bed.
- Be patient and understanding with the child.
- Respect your child privacy and do not talk about the bed-wetting in front of others.
- Use a reward system, such as a sticker chart on the bedroom wall for dry nights, put the focus on being dry, to keep the tone positive.
- Make sure your child drinks lots of water early in the day.
- Have your child go to the bathroom to empty the bladder right before bed time.
- Make sure your child is getting enough sleep.
- Reduce the fluid after dinner
- Wake your child up in the middle of the night, a little earlier than they usually wet the bed, and walk them to the bathroom to pee, then back to bed (called "night lifting")
- Try a bed-wetting alarm

Encopresis

- The condition of encopresis refers to a chronic disorder in which school children have bowel movement in unacceptable sites (usually their underwear) after the age of 4 years.

Causes

- Fear of school bathroom, prolonged or severe gastroenteritis, incomplete defecation, food intolerance or excess.
- Psychosocial stresses.

Treatment

- Consistency and support.
- A strong advice giving.
- Non-accusatory approach is most likely to be successful.

Selfishness or Possessiveness

Preschool children guard their belongings and may be bossy about them. They do not want to share the play materials or their property with other children but they may use others'.

Bad Language

Communication is the key to all family interaction and good communication with children requires listening and exchanging both words and feelings. Parents should be sensitive to the meanings behind children's words and action. Children will express the bad language for negative expression or feelings. It will be expressed when the children are felling hurt, angry, frightened and lonely. They learn bad language from their parents or family, friends in the school or in the community, they try to repeat the word without knowing the meaning of the language. The parents must understand the child's behaviours and help the child find safe, appropriate ways of expressing them. Parents should not encourage them to repeat, sometimes parents must ignore the children like not hearing anything. Parents must understand the child's cooperation, which is vital to effective, consistent parenting.

Destructiveness or Aggression

Destructiveness or aggression refers to behaviour that attempts to hurt a person or destroys property.

- Aggression differs from anger, which is temporary emotional state, but anger may be expressed through aggression.
- Hyperaggressive behaviour in preschool children is characterized by physical attack on other children and adults, destroying others' property.
- Increase in aggressive behaviour and frustration require modelling and reinforcement.

Hurting Others

- Preschool children due to frustration, may hurt others physically, may damage or throw the things in front of others to insult, and use bad language to scold others or parents.

Care Needs During the Preschool Period

- Physical care
- Sleep
- Safety measures (Prevention of accident)
- Health supervision
- Nutrition

Physical Care

- The preschool child needs daily care such as brushing the teeth, dental care, bath, dressing and toilet training, etc.

Sleep

- Sleep patterns vary widely, but the average sleep for preschooler is around 12 hours in night and he/she frequently takes daytime naps.
- Observe the preschoolers to identify the sleep disturbances like bedtime fear, waking during night, or having nightmares, etc.
- Interventions can also differ according to the problems.
- Other measures that may be helpful include keeping a light on in the room, providing transitional objects such as a favourite toy or leaving a drink of water by the bed.
- Encourage the parents to tell a story which is an inspiration to the child to go for sleep.
- Sleep problems are common. It is related to fears of separation and the dark.
    - Bedtime rituals help to decrease insecurity.
    - Security objects, such as blanket or favourite toys are helpful to reduce fear and separation.

Safety Measures (Prevention of Accident)

- Use locks or latches on cabinets; keep dangerous products in their original containers.
- Teach the parents or care taker that they should not leave the children alone.

Health Supervision

- Educate the parents to have a health check up like dental check, eye check up, hearing capacity for every 6 months to one year.

Nutrition

- They may have strong food preferences, so parents or caregiver has to assess the preferences of daily food (identify the likes and dislikes of the child).
- Provide small and frequent meals with nutrient content, do not mix the food together.
- Schedule the regular mealtimes, allow the children to participate in planning, preparing, serving and cleaning up.
- Maintain variety in the diet.
- Keep nutritional snacks in home which can be used instantly.
- Parents or caregiver should make sure that the child eats breakfast.
- Encourage the child to do the physical activity like playing to increase the appetite.

SCHOOL-AGE CHILD (AGES 5 TO 12)

Introduction

- School shapes the cognitive and social development of the children.
- Accidents are a major cause of death and disability during this period.

Psychosocial Development

- The teacher, perhaps the first important adult in the children's life, besides the parents, may be a major influence.
- The child plays with peers
    - The child develops a first true friendship.
    - The child develops a sense of belonging, cooperation, and compromise.
    - Groups offer a testing ground for the children's interpersonal interaction, development of self-concept and sex-role behaviour.

- Groups encourage competition through fair play.
- Groups relieve the child to make decisions.

- The child develops a sense of morality
  - The early school-age child sees actions as either right or wrong.
  - After age 9, the child understands intent and differing points of view; the child's super-ego matures.
- The child compares its own body to others and may become modest.
- The child participates in family activities.
- The child becomes aware of social roles.
- The child engages in fantasy play and day-dreaming.
- The child may exhibit a fear of death and school phobias; these fears may cause psychosomatic illness.

Cognitive Development

- The child develops concepts of time and space, cause and effect, nesting (building blocks, puzzle pieces), and numbers.
- The child understands the relation of parts to the whole (fractions).
- The child learns to classify objects in more than one way.
- The child learns to read and spell.
- The child becomes interested in board games, cards, and collections (stamps, coins from different countries).

Physical Development

- Slow growth continues during this period; height increases about 2" (5 cm) per year, and weight doubles between ages 6 and 12.
- The first primary tooth is displaced by a permanent tooth at age 6 and permanent erect by age 12, except for the final molars; the jaw.
- Grows to accommodate permanent teeth
  - This is a prime time for the development of dental caries.
  - Nutrition and dental education should be reinforced in the home and school.
- Vision matures by age 6.
- Both sexes are about the same size until about age 9, when some females begin puberty and grow faster.
- Bones grow faster than muscles and ligaments; therefore, the child is limber and prone to bone fractures.
- Large and small muscle groups are refined.
- Lymphoid tissue hypertrophies to maximum size.

Social Development is Perfect

- The child participates in group activities
  - The child likes to accomplish tasks.
  - The child engages in cooperative play.
  - The child's play involves group goals with interaction.
  - The child plays by the rules but often cheats.

Problems of School-Age Children

- Limit-setting and discipline
- Dishonest behaviour
- Coping up with stress
- Fears
- Latchkey children
- Accident
- Sleep problem

Limit-setting and Discipline

School children have a less or limited and no manager of discipline due to the psychosocial maturity of the parents,

- The childhood children rearing experience of the parents.
- The temperament of the children.
- The context of the children's misconduct and the response of the children towards rewards and punishments.

Dishonest Behaviour

Children may engage in what is considered to be antisocial behaviour, like lying, stealing and cheating which may become manifest in previously well-behaved children. It is especially disturbing to the parents, who may have difficulty coping with this behaviour.

Coping up with Stress

School children are getting stress from many sources like identifying friends from peers, eating, dressing and talking etc. Also they are pressed by the parents about their education, sports, games, extra-curricular activities and overloaded curriculum of the school. Quite early children produce capability to cope up with these stresses caused by the very near environment of their parents, teachers and peers.

Fears

A wide variety and degree of anxiety causes fear in the children. It includes fear of dark, excessive worry about the study or past behaviour, social withdrawal, self consciousness, etc.

Latchkey Children

The term latchkey children is used to describe children who are left to care for themselves or whose care arrangement is so loose that it is ineffective. This problem in children is due to single parent families and working mothers. The lack of childcare causes a stress provoking situation for the school age children.

Accident

School age children are prone to get accidents due to stress and over workload, aggressive behaviour, sleep disturbance, confusion and competition, etc.

Sleep Problem

School children will have sleep problem due to parents and teachers expectations, fear, anxiety, confusion and loneliness. Moodiness and stress also cause sleep disturbance to the children.

Care Needs During School-Age Period

- Promoting healthcare behaviour
- Nutrition
- Sleep and rest
- Injury prevention

Promoting Healthcare Behaviour

- Parents should encourage the children to assume the personal responsibility for selfcare in the areas of hygiene, nutrition, exercise and recreation, sleep and safety.
- Health education is a primary component of comprehensive healthcare and programmes should be designed to promote desired health behaviour through guided learning and modelling.
- Arrange an optimum programme which should help children learn that their behaviour affects their health.
- The behaviour should be encouraged in the children by:
  1. Asking questions
  2. Telling about themselves
  3. Listening and learning about new ways to take care of themselves
  4. Helping to decide what to do and
  5. Doing those things that promote health.

Nutrition

- In school age calorie needs are different according to body size. Resources are being laid down for the increased growth needs of the adolescent period.
- Encourage the parents and children to follow a balanced diet to promote growth.
- Encourage school-based intervention to promote nutrition education to the children.
- Children need to be educated about food selection and the importance of body-building nutrients as opposed to empty caloric intake.

Sleep and Rest

- The amount of sleep and rest required during school children is a highly individual matter.
- There is no specific amount of sleep needed at this age. Depends on age, activity level and other factors may change according to the health status.
- During this age nap is not required, but children sleep approximately nine and a half hours.
- Parents should identify the sleep problems in their children like:
  - Bedtime resistance due to normal fears of this age, fear of dark, strange noise, nightmares other imagined phenomena.
  - Sleep walking occurs in the first 3 to 4 hours of sleep.
  - Sleep walking is not a purposeful activity.
  - Preventive measures include avoiding over fatigue, getting adequate rest, employing relaxation techniques for relieving the stress.
  - Sleep walking is usually self-limiting and requires no treatment.
  - In more troublesome cases, it may require low doses of sedation.

- ❍ Nightmares are common in children. The current external stresses, movies, or stories may also precipitate a nightmare by reactivating old traumas. So avoid all external stress for the children.
- ❍ Do not encourage the children to watch stressful movies.

Injury Prevention

- School age children are more prone to get an injury like a motor vehicle accident, drowning, burns, poisoning, body damage, etc.
- Educate and make them follow the safety rules to avoid accidents.
- Teach the child to swim.
- Use an approved floating device in water or boat.
- Instruct child to behave properly in areas involving contact with potential burn hazards.
- Instruct child to behave properly in the event of fire.
- Educate the child regarding hazards of taking non-prescription drugs and chemicals including aspirin and alcohol.
- Keep potentially dangerous products in properly labelled receptacles – preferably locked and out of reach.
- Provide facilities for supervised activities.
- Encourage to play in safe places.
- Teach danger safety.
- Teach name, address and phone numbers and to ask for help from appropriate people.
- Injury prevention is directed towards safety education, provision of safe play areas and equipment, well supervised sport activities.

ADOLESCENT (AGES 12 TO 18)

Introduction

- Adolescence is a rapid growth period characterized by puberty-related changes in body structure and psychosocial adjustment. Nutritional needs increase significantly.
- Vital signs approach adult values in this period.

Psychosocial and Cultural Development

- Early adolescence is spent in coping up with changes in the physical self and becoming aware of the bodies of others.
  - ❍ Fantasy thoughts and daydreams allow the adolescent to role-play different social situations.
  - ❍ The adolescent may find that keeping a diary helps to express feelings.
  - ❍ The adolescent may diet excessively to attempt to attain a desirable body image.
- Middle adolescence involves exploring and identifying one's values and defining oneself.
  - ❍ Peers may influence bad behaviour, values or conformity.
  - ❍ Interest in the opposite sex increases; some adolescents may experience same-sex attractions.
  - ❍ Eating is a social event and influenced by peers.
- Late adolescence involves maturation, expressed by independence from parents and participation in society.
  - ❍ Self-identity and personal morality develop.
  - ❍ The adolescent beings tend to plan for the future.
  - ❍ Concerns at this stage may range from acne and obesity to sexual identity and major social issues.

Cognitive Development

- The adolescents develop abstract thinking and an increased ability to analyze, synthesize, and use logic.
- The late adolescent reaches the cognitive level of an adult.

Development of Secondary Sexual Characters

- Developments in the female:
  - ❍ The hypothalamus induces the pituitary gland to release gonadotropins.
  - ❍ This increases secretion of luteinizing hormone (LH) and follicle stimulating hormone (FSH), which stimulate ovarian development and oestrogen production.
  - ❍ Oestrogen induces all secondary sexual characters except auxiliary and pubic hair, which are controlled by adrenal androgens.
- Breast development, or thelarche, is the first sign of puberty and begins at about age 9 with the bud stage:
  - ❍ Breast development takes about 3 years to complete.

- Breast development ends shortly after the first menses.
- Fatty tissue in the thighs, hips and breast increases; the hips broaden.
- The onset of menses occurs between ages 8 and 16, menses initially may be irregular.
- Pubic hair growth increases continuously for several years after menses begins.
- The female grows up to 7.6 cm a year and stops growing at about age 16.
- The sweat glands and sebaceous glands become more active; body odour and acne increase.

- Developments in the male
  - The hypothalamus signals the pituitary and the development of release of LH and FSH.
  - LH results in testicular enlargement and the development of Leydig's cells in the testes, which produce testosterone.
  - FSH stimulates the development of the seminiferous tubules of testis, leading to spermatogenesis and fertility.
  - Testicular enlargement signals the start of puberty.
  - The scrotum enlarges and the penis elongates and widens.
  - The penis reaches adult size at about age 17.
  - Muscle mass increases, the chest broadens, facial and body hair proliferates and laryngeal cartilage growth deepens the voice.
  - Pubic hair growth continues until age 20.
  - Sweat glands and sebaceous glands become more active; body odour and acne increases.
  - Nocturnal emissions are common; many males who ejaculate for the first time in a nocturnal emissions think that they have wetted the bed.
  - Masturbation with ejaculation is common.

High Risk Behaviours

- Motor vehicle accidents are the primary cause of mortality and morbidity, car safety information is essential at this age.
- One-half of all adolescents have had sexual intercourse by high school graduation.
- Smoking, drug and alcohol abuse are common risk-taking behaviours.
- Suicide is the third leading cause of death among adolescents.

Health Concerns of Adolescence

Risk behaviours are voluntary actions that threaten to harm an individual's mental or physical health, or increase the likelihood of illness, injury, and premature death. WHO identified six categories of risk behaviours in today's adolescent students. These include:

- Unintentional and intentional injuries
- Substance use
- Mental health
- Violence
- Sexual and reproductive health
- Dietary patterns and nutrition

The following provides information on each of these categories, as well as familiarizes mentors with the issues teenagers face on a daily basis and how involvement in these activities can harm youth.

Unintentional and Intentional Injuries

Approaches for reducing road traffic crashes, and the occurrence of serious injuries if and when crashes occur, are important for safeguarding adolescent health. These include:

- Enforcing speed limits.
- Combining education with laws to promote seat belt (and helmet) use and to prevent driving under the influence of alcohol or other psychoactive substances.
- Providing alternatives to driving by increasing the availability of safe and inexpensive public transport.

Actions to make the environment safer and to educate children and adolescents on how to avoid drowning, burns and falls can help reduce the likelihood of their occurrence. When someone is injured, prompt access to effective trauma care can be life saving.

Substance Use

In addition to laws that limit the availability of illicit substances, tobacco and alcohol, interventions to reduce demand for these substances improve the conditions for healthy development. Increasing their awareness of the dangers of substance use, building their competence to resist peer pressure and to manage stress in a healthy manner is effective in reducing adolescents' motivation for substance use.

Tobacco

Tobacco consumption includes the use of cigarettes, pipes, cigars, and smokeless tobacco. A type of central nervous system stimulant, tobacco makes a first-time user feel dizzy, light headed, excited, or nauseous. Over time, regular users develop a craving for nicotine, followed by relief and relaxation. when the product is used. Tobacco use affects both mind and body. It increases feelings of alertness and relaxation, and lowers stress and irritability. Tobacco also raises blood pressure, breathing, and heart rate; increases muscle relaxation; reduces pain; and decreases appetite. In addition, tobacco use can lead to chronic illnesses such as:

- Heart disease
- Cancer of the throat, mouth, and lungs
- Bronchitis
- Lowered resistance to colds, flu, and other infections

Alcohol and Other Drug Use

Alcohol is a psychoactive drug that depresses the central nervous system. Alcohol comes in many forms including clear, absolute liquid diluted and blended as beer, wine, or liquor. Alcohol initially makes individuals feel relaxed and sociable, but with prolonged use, these feelings will be replaced by feelings of depression, anger, loss of control, and drowsiness. Because of the large variance of tolerance levels, alcohol can have differing effects on individuals. Like tobacco, alcohol is a drug that affects both the mind and the body. Alcohol lowers the ability of the brain to control behaviour and impairs the ability to perform motor skills. In addition, alcohol lessens an individual's ability to move and speak.

Alcohol can also cause the following:

- Memory loss
- Addiction
- Liver, kidney, stomach, and intestine damage
- Brain damage
- Death from breathing or heart failure, and interactions with other drugs

Mental Health

Many mental health problems emerge in late childhood and early adolescence. Enhancing social skills, problem-solving skills and self confidence can help prevent mental health problems such as conduct disorders, anxiety, depression and eating disorders as well as other risk behaviours including those that relate to sexual behaviour, substance use, and violent behaviour. Health workers need to have the competencies to relate to young people, to detect mental health problems early, and to provide treatments which include counselling, cognitive-behavioural therapy and, where appropriate, psychotropic medication.

Violence

Life skills and social development programmes for children and adolescents are important for reducing violent behaviour. Supporting teachers and parents to build skills in problem solving and non-violent disciplining is also effective in reducing violence. If and when violence does occur, actions to make health systems more responsive, and to build the empathy and competence of health workers, can help ensure that adolescents who experience violence, including sexual violence, get effective and sensitive care and treatment. Ongoing psychological and social support can help adolescents deal with the long term psychological effects of violence, and to reduce the likelihood of their becoming perpetuators of violence in the future.

Sexual and Reproductive Health

Programmes that aim to educate adolescents about sexual and reproductive health need to be combined with programmes aimed at motivating them to apply what they have learnt in their lives. They should also be combined with efforts to make it easier for adolescents to obtain any preventive or curative health services they might need from competent and empathetic health workers. Sexual coercion in adolescence needs to be fought at different levels. Laws requiring severe punishment for this crime should be passed and energetically enforced, and public opinion should be mobilized to become fiercely intolerant of it. Girls and women should be protected from sexual harassment and coercion in educational institutions, work places and in other community settings.

Preventing too early pregnancy may require the enactment and enforcement of laws that specify a minimum age for marriage, as well as actions to mobilize families and communities to give their daughters the additional time they need to grow and develop from girlhood into womanhood before becoming wives and mothers. Alongside this, health services should be ready to provide adolescents who are pregnant with the antenatal care they need, or to obtain a safe abortion where this is permitted by law. Effective care during child bearing is important to ensure the survival of mothers and their babies, and the prevention of problems such as fistulas.

HIV

Young people's risk of HIV infection is closely correlated with age of sexual debut. Abstinence from sexual intercourse and delayed initiation of sexual behaviour are among the central aims of HIV prevention efforts for young people. Decreasing the number of sexual partners and increasing access to, and utilization of comprehensive prevention services, including prevention education and provision of condoms, are essential for young people who are sexually active. Programmes should also focus on prevention and early intervention in other health risk behaviours, such as substance use. Young people need HIV testing services that are accessible and appropriate. Young people living with HIV need treatment, care, support and positive prevention services. All HIV services for young people should involve young people living with HIV in their planning and provision

Dietary Patterns and Nutrition

Chronic malnutrition in earlier years is responsible for widespread stunting and to adverse health and social consequences throughout the life span. This is best prevented in childhood but actions to improve access to food could benefit adolescents as well. Anaemia is one of the key nutritional problems in adolescent girls. Preventing too-early pregnancy and improving the nutritional status of girls before they enter pregnancy could reduce maternal and infant mortality, and contribute to breaking the cycle of intergenerational malnutrition. This will involve improving access to nutritious food, to micronutrient supplementation and in many places to preventing infections as well. Adolescence is a timely period to shape healthy eating and exercise habits which can contribute to physical and psychological benefits during the adolescent period and to reducing the likelihood of nutrition-related chronic diseases in adulthood. Promoting healthy lifestyles is also crucial to halting the rapidly progressing obesity epidemic.

Chapter 2 PAEDIATRIC ASSESSMENT

OVERVIEW

Health assessment includes a discussion of growth pattern and nutrition as well as an examination of body systems. Our first task is to establish a good rapport with the child and his parents. When you talk to the child, you should show the empathy, understanding and use appropriate language according to the age. Children who comes to the hospital or clinic are frightened at first, then you play with the children for a while so that they may become calm and fearful. So nurses consider using toys or other play materials to communicate with the child. Before examining the child talk to him about toys, hobbies, pets or other subjects he is interested in and encourage his friendship with compliments.

ASSESSMENT OF GROWTH PATTERN AND NUTRITION

Purpose of Assessment

- To monitor changes in a child growth pattern
  - Failure to thrive
  - Obesity
- Assess a child's nutritional status.

Approaches to Assess the Child

- Plot the child height, weight, head circumference, and BMI (Body Mass Index) on growth grids, wrist circumference, Mid Upper Arm Circumference (MUAC) and Triceps Skin Fold (TSF). This allows you to screen the children growth pattern.
- The national center for health statistics has developed growth grids for children upto the age of 18.
  - Plot a children's height and weight of under five years in Harvard standard growth chart at each visit.
  - Plot an infant's head circumference until the age 2.
  - Calculate the children's BMI and plot on a gender-appropriate grid from the age of 2 to 20.
- Grids use percentiles to evaluate the children's growth.
  - The 50th percentile indicates an average height, weight, or head circumference for a child.
  - A child usually remains in the same percentile throughout his growth period; consider a large deviation (such as decrease from 50th to 5th percentile) as abnormal.
  - A BMI between 85th and 95th percentile for age and sex is considered a risk for the child to be overweight; a BMI over 95th percentile is considered overweight or obese.

TABLE 2.1: Expected Growth Rates at Various Ages

Age	Expected Growth Rate (cm/year)
1 to 6 months	18–22
6 to 12 months	14–18
2nd year	11
3rd year	8
4th year	7
5th to 10th years	5–6

Dietary History

- Obtain the child's diet history from the parents or child depending on age.

  For all paediatric age-group children to be assessed for
  - Daily nutritional plan (number and types of meals and snacks).
  - Special and modified diet.
  - Behavioural peculiarities associated with mealtimes.
  - Feeding problems.

- Assess for sugar intake: related to dental caries and obesity.
- Assess for iron intake: iron deficiency anaemia is a major childhood problem.
- Protein intake: protein is essential for growth
- Fat intake: it is needed in a balanced diet
- Calcium intake: it is needed to strengthen teeth and bones.

- Ask if the child was breast-fed and how long (how many months) and frequency of breast feeding.
- Ask how much water, milk, juice the child drinks.
- Ask if the child takes vitamins; ascertain the type and amount.
- Ask how many fruits and vegetables the child eats daily.
- Find out what type of snacks the child eats.

PHYSICAL EXAMINATION OF BODY SYSTEM

Goals of Physical Assessment

- Minimizes stress and anxiety associated with assessment of various body parts.
- Fosters a trusting nurse-child-parent relationship.
- Allows for physical and psychological preparation of the child.
- Preserves the essential security of the parent-child relationship especially with young children.
- Maximizes the accuracy and reliability of assessment findings.

Preparation of the Child for Physical Assessment

Physical examination consists of painless procedures. Using a tight arm cuff, probing in the ears and mouth, pressing on the abdomen and listening to the chest with cold piece of metal can be considerably stressful to the child, therefore some consideration is needed while preparing the child for physical examination procedures.

Guidelines for Performing Physical Examination

- Perform examination in an appropriate, non-threatening area
  - Prepare the room temperature comfortably warm, keep potential frightening equipment out of the children's sight, have some toys, stuffed animals and games for the different age groups of children.
  - Provide privacy especially for school age children and adolescents.
- Provide time for play to adjust with the environment.
- Observe the behaviour of the child for readiness to cooperate for the examination,
  - Talking to the nurse.
  - Child is accepting the equipment if she provide it to the child.
  - Allowing the physical touch to the child's body.
  - Accept to sit on the examination table.
- If the child is not cooperative, use the following techniques to do the examination,
  - Assess reason for uncooperative behaviour.
  - Try to involve child and parents in process.
  - Avoid prolonged explanations about examination procedure.
  - Perform examination as quick as possible.
  - Minimize any disruptions or stimulation.
- Start the examination in a nonthreatening manner for young children or children who are fearful.
- Involve the child in examination procedure,
  - Provide choices such as to sit on the examination table or parent's lap.
  - Allow the child to handle or hold the equipment.
  - Encourage the child to use the equipment on a toy or doll, family members or nurse or doctor.
  - Explain the procedure in simple language.
- Examine the child in a comfortable, secure and in child's preferable position.
  - Make the child to sit on parent's lap.
  - Sitting upright position if the child is in respiratory distress.
- Proceed to examine the body in an organized sequence usually from head to toe, alter sequence to accommodate needs depending upon children's age.
- Examine painful areas at last.
- In emergency situation examine vital functions (airway, breathing, temperature, circulation-pulse, blood pressure) and injury area first.

- Reassure the child throughout examination, especially about bodily concerns that arise during puberty.
- Discuss the findings with the family at the end of the examination.
- Praise the child for cooperation during examination; give rewards such as a small toy or sticker, etc.

Birth History and Early Development

- Ask the mother about the history of pregnancy and any complication during the pregnancy (Antenatal history).
- Ask the mother about delivery, history-mode of delivery, place of delivery and also the complication during delivery such as prematurity, birth trauma (Intranatal history).
- Assess the child's developmental milestones such as turning over, sitting up, crawling, and walking on correct age.
- Ask the mother about childhood diseases, injuries and known congenital abnormalities.
- Ask more specific questions depending on which body system is being assessed.
- Check the child height, weight and other developments according to the age, identify the deviation.

General Appearance

The general appearance of the child is a cumulative, subjective impression of the child's physical appearance, state of nutrition, behaviour, personality, interaction with parents and nurse, posture, development and speech. It should be recorded at the beginning of the physical examination; it encompasses all the observation of the child during the interview and physical examination.

- **Face**: The facial expression and appearance of the child gives clues regarding pain; have difficulty in breathing; feels frightened, discontent or happy; or mentally deficient or acutely ill.
- Observe **posture, position** and types of **body movement**. The child with hearing or vision loss may characteristically tilt the head in an awakened position to hear or see better.
- Check the child's **hygiene** in terms of cleanliness; any unusual body odour; the condition of the hair, neck, nails, feet; and the condition of clothing, etc. Such observation gives excellent clues for negligence, poor socioeconomic conditions, or lack of knowledge concerning child's needs.
- General appearance includes an overall impression of children's status of **nutrition**. The physical appearance like body weight and structure such as tall and slender, or it may estimate the quality and quantity of nutritional intake. According to the child's body build we can identify the nutritional status of the child (nutritional deficiencies).
- **Behaviour** includes the children's personality; levels of activity, reactions to stress, requests, or frustration; interaction with others.
    - Check the overall calm, anxious, tense, shy, talkative, aggressive, stable or mood.
    - Check whether the child has a long attention span or easily distracted.
    - Check whether the child uses eye to eye contact during conversation.
    - Observe whether the child is interested in the surroundings, does a child look in the room, asks questions related to unfamiliar objects, seems to explore the things to enjoy or destroy the things.
    - Observe whether the child is able to follow the instructions to use the instruments. Is the child quick or slow to grasp explanations?

Skin

Skin is assessed for colour, texture, temperature, moisture and turgor. Examination of the skin and its accessory structures primarily involves inspection and palpation.

- Assessing the skin colour is very important in newborns and infants.
- Reduced levels of oxygen (desaturated) or haemoglobin reach atleast 5 mg/dl reflects a bluish tone through the skin **(Cyanosis)**.
- **Pallor** or paleness of the skin may be a sign of anaemia, chronic diseases, oedema, or shock.
- **Erythema** or redness of the skin may be the result of increased temperature from climatic conditions, local inflammation or infection.
- **Ecchymosis and Petechiae** are caused by extravasations or haemorrhage of blood into the skin. **Ecchymoses are** large, diffuse areas usually black and blue in colour; strike off typically the result of injury. **Petechiae** are small, distinct pinpoint haemorrhage 2 mm or less in size and can denote some type of blood disorder, such as decreased platelets in leukaemia.

- **Jaundice** is a yellow staining of the skin usually caused by bile pigments, strike off always a significant finding.

Texture: Palpate the skin for texture and noting moisture. Normally the skin of young children is smooth, soft, and slightly dry to touch, not oily and clammy. Any variation from these findings is due to common problems like cradle cap, eczema, diaper rashes, or extra dryness (xeroderma), exposure to the weather or vitamin A deficiency. Excessively moist, clammy skin may indicate serious health problems particularly heart diseases.

Temperature: Evaluate temperature by symmetrically feeling each part of body and compare the upper ones. Note any distinct difference in temperature.

Turgor: Tissue turgor refers to the amount of elasticity in the skin. To assess turgor, grasp the skin on the abdomen between the thumb and index finger, pull it taut and quickly release it. Elastic tissue immediately returns to normal position. In children with poor tissue turgor it remains suspended or tented for a few seconds. Before slowly falling back on the abdomen it indicates dehydration.

- While evaluating tissue turgor, inspect for signs of **oedema**, which is normally evident as swelling or puffiness.
- Evaluate for changes in oedema according to position, specific location and response to pressure. For example in **pitting oedema**, pressing a finger into the oedematous area causes a temporary indentation.
- Neonates and infants
  - Jaundice occurs in approximately 50% of all babies.
  - Birth marks.
  - Bacterial and candidal infections may occur with diaper rash, check the papules, pustules (with vesicles satellite lesions).
  - The scaling and crusting of cradle cap may entirely cover an infant scalp.
- Preschool and school age children
  - Younger children are susceptible to common disorders such as allergic contact, dermatitis, warts, scabies, impetigo, eczema, ring worm infection and skin reactions to food allergies.
  - They typically have bruises on their lower extremities resulting from active play.
- Adolescents
  - At puberty, hormonal changes affect the children's skin and hair.

    Androgen level increases, causing sebaceous glands to secrete large amount of sebum which can clog hair follicle openings.

    Coarse hair appears on the face, axillae, pubic area in boys and on the axille and pubic area in girls.
  - Common dermatoses that occur during adolescence include acne, warts, sunburn, scabies, dermatitis, pityriasis rosea, contact dermatitis, and fungal infections.
  - For all age-groups, be aware of skin deviation that may indicate abuse.

Head

- In neonates general appearance, size, movement, head circumference (normal 33–35 cm), common variation like molding, fontanelles (anterior fontanelle: 3–4 cm long, 2–3 cm wide, diamond shaped and posterior fontanelle: 1–2 cm at birth, triangle–shaped), hair texture and distribution.
- Check for cephalhematoma (trauma during birth persists upto 3 weeks), Caput succedaneum (long labour and birth, disappears in 1 week).
- Assess for premature closure of sutures (craniostenosis), and late closure (hydrocephalus).
- At the age of one year head and chest circumference are equal, then chest circumference will increase. If head circumference will be increasing you have to identify the abnormality (hydrocephalus).
- Check the fontanelle for bulging (increased intracranial pressure, meningitis), sunken (dehydration).

Neck

When you assess head and neck, inspect the size of the neck and palpate it for associated structures.

- During infancy the neck is short, with skin folds between the head and shoulders; it lengthens during the next 3 to 4 years.
- A short or webbed neck is associated with various anomalies, such as Turner syndrome.
- Marked oedema of the neck may indicate mumps, local or mouth infections or diphtheria.
- Distended neck veins often indicate difficulty on expiration such as asthma or cystic fibrosis.
- Palpate the trachea by placing the thumb and index finger on each side and sliding them back and forth to note any masses. Normally the

trachea is in the midline or slightly to the right of the midline. Note any shift, because it can signify serious lung problems such as a tumour or foreign body in the lung.

- Palpate the thyroid gland which is located at the base of the neck, whose neck is short and thick. If any masses are detected in the neck, record and report them for further investigation.

Eyes and Vision

Examination of the eyes involves inspection of all exterior structure for size, symmetry, colour and motility as well as inspection and surface examination of retinal structure. Accurate examination of each structure requires the use of an ophthalmoscope and is a highly skilled procedure. The nurse should know the normal findings to differentiate from abnormality.

The third part of the examination involves vision testing.

- Behaviour problems or poor performance in school may relate to difficulty in seeing the blackboard.
- History questions
  - Look for clues to familial eye disorders, such as refractive errors and retinoblastoma.

    Refer a child with family history of glaucoma to an ophthalmologist, even if there are no obvious symptoms.
  - Ask the parents if the child has difficulty reading the blackboard in school or squints, which may be a sign of myopia, or near sight (the ability to see objects at close range but not at a distance); children usually do not have a difficulty with reading or other work.

Inspection of External Structure of Eye

Observe the eyes for relative placement on the face, symmetry of location, and general slant of the palpebral fissures or lid.

- If any abnormality of placement is observed, measure the interpupillary distance, which is approximately 4.5–5.5 cm or inner canthal distance is approximately 2.5 cm. Large spacing between the eyes is called **hypertelorism**. It suggests mental retardation.
- Determine the general slant of the **palpebral fissures** or lid by drawing an imaginary line through the two points of the medial canthus and across the outer orbit of the eyes and aligning each eye on the line. Normally the palpebral fissures lie horizontally but slant is normally upward. Eye abnormalities are common in many chromosomal disorders so carefully we have to observe and record the deviation. In a child with Down syndrome we can find hypertelorism, epicanthal folds and upward palpebral slant.
- Inspect the **lids** for proper placement of the eye. **Ptosis** refers to a lid that covers part of the pupils or the lower part of the iris. The term **sunset eyes** indicates an upper lid that covers no part of iris, allowing some of the sclera or the "white of the eye" to show.
- When the eyes are closed, the lid should completely cover the cornea and sclera. Incomplete closure of lid results in chronic irritation and infection to the eye. Malposition of eyelids indicates **extropion** a rolling out of the eyelid with exposed conjunctiva and **entropion** a turning-in of the lid.
- Observe the lids for blinking movement. Excessive blinking movement can indicate eyestrain or nervous habits. Test the **blinking reflex.**
- Inspect the **eyelashes** for distribution, lashes that turn inward the eyeball can cause conjunctival irritation.
- The **Sclera** or the write covering of the eyeball, should be clear, if it is yellow this may indicate **jaundice**. A bluish tone may indicate the disorder of **oesteogenesis** imperfect or **glaucoma.**
- Check the **cornea** or covering of the iris and pupils. These should be clear and transparent. Record any opacity, it can be a sign of scarring or ulceration and can interfere with vision.
- Compare the pupils for size, shape and movement, they are round, clear and equal.
- Test the pupils for **reaction to light** and test for **accommodation.**
- Check the **iris** for size, colour, and clarity. Black and white speckling of the iris is known as **Brush field spots.**

Inspection of Internal Structures of Eye

Internal structure to be checked by special instruments like ophthalmoscope, funduscope.

- Ophthalmoscope permits visualization of the interior of the eyeball with a system of lens and high-intensity light. This examination is used to inspect the cornea, iris, lens, retina, to inspect the blood vessels, macula or optic disc.

- Funduscope shows the structure of the back of the eyeball or the fundus. This examination can assess disc diameter, central retinal artery and vein, arteriolar light reflex,

Vision Test

Several tests are available for assessing the vision, they focus on four areas.

1. Binocularity
2. Visual acuity
3. Peripheral vision
4. Colour vision

- At the age of 3 to 4 months children normally achieve **binocularity**. This test is important for binocularity strike off alignment of the eyes to detect nonbiocular vision or **strabismus**. If strabismus is not detected and corrected by age 4 to 6 years, a type of blindness known as **amblyopia** may result.
- **Visual acuity test** refers to the ability to see near and far objects clearly. The most commonly used test for measuring acuity is the **Snellen letter chart**, which consists of lines of letter in decreasing size. Each line is given a value; for example, line 7 has a value of "20".
- **Snellen symbol chart** is often used to screen preschool children; however, children have confusion in identifying the direction of the E, rather than inability to see the symbol clearly. To avoid problem, a nurse developed the **Blackbird preschool Vision Screening Test**. This is a test done with flash cards or a wall-mounted chart and the child is instructed to indicate the direction of the bird flight.
- **This Snellen Chart test** is used for checking the Visual acuity to detect Myopia (near sight) and **Hyperopia** (far sight).
- Visual acuity testing in infant is easy and difficult to test in the children. In newborn the vision is tested mainly by checking for light perception by shining a light into eyes and noting responses such as papillary constriction, blinking, increased alertness or refuse to open the eyes after exposer to light.
- **Peripheral vision.** In children who are old enough to cooperate, estimate peripheral vision. Limitation in peripheral vision may indicate blindness from damage to structure within the eyes or any of the visual pathways.
- **Colour vision.** It is an important test for colour vision to identify the colour blindness.

Ears

Ear examination involves inspection of the internal and external auditory structures and screening for hearing ability.

Inspection of External Structures

- The external earlobe is called the **Pinna**. Measure the height alignment of the pinna by drawing an imaginary line from the outer orbit of the eye to the occiput, the top of the pinna should meet or cross this line. Low set ear are commonly associated with renal anomalies or mental retardation.
- Inspect the **skin** around the ear for small openings, extra tags of skin or sinuses.
- Inspect the ear for general **hygiene**. An otoscope is strike off necessary to look into the external canal to note the presence of **cerumen**, a waxy substance produced by the ceruminous glands in the outer portion of the canal.
- Inspect for any ear discharge from the aural canal.

Inspection of Internal Structures

- Inspection of internal structure of ears is carried out by the instruments like **otoscope** to inspect the walls of the canal, the colour of the tympanic membrane, the light reflex and usual landmarks of the bony prominences of the middle ear.
- **Auditory Testing:** Several types of hearing test are available. Audiometric testing involves specialized equipment that measures the degree of hearing loss.
- One of the commonly used tests is **audiometry,** which measures the threshold of hearing for pure-tone frequencies (measured in hertz (Hz)).
- **Pneumatic Otoscopy:** To measure the pressure of the tympanic membrane.
- **Vestibular Testing:** Vestibular testing is for inner ear function concerning equilibrium.
    - Some have mandated Auditory Brainstem Response (ABR) Test as part of newborn screening.
    - An infant younger than age 6 months should respond to a spoken voice, by age 6, an infant can localize the direction of sound; and by age 5, a child's hearing is fully developed.
    - Investigate the child's speech development by listening to him carefully, speech development sometimes reflects hearing acuity during childhood.

- Observe the behaviour for possible sign of ear disorder.
  - Does the child rub his ear as though it hurts?
  - Does he tilt his head when listening?
- The parents birth history may provide clues to possible hearing disorder.
  - Prenatal causes of congenital hearing defect include maternal infection especially rubella during the first trimester, and maternal use of ototoxic drugs.
  - Events at birth that may cause hearing loss include hypoxia, jaundice and trauma.
  - If the child has a craniofacial deformity, such as cleft palate, he has an increased risk of developing otitis media, which can lead to hearing loss.
- When asked about daily activities, child may relate observations that indicate possible hearing loss.
  - The child does not startle or wake up in response to a loud stimuli.
  - The child has to be told several times to do something, even though he is old enough to understand.
- Evaluating hearing in an infant
  - Acoustic blink reflex
  - Make a sudden loud noise, clapping your hands or snapping your fingers about 12″ from his ear.
  - The infant should respond with the startle reflex or by blinking.
- Screening hearing in a child between ages 2 and 5
  - Use play techniques.
  - Routine screening with an audiometer usually begins at age 3.
- Screening hearing in an older child
  - Use the whisper test, making sure to use words he knows and taking care to prevent him from lip reading.
  - The child should hear a whispered question or simple command at 8.

Mouth and Throat

The mouth is the beginning of the passageway to the digestive tract, but it also functions as the entry or exit of air. The major structure of the exterior of the mouth is the **lips**.

- Inspect the lips for colour, check any deviation like **cheilitis**—which is the presence of painful, inflamed, dried cracks or fissures of the lips. **Cheilitis** is caused by exposure to harsh climate condition, mouth breathing from respiratory distress or dehydration, due to fever.
- Check for **cheilosis** or angular stomatitis which is a fissure at the angles or corner of the lips, it may be due to deficiency of riboflavin or niacin.
- Observe for lesion on the lips. The herpes simplex virus produces singular or cluster of vesicular eruptions, often called **cold sore**.
- Visual examination within the oral cavity and oropharynx are the mucosal lining of the lips, cheeks, gums, teeth, tongue, palate, uvula, tonsils and posterior oropharynx.
- Inspect all areas lined with mucous **membranes**. Note any deviations such as colour, white patches or ulcerations, bleeding and sensitivity.
- Check for any candidiasis in the mucous membranes of the palate and gums and surface of the tongue.
- Inspect the **teeth** for number in each dental arch, hygiene and occlusion or bite, discolouration of teeth enamel with obvious plaque. It is a sign of poor hygiene.
- Examine the gums surrounding the teeth. The colour of the gum is normally pink and the surface texture is stippled. Note if the gum is inflamed, redness, puffiness along the gum line. Bleeding is a sign of gingivitis.
- Inspect the **Tongue** for the presence of papillae, small projections that contain several taste buds. Note changes in the surface texture, such as
  (1) "geographic tongue," unusual patterns of papillae formation and denuded areas;
  (2) coated tongue, such as in candidiasis; or
  (3) an exceptionally beefy red and swollen tongue, which is a sign of various systemic diseases.
- Inspect both **soft palate** and **hard palate** carefully to be sure they are intact. Sometimes there is a pinpoint cleft in the soft palate that may go undetected unless carefully inspected. Such a cleft is especially important if the uvula is bifid, or separated into two appendages.
- While inspecting the recesses of the oropharynx, note the size and colour of the **palatine tonsils**.

Enlargement, redness, and white patches on the tonsils and surrounding area may indicate suppurative tonsillitis or pharyngitis. Report these findings for further evaluation.

Chest-Lung

Upper respiratory tract infection commonly occur in children because a child's respiratory tract is immature and the mucous membranes cannot produce enough mucous to warm and humidify inhaled air.

The thoracic cavity has two vital organs, the heart and the lung. The anatomical structure of the chest wall is an important source of information concerning cardiac and pulmonary function. Inspect the chest for size, shape, symmetry, movement. Inspection of lungs involves observation of respiratory movement, palpation, percussion, auscultation of breath sound.

- History collection
  - Ask parents how often the child has upper respiratory tract infections.
  - Find out if the child has had other respiratory signs and symptoms such as cough, wheezing, rhinorrhea, or a stuffy nose; ask if they appear related to the child's activities or to seasonal changes.
- Normal respiratory rates
  - Newborn babies: 30–70 breaths/minute.
  - Young infant (2 months up to 12 months) 30–60 breaths/minute.
  - Toddlers: 20–40 breaths/minute.
  - Preschoolers: 20–30 breaths/minute.
  - School age children: 15–25 breaths/minute.
  - Adolescents (about age 15) 12–20 breaths/minute.
  - The best time to obtain a child's respiratory rate is when he is awake and sitting quietly or when he is sleeping.
  - Child's respiratory rate doubles in response to exercise, illness, or emotion.
- While doing a physical assessment the sitting position allows you the easiest access to the child's thorax.
- If the child is quiet, auscultate the lung first.
- Use a flashlight and tongue blade to examine the child's mouth and throat.
  - Never test the gag reflex or examine the pharynx in a child suspected of having epiglottiditis; this procedure can cause complete laryngeal obstruction.
- The thoracic cavity is also divided into segments by drawing imaginary lines on the chest and back to illustrate the anterior, lateral and posterior division.
- Measure the size of the chest by placing the tap around the rib cage at the nipple line. It is important to compare with the head circumference.
- Inspect the shape of the chest to identify the abnormality.

Inspection

Inspection of the lung primarily involves observation of respiratory movement. Evaluate the respiration for

1. Rate (number per minute)
2. Rhythm (regular, irregular, or periodic)
3. Depth (deep or shallow)
4. Quality (effortless, automatic, difficult or labored)

The usual ratio of breaths to heart beats is 1 : 4.

When examining a child, note these structural abnormalities of the chest.

- Barrel chest may indicate chronic respiratory disease, such as cystic fibrosis or asthma.
- Funnel chest may indicate rickets or marafan syndrome.
- Localized bulges may indicate underlying pressure, such as cardiac enlargement or an aneurysm.
- Pigeon chest may indicate marfan or morquio's syndrome or a chronic upper respiratory tract condition.
- Rachitic beads (bumps at the costochondral junction of the ribs) may indicate rickets.
- An unusually wide space between the nipples may indicate Turner's syndrome (the distance between the outside areolar edges should not be more than one-fourth of the child's chest circumference).

- While examining the posterior thorax of the older child, make sure you check for scoliosis.
- Intracostal, subcostal, and suprasternal retractions and expiratory grunts are always serious signs in children.
  - Refer an infant or a child with these signs for further evaluation and treatment immediately.
  - He may have pneumonia, respiratory distress syndrome or left-side heart failure.

Palpation

- Evaluate **respiratory movement** to assess the amount of respiratory excursion and note any asymmetry of movement.
- Palpate for **vocal fremitus** which is the condition of voice sounds through the respiratory sound
  - Decreased vocal fremitus in the upper air way may indicate several gross pulmonary changes.
  - The absence of fremitus usually indicates obstruction of major bronchus—result of foreign body aspiration.
- Check for **crepitation and plural friction-crepitation** which is a course, crackling sensation felt as the hand is pressed over the affected area, results from air escaping the lungs into the subcutaneous tissues as a result of injury or surgical intervention. **Plural friction rubs** which is a grating sensation due to inflammation of pleural lining rubbing against one another. Both conditions can be heard and felt.

Percussion

The lungs are percussed in order to evaluate the densities of underlying organ.

Expected sounds on percussion are:

1. **Resonance** is heard over all the lobes that are not adjacent to other organs.
2. **Dullness** is heard beginning at the fifth interspace in the right midclavical line, percussion downward to the end of the liver.
3. **Flat sound** is heard because the liver no longer overlies the air-filled lung.
4. **Cardiac dullness** is felt over the left sternal border from the second to the fifth interspace and medially to the midclavicular line.
5. **Tempany** below the fifth interspace on the left side, tempany results from the air-filled stomach.

Note: Always record and report deviations from these expected sounds.

Auscultation

Auscultation involves using the stethoscope to evaluate breath and voice sounds.

- Breath sound in the lungs is classified as vesicular, bronchovesicular or bronchial.
- **Absent or diminished breath sound** is always an abnormal finding and warrants investigation.
- Fluid, air or solid masses in the plural space interfere with the conduction of breath sounds.
- **Voice sounds** are also part of auscultation of the lung, vocal resonance or voice sounds are normally heard, but the syllables are indistinct. Elicit them in the same manner as for vocal fremitus, expect to listen with the stethoscope.
- Consolidation of lung tissue produces three types of abnormal voice sound:
  1. Whispered pectoriloquy words are whispered and syllables are heard.
  2. Branchophony spoken words are not distinguishable, but the vocal resonance is increased in intensity and clarity.
  3. Egophony "ee" is heard as the nasal sound "ay" through the stethoscope.
  4. Decreased or absent vocal resonance is caused by the same conditions that affect vocal fremitus.

Abnormal Lung Sounds

1. **Coarse crackle:** Discontinuous, interrupted explosive sounds, loud and low in pitch.
2. **Fine crackle:** Discontinuous, interrupted explosive sounds. Less loud than above and of shorter duration; higher in pitch than coarse crackles.
3. **Wheeze:** Continuous sound of high pitch, a hissing sound.

Heart

The nurses should have knowledge of the anatomy and physiology of the normal heart. It is essential in order to properly evaluate the findings.

The heart is positioned in the thorax like a trapezoid:

- **Vertically** along the Right Sternal Border (RSB) from the second to the fifth rib.
- **Horizontally** (**long side**) from the lower right sternum to the fifth rib at the Left Midclavicular Line (LMCL).
- **Diagonally** from the Left Sternal Border (LSB) at the second rib to the LMCL at the rib.
- **Horizontally** (**short side**) from the RSB and LSB at the second Intercostals Space (ICS) base of the heart.

The most important skill in examining the heart is auscultation, which is performed when the child is quiet. Inspection and palpation also yield important information. However, percussion is of little value in assessing cardiac size or function.

Inspection

- When examining the chest, note any obvious bulging, especially on the left side, which may indicate cardiac enlargement.
- Comprehensive evaluation of cardiac function is not limited to the heart, also consider other findings such as the presence of pulse (Especially the femoral pulse), distended neck veins, clubbing of the fingers, peripheral cyanosis, oedema, blood pressure and respiratory status.

Palpation

- Palpation to determine the location of the **apical impulse (AI)**. AI gives a general idea of the size of the heart (with enlargement, the apex is lower and more lateral). The AI is found:
  - Just lateral to the LMCL and fourth ICS in children < 7 years of age.
  - At the LMCL and fifth ICS in children > 7 years of age.
- The **Point of Maximum Intensity (PMI)** is an impulse, strike off an area of most intense pulsation. Usually the PMI is located at the site as the AI.
- **Thrills** are palpable vibrations most commonly produced by the flow of blood from one chamber of the heart to another through a narrowed or abnormal opening, such as a stenosis valve or a septal defect. Thrills are felt with palmar surface at the base of the fingers and during expiration.
- **Pericardial friction ribs** are scratchy, high-pitched grating sounds; but they are not affected by changes in respiration. Both thrills and ribs are abnormal. Report them for further evaluation.
- **Capillary refill time**—an important test of peripheral circulation. Blanch the nail bed with sustained pressure for a few seconds and then release the pressure. The time it takes for the nail to return to its original colour is the capillary refill time.
  - Capillary refill should be brisk – in less than 2 seconds; prolonged refill may be associated with poor systemic perfusion.

Auscultation

The heart sounds are produced by the opening and closing of the valves and the vibration of blood against the walls of the heart and vessels.

- Normally two sounds S-1 and S-2 are heard, "LUB-**DUB**" often describe the 4 sounds.
- S_1 is caused by closure of the **atrioventricular valves.**
- S_2 is the result of closure of **pulmonic** and **aortic valves.**
- Normally the split of the two sounds in S_2 is distinguishable and widens during inspiration.
- "Fixed splitting" in which the split in S_2, does not change during inspiration, is an important diagnosis sign or atrial septal defect.
- Two other heart sounds are S_3, S_4.
- S_3 is the result of vibration produced during ventricular filling. It is normally heard in some children and young adult but it is considered abnormal in old individuals.
- S_4 is caused by the recoil of vibrations between the atria and ventricles following atrial contraction at the end of diastole. It indicates that the child needs for further evaluation.

Murmurs

Murmurs are an important category of the heart sound which are produced by vibrations within heart chambers or in the major arteries from the back and forth flow of blood.

In general recognize murmurs as distinct swishing sound that occurs in addition to the normal heart sounds and record the:

1. Location
2. Time
3. Intensity
4. Loudness

Other abnormal sounds, such as ejection clicks, snaps, gallops and hums are beyond the scope of this discussion.

Abdomen

Examination of the abdomen involves the usual four skills, except that the order is altered. Start with inspection and follow with auscultation percussion and palpation because the latter three manoeuvres may distort the normal abdominal sounds. Abdominal cavity is divided into four quadrants, they are

1. Right upper quadrant
2. Right lower quadrant
3. Left upper quadrant
4. Left lower quadrant

Inspection

- Inspect for **contour**—Normally the abdomen of the infant and young children is quite cylindrical in the erect position.
- Check for the **size and tone** of the abdomen, it gives indication of general nutritional status and muscular development.
  - A large and prominent, flabby abdomen is seen in obese children.
  - Concave abdomen suggests undernutrition.
  - Carefully note a protruding abdomen which may indicate any pathological condition like abdominal distension, ascities, tumours or organomegally. A protuberant abdomen flat extremities, wasted buttocks indicate severe malnutrition.
- The **Skin** covering of the abdomen should be uniformly taut without any wrinkles or creases. Skin may be stretched due to ascities. Superficial vein may be visible in thin, light colour children, but distended vein in abnormal finding that suggests vascular or abdominal obstruction or abdominal distension.
- Observe **movement** of the abdomen, Infant and thin children may have visible peristaltic waves. Nurses should assess properly and report this finding; it indicates pathologic states like intestinal obstruction such as pyloric stenosis.
- Inspect the **umbilicus** for herniation, discharge, hygiene, and fistula. Instruct the child to cough to identify the protrusion of the umbilicus, if the child is too young to cough tell the child to blow the balloon, it increases the intraabdominal pressure sufficiently to demonstrate the presence of an Umbilical hernia.
- Inspect for the **Inguinal hernia** in the inguinal or femoral region.

Auscultation

Auscultate each of the four quadrants using the stethoscope, the most important sound to listen for it is **peristalsis**, or **bowel sound,** which sounds like short metallic clicks and gurgles. Normally bowel sounds may be heard every 10 to 30 seconds. Always report hyper peristalsis or an absence of bowel sound, it indicates that there is some abdominal disorder.

- Various other sounds may be heard in the abdominal cavity. Normally the pulsation of the aorta is heard in the epigastrium. Always refer the case if you hear the sound that resembles murmurs, hums for further evaluation.

Percussion

Percussion should be done in the abdomen same like lung percussion. Normally dullness or flatness is heard on the right side at the lower costal margin because of the location of the liver. Tympany is typically heard over the stomach on the left side and in the rest of the abdomen.

- An unusually tympanic sound, like the beating of a tight drum denotes air in the stomach, which is commonly due to mouth breathing. However, this sound can indicate a pathologic condition like low intestinal obstruction or paralytic ileus.

Palpation

Palpation is performed by two types: Superficial and deep.

- Palpate the pain area of the abdomen at last.
- Clues to a child's pain include facial grimacing, and a change in the pitch of the child's cry.

Superficial palpation: Place the hand lightly against the skin and feel each quadrant, noting any areas of tenderness, muscle tone, and superficial lesion such as cysts.

- Always note tenderness or pain anywhere in the abdomen during superficial palpation.
- Identify the types of pain like visceral and somatic pain.
- **Visceral pain:** Which arises from the viscera or internal organ like intestine. Child usually has pain dull, poorly localized and difficult for the child to describe
- **Somatic pain:** Which arises from the walls or linings of the abdominal cavity, such as peritoneum. Pain is generally sharp, well-localized and more easily described.
- When assessing the abdominal pain inform the child to respond like either there is pain or there is great pain. Assess the intensity of the pain.
- Elicit **rebound tenderness** or **Blumberg sign**, if the child complaints of abdominal pain. Press firmly over the part of the abdomen distal to the area of tenderness and release the pressure suddenly.
  - **If rebound tenderness** is present, the child feels pain in the original area of the tenderness. This response indicates that a small organ is inflamed such as appendicitis.

Deep palpation: It is used for palpating organs and large blood vessels and for detecting masses and tenderness not identified during superficial palpation.

- Palpate the abdominal organ by pressing it against your free hand, which is placed on the child's back.
- Begin the palpation in the lower quadrant and proceed upward to avoid missing the edges of an enlarged **liver** and **spleen.**
- If the liver is palpable 3 cm below the right costal margin or the spleen is palpable more than 2 cm below the left costal margin, it indicates that these organs are enlarged.
- Other anatomic structures that are sometimes palpable in children include the kidney, bladder, caecum and sigmoid colon.
- The **Bladder** may be palpated slightly above the symphsis in infant and children.
- The **Caecum** is a soft, gas-filled mass in the right lower quadrant.
- The Sigmoid colon is felt as a sausage-shaped mass that is freely movable over the pelvic brim in the left lower quadrant; it is normally tender.
- Locate the femoral pulses by placing the tips of two or three fingers (index, middle and/or ring finger) along the inguinal ligament about mid way between the iliac crest and pubic symphysis. Feel both pulses simultaneously to make certain they are equal and strong.
- Examine the **abdominal reflexes** by scratching the skin toward the umbilicus. The normal response is umbilicus moves towards the stimulus. Normally in children under one year of age these reflexes may be absent. These reflexes to identify the asymmetry or absence of response.
- Absence of femoral pulse is a significant sign of coarctation of the aorta, it needs referral for future evaluation.
- High-pitched abdominal sound may indicate intestinal obstruction or gastroenteritis.
- Venous hum may indicate portal hypertension.
- Splenic or hepatic friction rub may indicate inflammation.
- Double sound in the femoral artery may indicate aortic insufficiency.
- Absence of bowel sound may indicate paralytic ileus and peritonitis.
- Causes of acute abdominal pain may indicate appendicitis, incarcerated inguinal hernia, intussusception.

Genitalia

Examination of genitalia is carried out to identify the opening of Vulva and Vagina in female children, size and orifice urethral meatus for location, size of the scrotum and testes in males

Male Genitalia

- Examination of penis is for size, fold of the skin, gland and shaft for the sign of swelling, skin lesions, inflammation or other irregularities. Any of these signs may indicate underlying disorders, especially sexually transmitted diseases.
- The urethral meatus is carefully inspected for location and evidence of discharge. Normally the meatus should be in the center of the shaft.
- Location and size of the scrotum are noted. The scrotum hangs freely from the perineum behind the penis, the left scrotum normally hangs lower than right. The skin of the scrotum is loose and highly rugated (wrinkled).

Palpation of the scrotum identifies the testes, epididymis and inguinal hernia. The two testes are felt as small ovoid bodies about 1.5 to 2 cm long, one in each scrotal sac. Check for the presence of testes. (Avoid cremasteric reflex which is stimulated by cold touch. This reflex pulls the testes into the pelvic cavity).

- Check for undescended testes, absence of testes, or any hydrocele (unilateral or bilateral), it should be reported.
- Identify location of urethral opening on the dorsum of the shaft epipadias or urethral opening on the underside of the penis or on the perineum hypopadias.

Female Genitalia

The examination of female genitalia is limited to inspection and palpation of external structures.

- Examine the female genitalia for size and location of the structures of the Vulva or Pudendum. The mons pubis is a pad of adipose tissue over the symphysis pubis.
- Note the size and location of the Clitoris.
- Examine the Labia majora and Labia minora
- Inspect for the urethral meatus which is located posterior to the clitoris. Note its location, especially if it opens from the clitoris or inside the vagina. Gently palpate the glands for cysts and sexually transmitted lesions.

- Inspect the vaginal orifice which is located posterior to the urethral meatus. Ordinarily, examination of the vagina is limited to inspection. In virgins a thin crescent shaped or circular membrane, called hymen is present.
- Check for vasico vaginal fistula, irritation, swelling or abnormal vaginal discharge in female children.

Anus

After examination of genitalia, the anal area is easily examined; the children should be placed on the abdomen.

- Note the general firmness of the buttocks and symmetry of the gluteal folds.
- Assess the tone of the anal sphincter by eliciting the anal reflex.
- Gently scratching the anal area results in an obvious quick contraction of the external anal sphincter.
- Inspect for any abnormality like imperforated anus, absence of sphincter control or reflex or fistula.

Back and Extremities

History Collection

- Determine the ages at which the child reached major development milestones.
- For infant, these include the age at which he held up his head, rolled over, sat unassisted, and walked alone, jumped, walked upstairs, and pedalled a tricycle.
- Ask about a history of repeated fractures, muscle strains or sprains, painful joints, clumsiness, lack of which may indicate a musculoskeletal problem.
- Range of motion (ROM) and muscle strength:
  - For children who can follow instructions and do active ROM movements, demonstrate what you want the child to do and ask him to mimic you.
  - Observe the child's muscles for size, symmetry, strength, tone, and abnormal movements.
  - Test muscle strength in a preschool or school-age child by having the child push against your hands or arms.
  - To test muscle strength in an infant or a toddler who cannot understand directions, observe his sucking as well as general motor activity.

Examination of Back and Extremities

It includes spine, extremities, joints and muscles (Whole Musculoskeletal system) in this:

- Observe the child's muscles for size, symmetry, strength, tone, and abnormal movement.
- Test muscle strength.
- Check for scoliosis by asking the child to bend over and touch her toes without bending her knees.
- Ask the child to walk, run, and skip away from you and then return to check gait, balance and stance.
- Observe the child's legs for shape, length, symmetry and alignment.
- Inspect the child's feet for club foot, outward-turned toes and pigeon toes.
- Test the child for tibial torsion.

Spine

The general curvature of the spine is noted. Normally the back of a newborn is round or C shaped from the thoracic and pelvic curve.

- Marked curvatures in posture are abnormal. Scoliosis, lateral curvature of the spine, is an important childhood problem. It is more common in girls than in boys. Ask the child to bend over and touch her toes without bending her knees and observe for lateral curves and differences in the height of the shoulders and the iliac crests. A slight limp, a crooked hemline or complaints of sore back are other signs and symptoms of scoliosis.
- Kyphosis and lordosis usually from poor posture.
- Inspect the back, especially along the spine, for any tuffs of hair, dimples or discolouration to assess the neural tube defect.
- Mobility of the vertebral column is easily assessed in most children.
- Check the child's gait, balance and stance, ask her to walk, run, and skip away from you and then return.
- Assessment of the cervical spine is an important diagnostic sign of neurologic problems, such as meningitis.

- Hyperextension of the neck and spine, or opisthotones, which is accompanied by pain when the head is flexed, is always referred for medical evaluation.

Hip and Extremities

- Inspect hip and each extremity for symmetry of length and size, refer any deviation for orthopaedic evaluation.
- Neonates should be screened for developmental dysplasia of the hip using the Ortolani and Burlow tests (should be performed only by an experienced clinician).
- Observe the children's leg shape, length, symmetry and alignment.
  - **Genu varum** (bowlegs) is common in children between ages 1½ and 2½ years, to test for bowlegs, have the child stand straight with his ankles touching; in this position, the knees should not be more than 2.5 cm apart.
  - **Genu valgum** (Knock–Knees) is common in preschool age group of children, to test the knock-knees, have the child stand straight with his knees touching; the ankles should not be more than 2.5 cm in this position.
  - Look at the pattern of wear on the child's shoes—wear on the outside of the heel suggests bowlegs; on the inside knock-knees.
- Observe the child's feet for **club foot** (equinovarus), outward-turned toes (toeing out or pes valgus) and pigeon toes (toeing in or pes varus).
- Test the child for **tibial torsion**, internal and external tibial torsion.
- Observe for **Polydactyly** (extra digit of fingers or toes) or fusion of digits of fingers or toes (**Syndactyly**).

Neurologic Assessment

The assessment of the nervous system is the broadest and most diverse because every human function is controlled by neurologic impulses. This discussion focuses primarily on a general appraisal of behaviour, cognitive-perceptual development, sensory and cerebella functioning, deep tendon reflexes, the cranial nerves, and "soft" signs.

Nervous System

- History questions
  - Ask if the child has experienced head or neck injuries, headaches, tremors, seizures, dizziness, fainting spells, or muscle weakness.
  - Determine if the child has ever seen spots before his eyes, and if so, note the age this occurred.
- Physical assessment
  - Head and neck.

    Watch a young child as he plays or interacts with his parents.
  - Check for head and facial symmetry.
  - Observe how he cries, laughs, turns his head and wrinkles his forehead.
- To examine an infant's cranial bones, gently run your fingers over his head, checking the sutures and fontanel; look for fullness, bulging, or swelling, which may indicate an intracranial mass or hydrocephalus.
- Note the shape and symmetry of his head; abnormal shape accompanied by prominent bony ridges and poor head growth accompanied by prominent bony ridges and poor head growth may indicate craniosynostosis (premature suture closure).
- Assess the child's head and neck muscles
  - Decreased neck mobility is an important indicator of neurologic disorders such as meningitis.
  - With the child in a supine position, test for nuchal rigidity by cradling his head in your hands; supporting the weight of his head, move his neck in all directions to assess ease of movement.

Cerebral Function

- To assess level of consciousness (LOC) in a young child, use motor cues:
  - Observe for lethargy, drowsiness, and stupor.
  - Observe for hyperactivity.
  - Assess orientation to; person and place.
- To test attention span and concentration, ask the child to repeat a series of numbers after you.
- To test a child's recent memory, show him a familiar object and tell him that you will ask him later what it was; wait 5 minutes and then ask him to recall the object.

Cranial Nerves (CNs)

CN assessment can be difficult in a child younger than age 2, but by simple observation, you can check for symmetry of muscle movement, gaze, sucking strength, and hearing.

In a child older than age 2, assess the cranial nerves as you would in an adult, making these alterations:

- CN I (olfactory): Ask the child to identify familiar odours, such as chocolate, peppermint, candy; for a very young child who may not be able to identify a smell, try a same-different game to determine whether he can distinguish one smell from another.
- CN II (optic): Test a child's visual acuity as you would for an adult, but use Allen cards for a very young child or preschooler; for visual field testing, also follow the procedure for an adult but hold a bright object near the tip of your nose to help the young child keep his eyes focused.
- CN V (trigeminal): Test the sensory division of this nerve as you would for an adult, but make a game out of it by telling the child that a gremlin is going to brush his cheeks, pinch his forehead, and so on; test the motor division by having the child bite down hard on a tongue blade as you try to pull it away and at the same time palpate his jaw muscles for symmetry and contraction strength.
- CN VII (facial): Test the muscles that this nerve controls as you would for an adult, but instead of asking the child to perform certain movements, have him mimic your facial expressions; test the sensory division of the facial nerve with salt and sugar as for an adult.
- CN VIII (acoustic): Test the cochlear division of the acoustic nerve in a child by checking his hearing, acuity and sound conduction.
- CN IX, X, XI, and XII (glossopharyngeal, vagus, spinal accessory, and hypoglossal): Test these nerves as you would for an adult, using games to facilitate the examination when necessary.

Motor Function

- Assess balance and coordination in a child by watching motor skills such as dressing and undressing; you can also have the child stack blocks, put a bead in a bottle, or draw a cross.
- A child may demonstrate a preference for one-hand dominance between ages 12 and 24 months; handedness is well established by the school-age years.
- A child at age 4 should be able to stand on one foot for about 5 seconds; a child age 6 along with his arms folded across his chest for 5 seconds; and a child age 7 along with his eyes closed for 5 seconds.

Sensory Function

- Test the sensations of pain, touch, vibration and temperature in an older child as you would in an adult.
- Most of these tests are not applicable to an infant or a very young child; younger children may respond to pain or touch, but their responses may be unreliable.

Reflexes

Testing reflexes is an important part of the neurologic examination. Primitive reflexes, loss of reflexes or hyperactivity of deep tendon reflexes are usually the result of a cerebral insult.

Several **superficial reflexes** such as the abdominal, cremasteric, anal and plantar are present.

Deep tendon reflexes are stretch reflexes of a muscle. The most common deep tendon reflexes are the knee jerk or patellar reflex (sometimes called quadriceps reflex). Use the grading system to evaluate the reflexes. Report absent or hyperactive reflexes for further evaluation.

Grading of Reflexes

The various grading of reflexes have been depicted in the following table.

TABLE 2.2: Grading of Reflexes

Grade	Description
4+	Extremely brisk, hyperactive
3+	Brisker than normal
2+	Average, normal
1+	Diminished
0+	Absent

- Many children and some adults tighten their muscles, making reflex testing almost impossible.
  - Make a special effort to relax a child when assessing his reflexes; ask him to interlock the fingers of both hands and pull them tight

or clench his teeth on the count of three; meanwhile, you tap the tendon.

- Keep in mind that these actions may artificially magnify the reflex.

- A positive Babinski's sign may normally be present up to age 2.

NEUROLOGIC "SOFT" SIGNS

1. Short attention span
2. Unusual body movement, such as mirroring
3. Poor coordination and sense of position
4. Excessive, sustained and purposeless movement (hyperactivity)
5. Hypoactivity
6. Impulsiveness
7. Labile emotions
8. Distractibility
9. No established handedness
10. Language and articulation problems
11. Perceptual deficits (space, form, movement, time)
12. Problems with learning, especially reading, writing and arithmetic.

Test for Cerebellar Function

- **Finger-to-nose test:** With the child's arm extended, ask child to touch the nose with the index finger, both with the eyes open and then closed.
- **Heel-to-shin test:** While standing, have child run the heel of one foot down the shin or anterior aspect of the tibia of the other leg. Both with the eyes opened and then closed.
- **Roberg test:** With the eyes closed, have child stand with the heels together; falling or leaning to one side is abnormal.

Chapter 3

CARE OF NEONATES WITH COMMON HEALTH PROBLEMS

CARE OF THE PRETERM NEWBORN (PREMATURE BABY)

Definition

Preterm infant is an infant born before the end of 37 completed week gestation (child born prior to the estimated date of delivery).

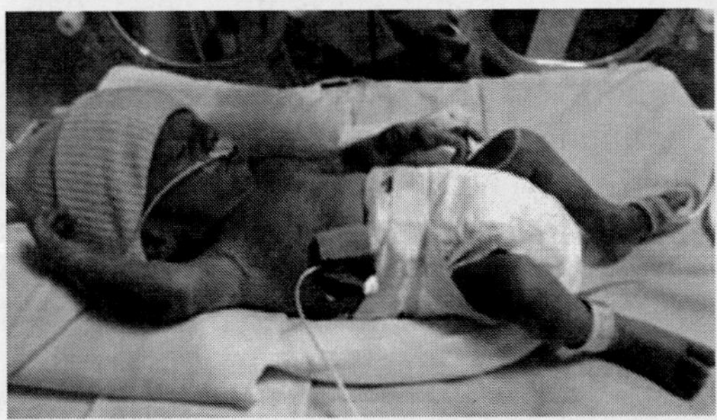

Fig. 3.1: Preterm baby (See Pl. 24)

Cause

There is no actual cause for premature birth, but following may attribute to it in one way or the other.

Predisposing Factors

1. Maternal Factors
   - Low socioeconomic classes
   - Excessive exercise and long hours of maternal activity
   - Pregnancy induced hypertension
   - Chronic medical illness (Heart disease, Kidney disease)
   - Infection—Genitourinary tract infections
   - Drug abuse
   - Abnormal structure of the uterus
   - Cervical incompetence
   - Mothers with previous preterm birth
   - Women under the age of 16 and over 35 years
   - Placental accident
   - Anaemia of mother.
2. Foetal factors
   - Foetal stress
   - Multiple gestation
   - RH/Blood group incompatibility
   - Congenital malformation.
3. Factors related to the pregnancy
   - APH: Placenta previa, placenta abruption
   - Premature rupture of membrane
   - Polyhydramnions
   - Abnormal or decreased function of the placenta.

Clinical Characteristics

Appearance

- Infant is very small in appearance
- Lack of or minimal subcutaneous fat deposits
- Proportionately large head in relation to the body.

Skin

- Colour-bright pink, smooth and shiny
- Small blood vessels clearly visible underneath the thin, transparent epidermis
- Fine lanugo hair in forehead and back.

Ear

- Cartilage is soft and pliable.

Extremities

- Soles and palms have minimal creases
- Bones are very soft.

Eye

- Eyes are prominent but closed.

Abdomen

- Protruded, visible vein.

Genitalia

- Male—Few scrotal rugae and testes are undescended
- Female—Labia and clitoris are prominent.

Reflex

- Partially developed
- Sucking reflex absent, weak, ineffective
- Swallowing, gag and coughing reflexes—weak

Neurological signs are absent or diminished.

Common Complications of Prematurity

- Apnea
- Hypothermia
- Patent ducus arterious
- RDS—Respiratory results from inadequate surfactant production
- Intraventricular haemorrhage
- Hypocalcaemia
- Hypoglycaemia
- Necrotizing enterocolitis
- Anaemia
- Hyperbilirubinemia
- Infection.

Treatment

- Maintain adequate temperature by keeping the baby in a warmer or incubator or immediate skin to skin contact or KMC should be started immediately.
- Initiate breastfeeding to the baby as early as possible and give feeding every two hours.
- Prevent infection by minimizing atraumatic care and avoid too many visitors to maintain proper hygiene.
- Early assessment of complication and treatment.

Kangaroo Mother Care (KMC)

Kangaroo care seeks to provide restored closeness of the newborn with mother and/or father by placing the infant in direct skin-to-skin contact with one of them. This ensures physiological and psychological warmth and bonding. The Kangaroo position provides ready access to nourishment. The mother's body responds to the needs of the infant directly, helps regulate temperature more smoothly than an incubator, her milk adjusts to the nutritional and immunological needs of her fragile infant, and the baby sleeps more soundly.

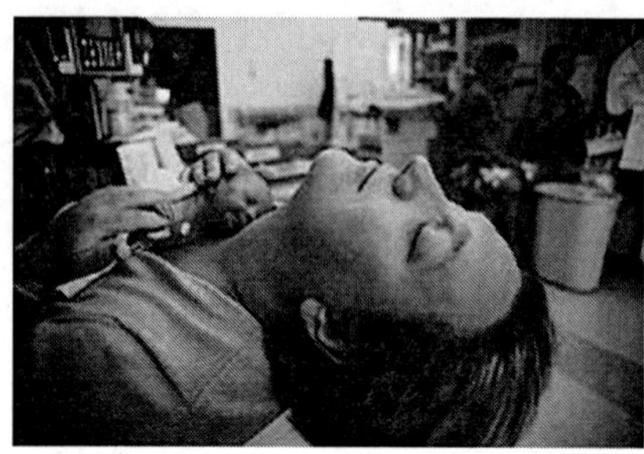

Fig. 3.2: Kangaroo mother

Eligibility Criteria

Originally babies who are eligible for Kangaroo care include preterm infants weighing less than 1500 grams, and breathing independently. Cardiopulmonary monitoring, oximetry, supplemental oxygen or nasal Continuous Positive Airway Pressure (CPAP) ventilation, intravenous infusions, and monitor leads do not prevent Kangaroo care. In fact, babies who are in Kangaroo care tend to be less prone to apnea and bradycardia and have stabilization of oxygen needs (London, Ladewig, Ball and Bindler, 2006).

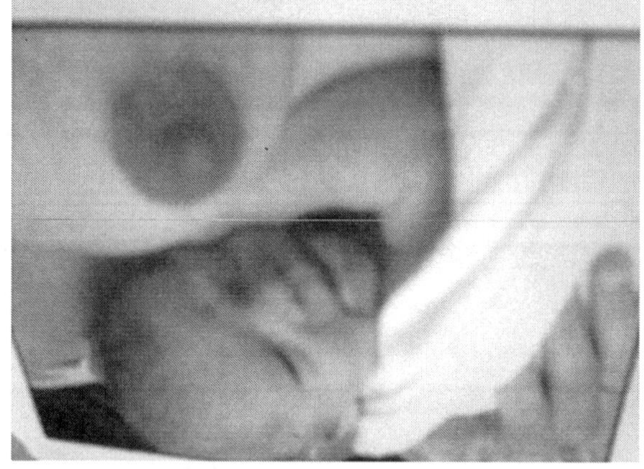

Fig. 3.3: Care of baby with Kangaroo mother

Principles of KMC

- Put all preterm and low birth weight babies on KMC regardless of the gestational age and birth weight.
- Warm the room using a radiant heater or any heat source including firewood in the rural set-ups.
- Continue breastfeeding and if baby is unable to feed put NGT and give expressed breast milk through NGT.

- Look meticulously for signs of infection.
- Monitor the temperature very closely at every one hour for the first day and twice a day thereafter until the baby is weaned off from KMC and if there was hypothermia, within one to two hours it should return to normal value.

Techniques

- Typically in Kangaroo care, the baby wears only a diaper and is tied in a head-up position to the mother's bare chest with a strip of cloth in a manner that extends the baby's head and neck to prevent apnea. The mother wears a shirt or hospital gown with opening to the front. The cloth wraps around and under the baby's bottom to create flexion.
- The tight bundling is enough for the mother's breathing and chest movement to stimulate the baby's breathing. Because of the close confines of being attached to its mother's chest, the baby is enclosed in a high carbon dioxide environment which also stimulates breathing. Fathers can also use the skin-to-skin contact method.
- Beginning Kangaroo care within the first 2 hours after birth seems to be the most effective time period for successful breastfeeding.
- Many advocates of natural birth encourage immediate skin-to-skin contact between mother and baby after birth, with minimal disruption.
- Babies must be kept warm and dry. This method can be used continuously around the clock or for short periods per day gradually increasing as tolerated for infants who are compromised by severe health problems.
- It can be started at birth or within hours, days, or weeks after birth. Proponents of Kangaroo care encourage maintaining skin-to-skin contact method for about six weeks so that both baby and mother are established in breast feeding and have achieved physiological recovery from the birth process. (London *et al.*, 2006).
- The practice of baby wearing is used by many parents of both preterm and full term newborns to facilitate Kangaroo care.
- A variety of slings and other carriers may be used, some are designed specifically for neonates and the classic "upright between the breasts" positioning, and some are intended for a wider variety of positions and ages.

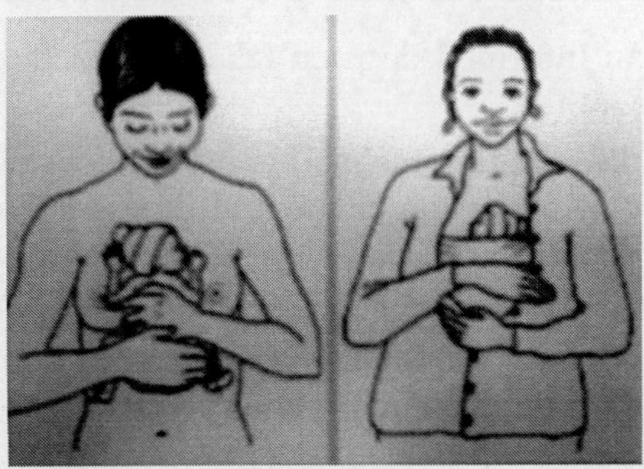

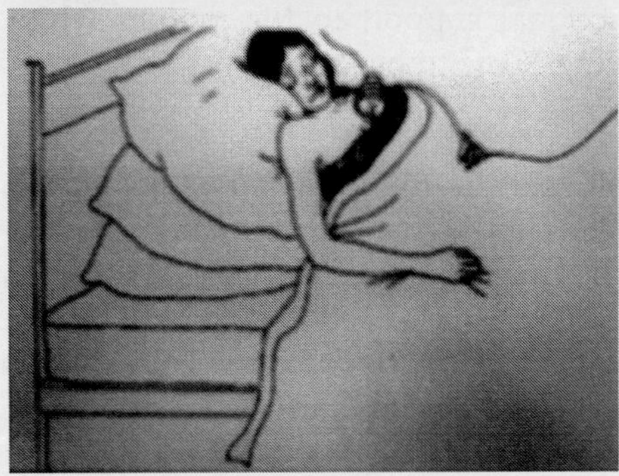

Fig. 3.4: Position of baby with Kangaroo parents

Benefits

Kangaroo care helps build basic trust for the community for:

- Reduced morbidity and mortality especially in developing countries.
- Opportunities for teaching during pregnancy and follow-up in preparation for postnatal implementation.
- Decreased hospital-associated costs.
- Promotion of total family health.

Counselling the Mother for KMC

Counselling is very important for the mother, how she has to maintain the temperature of the baby by KMC, so we need to counsel all mothers or caretakers who will have to put their babies on KMC. If you anticipate a preterm delivery, it is always important to start counselling KMC before delivery, so that mothers can prepare themselves mentally before delivery about their baby care especially about KMC.

There are important points to remember that we need to address during counselling.

- Give the mother the necessary information about KMC including the advantage and the problems that she may face during the whole period of KMC. Make sure that she is convinced about the importance of this mode of care to her baby and is willing to do it for some days continuously. It is an informed decision taken by the mother or the family.

- Make sure that the mother herself does not have any complication or medical illness during this period. If she has any close member of the family, she can replace her to put the baby on KMC.
- The family should also be informed about KMC and the detailed information about the procedure should be provided along with the necessary emotional support to the mother while she is giving KMC to her baby.

Setting

- KMC can be implemented at health facility, at home and during transportation to or from the health facility. It is only for the first 3–5 days that the mother may need to lie on the bed, until the baby is stabilized. Once the baby's condition is stable, the mother can walk and do even her routine work while the baby is inside the KMC.
- Measure axillary temperature by placing the thermometer in the auxilla for 3–4 minutes (or feel for low body temperature).

  Babies can receive most of the necessary care, including feeding while in Kangaroo care. They need to be removed away from the skin to skin contact only for:
  - Changing diapers hygiene and cord care.
  - To evaluate the baby for any medical problem.

Nursing Management

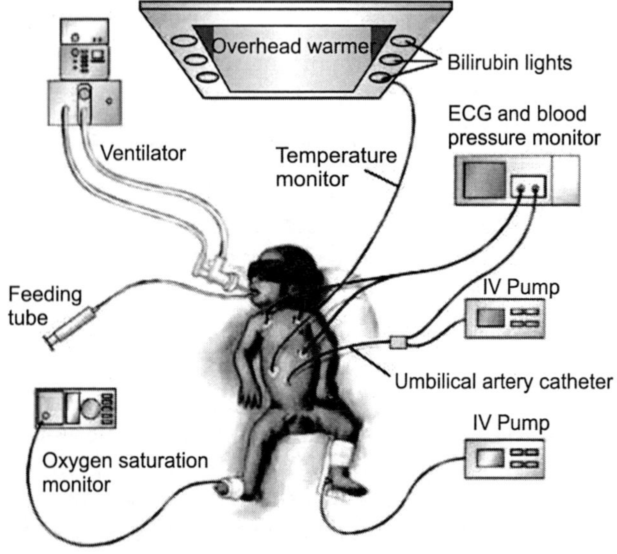

Fig. 3.5: Care of preterm baby in NICU

1. ***Maintenance of Respiratory Factors***
   - Positioning of the newborn head should be elevated to maintain the air way.
   - Avoid supine position to prevent aspiration.
   - Encourage prone position that facilitates chest expansion and improves air entry and oxygenation.
   - Suction to be done to clear the secretions.
   - Prevent aspiration-because of poor sucking reflex. Cardiac sphincter not developed.
   - Monitor heart rate and respiratory rate.
   - Observe the signs of respiratory distress which includes:
     - Cyanosis
     - Respiratory rate > 60/minute
     - Chest retraction
     - Flaring of nostrils
     - Apneic episodes
     - Inadequate breathing sound
     - Fatigue
   - Administer O_2, monitor the O_2 concentration by pulse oximeter.

2. ***Maintenance of Normal/Neutral Thermal Environment***
   - Maintain normal temperature of the baby.
   - Keep the baby warmer or in incubator.
   - Avoid placing or exposing the baby on cold surface.
   - Dry and cover the baby well to prevent heat loss.
   - Maintain the temperature of the baby between 36°C–37°C.
   - Use a skin probe to maintain the baby skin temperature if it is kept in incubator or in the radiant warmer.

3. ***Maintenance of Fluid and Electrolyte Status***
   - Encourage the mother to give only breastfeeding.
   - If the baby is unable to suck, give expressed breast milk through NG tube or intravenous fluid intake prescribed to the child, normally 60–80 ml/kg/day.
   - Insensible water loss can be minimized by providing a neutral thermal environment.
   - Evaluate the hydration status of the baby by assessing and recording signs of dehydration.
   - Check the weight of baby every day.

- Intake and output chart to be measured accurately.
- Check specific gravity of pH.
- IV fluids if needed to be administered.

4. ***Prevention of Infection***
   - Strict hand washing, reverse isolation and use of equipments for only one infant. It prevents cross infection (proper umbilical dressing).
   - IV solutions and tubing should be changed every 24 hours.
   - Administration of IV fluid in aseptic way.
   - Change the position of the baby every 2 hours.
   - Restrict the visitors, any one who has respiratory infection to avoid to handle the baby.
   - Minimal handling of infants.
   - Any procedure to be done in aseptic manner.

5. ***Provide the Adequate Nutrition***
   - Encourage the mother to feed breast milk if sucking reflex is poor, expressed breast milk to be given.
   - If first feedings are small amount given every 2–3 hrs then increase to 1–2 ml every hour.
   - Feeding method depends on the health status of the preterm newborn, cup feeding, 120–150 kcal/kg/day to be given.
   - If child is not sucking, feed the baby through NG tube.
   - Daily weight should be checked and recorded.
   - After feeding, the baby should be placed on the right side of the abdomen. It enhances gastric emptying and decreases the chance of aspiration. if regurgitation occurs (gastro oesophagus reflux is not common in preterm babies).

6. ***Promotion of Parent-Infant Attachment***
   - Nurse should take measures to promote positive parental feelings towards the newborn.
   - Photographs of the baby are given to parents to keep at home.
   - Encourage daily participation by early and frequent visits.
   - The nurse provides opportunities for parents to touch, hold and to take care for the baby.
   - Encourage the parents to give care to the baby.
   - Encourage breastfeeding also.

LOW BIRTH WEIGHT INFANTS

Introduction and Definition

Low birth weight infants are those born weighing less than 2500 g. These are further subdivided into:

- *Very Low Birth Weight* (*VLBW*): Birth weight < 1500 g.
- *Extremely Low Birth Weight* (*ELBW*): Birth weight < 1000 g.

Obstetrical history (LMP, sonographic data), newborn physical examination, and examination for maturational age are critical data to differentiate premature LBW from other infants. Survival statistics for ELBW infants correlate with gestation age. Morbidity statistics for growth retarded VLBW infant correlate with the etiology and the severity of the growth-restriction.

Causes

- Premature birth.
- Intrauterine growth retardation due to placental problem or birth defect.

Risk Factors

- **Race**—African-American babies are twice as likely as Caucasian to be VLBW. Black infants account for 37% of ELBW infant.
- **Age**—Teenage mothers (especially if < 15 years old) have a much higher risk of having VLBW infant.
- **Multiple birth**—Multiple birth babies are at increased risk of being VLBW because they often premature. More than 50% of twins and other multiple gestations are VLBW.
- **Maternal health**—Women exposed to drug, alcohol and cigarettes during pregnancy are more likely to have LBW or VLBW babies. Mothers of lower socioeconomic status are also more likely to have poorer pregnancy nutrition, inadequate prenatal care and complication of pregnancy. All are factors that can contribute to VLBW.

Complications

- **Hypothermia**—LBW infants have higher body surface area: body weight ratios, decreased stores of brown fat and glycogen, and may not be able to conserve or generate body heat. Clinical problems associated with hypothermia include hypoglycaemia, apnea, increased oxygen consumption and metabolic acidosis.

- **Prevention of hypothermia**—Increased survival of the infants, methods of preventing heat loss includes: drying the infants at birth to prevent evaporative heat loss.
  - Provide Kangaroo care to the baby. (see Fig. 3.4).
  - Warmed blankets or plastic wrap to prevent convective and radiant heat loss during transport.
  - Swaddling to preserve body heat in larger infants and radiant heater or a heated incubator to maintain a neutral thermal environment for smaller infants.
- **Hypoglycaemia**—Hypoglycaemia due to decreased storage of glycogen and fat in the baby's body. Hypoglycaemia and hypoxia aggravate this due to increased metabolic demands and anaerobic glycolysis.
- **Perinatal asphyxia**—Perinatal asphyxia especially among growth retarded infants because of compromised oxygen delivery in utero.
- **Respiratory problems**
  - Respiratory distress syndrome due to surfactant deficiency
  - Apnea of prematurity
- **Fluid and electrolyte imbalance**—Fluid and electrolyte imbalance due to increased insensible water loss due to increased surface area, thin skin, body weight ratio, impaired renal function. They are at risk of overload, hypernatremia, hyponatremia, hypokalemia, hypocalcemia.
- **Hyperbilirubinemia**—Hyperbilirubinemia due to bruising or haemorrhage decreases RBC survival, hepatic immaturity, delays enteric feedings and decreases gut motility, infection and polycythemia.
- **Anaemia**—Anaemia is due to small blood volume or prematurity.
- **Infection**—There is increased risk of infection due to immunologic immaturity, prolonged invasive treatment (*e.g.*, endotracheal tube, intravascular catheters), parental nutrition and prolonged, recurrent treatment with antibiotics.
- **Neurological problems**
  - Interventricular haemorrhage
  - Long-term risk for cerebral palsy, development delay, learning disabilities.
- **Ophthalmologic complications**—Ophthalmologic complications include retinopathy (due to oxygen toxicity) of prematurely, strabismus.
- **Hearing deficits due to**
  - Prematurity
  - Hyperbilirubinemia
  - Meningitis
  - Hypotension

Management

- Most of the LBW will require intubation at birth and assisted ventilation for a prolonged period for respiratory care.
- Maintain the temperature of the baby by keeping the infant in a radiant warmer or incubator to prevent hypothermia.
- Most VLBW and almost all ELBW infants require an umbilical arterial catheter for blood sampling and blood pressure measurement.
- For hypotension effective therapy is dopamine 5 mcg/kg/mt.
- Oxygen therapy is given to maintain O_2 level in the tissue.
- Check the oxygen saturation by pulse oximeter.
- Administration of fluid little higher than preterm babies 100–125 ml/kg/day. We should strictly follow the intake and output for first several days.
- Electrolytes should be maintained to avoid electrolyte imbalance on the 1st day, do not give Na^+ or K^+, to avoid hypocalcemia, start calcium gluconate at 200 mg/kg/day. Follow the serum electrolytes closely.
- Encourage breastfeeding or expressed breast milk to be given. In case baby has poor sucking and swallowing reflex present Ryle's tube feeding is preferable to the baby.
- Control the infection, obtain CBC and blood culture at birth, if there is any risk factors, start antibiotic therapy.
- Maintain the blood glucose level to avoid hypoglycaemia. Initial IV fluid should be dextrose water 10%. Some ELBW infants may become hyperglycaemic and require lower glucose intake and/or insulin.
- VLBW infants will need at least one transfusion because of anaemia, so discuss for donor blood, check for type and cross match of the infant. Administer packed cells for infant.

Outcome

Survival of VLBW babies is directly related to birth weight. Long-term outcome of VLBW and ELBW infants indicates increased risk for cerebral palsy, developmental delay, mental retardation, visual problem, hearing impairment, chronic lung diseases and sudden infant death syndrome.

MECONIUM ASPIRATION SYNDROME

Meconium aspiration is a serious condition that accounts for a substantial number of neonatal deaths. During deliveries, there is meconium in the amniotic fluid. Aspiration of meconium results in respiratory distress that, in severe cases, can be life threatening. It occurs when foetus has been subjected to foetal asphyxia or other intrauterine stress that causes relaxing of the anal sphincter and passage of meconium into the amniotic fluid. The majority of meconium aspiration occurs with the first breath. However, a severely compromised foetus may aspirate in utero. At delivery of the chest and initiation of the first breath, infants inhale fluid and meconium in the nasoorophagynx. It occurs in 5–10% of births.

Predisposing Factors/Causes

- Small for gestation age or immature baby/ preterm babies.
- Post term babies.
- Prolonged labour.

Pathophysiology

Due to prolonged labour or other causes (foetal distress in the uterus)

↓

Anal sphincter relaxes

↓

Meconium passed into the amniotic fluid

↓

Meconium it may be strain in the skin

↓

During gestation or at birth first breath, meconium is aspirated into the lungs

↓

Mechanical plug causes partial airway obstructed (infant struggles to take in more air during inspiration—air hunger)

↓

Child causes respiratory distress

(Due to hyperinflation, hypoxemia and acidosis results in increased pulmonary vascular resistance.)

Clinical Manifestations

- Baby released meconium in utero for sometime before birth are strained from green meconium stools, tachypenic, hypoxic and often depressed at birth.
- Low APGAR score.
- They may develop expiratory grunting.
- Nasal flaring and retractions of the chest.
- Baby initially may develop cyanosis or pallor, tachypenic.
- Severe meconium aspiration progresses very rapidly to respiratory failure.
- Baby has respiratory distress with gasping, ineffective ventilations, marked cyanosis and pallor and hypotonia.

Investigations

- At birth, meconium can be visualized via laryngoscopy in the respiratory passage and vocal cord.
- Chest X-ray shows uneven distribution of patchy infiltrates, air trapping, hyperexpansion and atelectasis.
- Echocardiography assists in the diagnosis of right-to-left shunting of blood away from the pulmonary system.

Treatment and Nursing Management

For all Infants Born with Meconium in the Amniotic Fluid

1. All infants with meconium in the amniotic fluid, should have their nose, mouth and pharynx suctioned as soon as the head is delivered regardless of whether the meconium is thin or thick.
2. If the amniotic fluid is merely coloured or stained with meconium but there is no particular meconium in the fluid, no further special intervention for meconium is indicated and the infant should receive route resuscitation as indicated by the infant's condition.
3. Administration of intravenous fluid.

For Infants Born with a Particle of Meconium in the Amniotic Fluid

1. Assess the infant immediately after birth before any drying or simulation, meconium strain on the baby's skin.

2. If the infant is depressed (absent or depressed respiration or HR <100/minute or decreased muscle tone in the 1st 15 seconds after birth), following treatment should be given.
   - Immediately perform direct laryngoscopy, before drying or stimulating the infant.
   - Suction any meconium that is in the hypopharynx.
   - Then intubate the infant's trachea, apply suction directly to the endotracheal tube as it is withdrawn from the trachea.
   - If meconium is obtained, repeat the intubation and suctioning until little meconium is recovered or the heart has < 60 beats/minute, and then proceed with normal resuscitation.

     Do not intubate and suction more than three times.
   - If infant has markedly depressed respiration, it may be necessary to give positive pressure ventilation and proceed with resuscitation. Infant should be intubated and suction must be done only one time before giving positive pressure ventilation.
   - Insertation of nasogastric tube and aspirate the stomach content because the baby may swallow the meconium content with aminiotic fluid.
   - Administration of systemic antibiotics.
   - Drugs like sodium bicarbonate given to correct acidosis.
3. If the infant is vigorous (baby has spontaneous respiration and HR > 100/minute and good muscle tones in the 1st 15 seconds after birth), use routine resuscitation procedures as by the infant's condition.

If Respiratory Distress Develops in an Infant Born through Meconium

Infant requires close observation and early intervention.

- Provide liberal amount of humidified oxygen to maintain adequate systemic and alveolar oxygenation and to correct acidosis, if present, to avoid development of persistent pulmonary hypertension.
- Obtain chest X-ray immediately.
- Consider early insertion of an umbilical arterial catheter to monitor arterial oxygenation and acid-base status.
- If the infant requires assisted ventilation, avoid high inspiratory pressure in an attempt to prevent pneumothorax.
- ET tube suctioning to remove the secretion—frequent suction causes bradycardia.
- Observe the colour of the baby, blood gas analysis to be done.
- Apply vibration to loosen the secretions.

Complications

- Pneumothorax—because overexpansion of lungs and rupture of alveoli
- Anoxia
- Persistent pulmonary hypertension
- Retrolental fibroplasias
- Broncho pulmonary dysplasia

Note: Hyperventilation causes rupture of alveoli.

ASPHYXIA

Asphyxia occurs due to impaired transfer of gases both between the mother and the foetus or due to delayed or ineffective onset of breathing at the time of birth with accompanying hypoxia, hypercarbia and acidosis.

Causes or Conditions that Increase the Risk of Asphyxia

1. *Maternal Conditions*

(*i*) Age < 16 and > 40

(*ii*) Placental or cord

Interfere with uteroplacental perfusion—Chronic illness, hypertension, preeclampsia, diabetes, hypotension, and anaemia.

(*iii*) Anaesthesia, maternal medication leads to apnea at birth.

(*iv*) Antepartum haemorrhage.

2. *Labour and Delivery Conditions*

(*i*) Forceps or vacuum extraction

(*ii*) Abnormal presentation or breech

(*iii*) Caesarean section

(*iv*) Cephalo-pelvic disproportion

(*v*) Maternal hypotension or haemorrhage

3. *Foetal Conditions*

(*i*) Premature or post mature birth

(ii) Meconium in amniotic fluid
(iii) Foetal growth retardation
(iv) Foetal malformation
(v) Hydrops foetalis
(vi) Oligo- or polyhydramnios
(vii) Multiple births
(viii) Sepsis
(ix) Birth trauma
(x) Difficult birth

Pathophysiology

- Hypoxia and hypercarbia—leads to respiratory acidosis.
- Hypoxia—causes metabolic acidosis.
- Acidosis—leads to mixed respiratory and metabolic acidosis.
- Acidosis and hypotension of asphyxia stimulates chemoreceptors and baroreceptors causing constriction of the arterioles and a shunting of blood to the brain, heart and adrenals at the expense of the other organs of the body.

Essential Precautions Assessment and Management

1. Assessment of apnoea
   (i) Heart rate
   (ii) Response to stimulation
   (iii) Need for positive pressure ventilation
2. Initial treatment goal
   (i) Eliminate hypoxic environment
   (ii) Correct metabolic and respiratory acidosis
   (iii) Stabilize blood pressure to maintain adequate cardiac output.
3. Neonates at risk immediate and initiation of care plan.

Resuscitation

Purpose or Indication

- To provide an adequate air way with expansion of the lungs to decrease the PCO_2, increase the PO_2.
- To support adequate cardiac output.
- To minimize oxygen consumption by reducing heat loss.

ABCD approach

A—Air way

B—Breathing

C—Circulation

D—Drugs

Assessment of newborn after birth, depends on the APGAR score, of the asphyxia are classified and management provided to the infant.

If APGAR score is:

- 7 to 10—No or mild depression/asphyxia
- 4 to 6—Moderate depression/asphyxia
- Below 3—Severe asphyxia

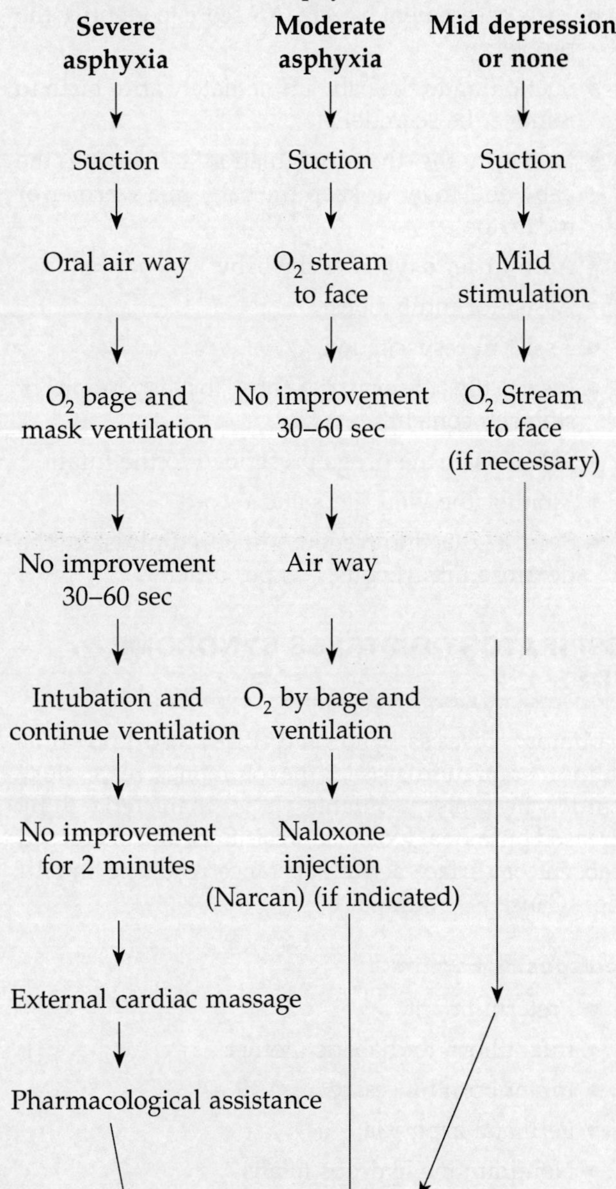

If it is severe asphyxia immediate cardio pulmonary resuscitation.

Medication

- Injection naloxone 0.25 ml/kg IV or IM or ETT
- Injection adrenaline 0.25 ml/kg at 1 : 10,000 solution
- Injection sodium bicarbonate slowly—5 ml of 4%, sodium bicarbonate through umbilical vein
- Dextrose water IV 5 ml slowly.

Nursing Management

- Early assessment by APGAR score to identify the problem.
- Suctioning to the baby immediately after birth to remove the secretion.
- Maintain the thermoregulation by drying the baby and cover or keep the baby in a warmer or incubator.
- Administer oxygen to the baby.
- Assist for intubations.
- Assist in resuscitation.
- Insert the nasogastric tube for aspiration of stomach content.
- Administer the drugs prescribed to the infant.
- Monitor the vital signs and record.
- Secure the intravenous line, administer the dextrose intravenously as per order.

RESPIRATORY DISTRESS SYNDROME (RDS)

Respiratory Distress Syndrome (RDS) also known as hyaline membrane disease, is the commonest respiratory disorder in preterm infants. It is characterized by increased pulmonary vascular resistance and decreased or absent of surface-active substance resulting in stiff lungs. Cause is unknown.

Predisposing Factors

- Preterm infant
- Infant born to diabetic mother
- Infant born by cesarean section
- Perinatal asphyxia
- Non-immune hydrops fetalis
- Low birth weight babies.

Pathophysiology

Surfactant is a surface-active phospholipid secreted by the alveolar epithelium. It acts as a detergent, this substance reduces the surface tension of fluid that lines the alveoli and respiratory passages resulting in uniform expansion and maintenance of lung expansion

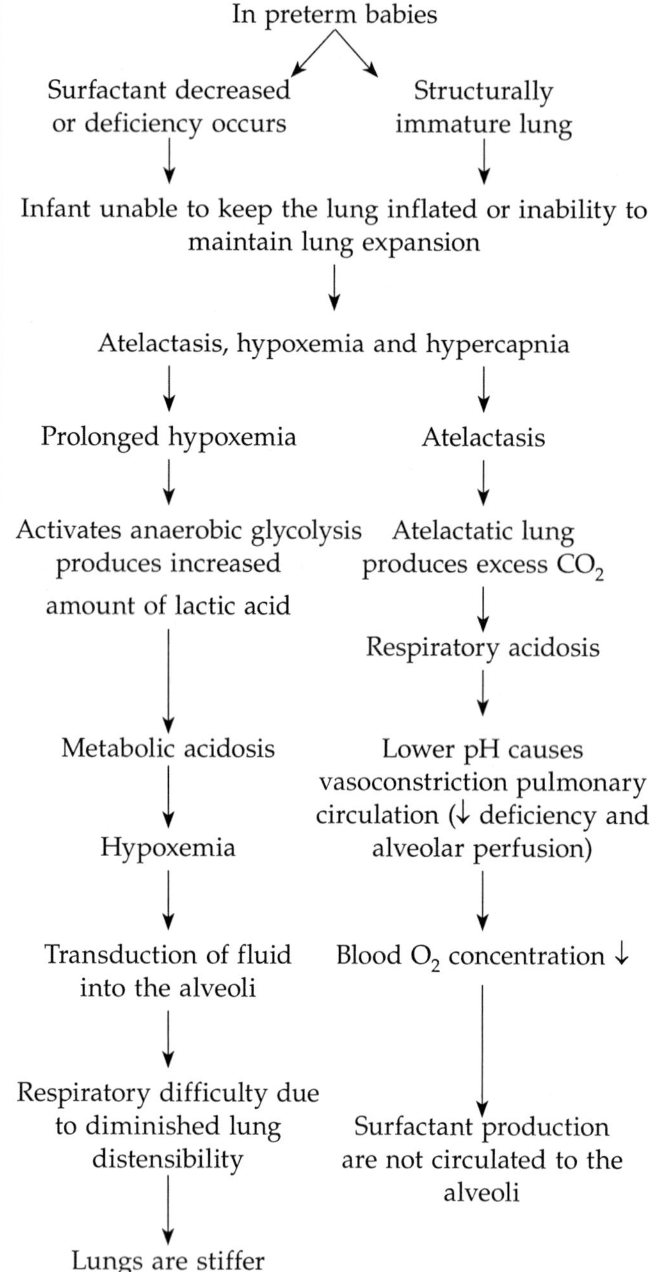

Clinical Manifestations

- Tachypnea (> 60 breaths/minute)
- Chest retraction
- Nasal flaring
- Grunting
- Cyanosis
- Poor air entry

- Later stage—abdominal distension
- Bowel sounds are poor or absent
- Oedema is common in hands and feet.

Diagnostic Test Findings

- Chest X-ray may be normal for the first 6 to 12 hours (in 50% of neonates with RDS), but 24 hours after birth X-rays show ground glass appearance and air filled bronchi.
- Arterial Blood Gas analysis (ABG)—Increased PCO_2, decreased PO_2, decreased arterial blood pH (from respiratory or metabolic acidosis both).
- Chest auscultation reveals normal or diminished air entry and crackles (rare in early stages).

Medical Management

- Provides effective respiratory support
  - Warm, humidified oxygen is administered by oxygen hood, or if such treatment fails, by continuous positive airway pressure (administered by nasal prongs or mechanical ventilation).
  - Special ventilation techniques are used on infants who don't respond to conventional mechanical ventilation.
    - High-frequency ventilation.
    - Nasal continuous positive airway pressure (CPAP) is used in less severe cases.
    - High-frequency oscillatory ventilation.
  - Extra corporeal membrane oxygenation
    - The last choice for ventilation.
    - Keep the baby in controlled ventilation usually positive end expiratory pressure (PEEP) if CO_2 is increased.
- Keep the baby in a radiant infant warmer or isolate for thermoregulation.
- Secure intravenous line to maintain fluid and electrolyte balance.
- Administer sodium bicarbonate 5 ml of 4% to control acidosis.
- Nasogastric tube feeding or TPN if the neonate is too weak to suck the breast or oral feeding.
- Administration of surfactant by an ET tube with in the first 24 hours after birth.
  - Time of surfactant administration—two approaches have been used for surfactant delivery:
    - Prophylactic and rescue treatment.
    - Prophylactic administration involves giving surfactant soon after birth, as soon as the infants has been stabilized.
    - Rescue administration involves giving surfactant to infants who have established RDS and require mechanical ventilation and supplemental oxygen.
  - Administration and dose of surfactant
    - Normally single dose therapy is administrated but several studies have shown that two doses therapy is better.
    - The dose of surfactant is

      Infasurf–3 ml/kg

      Survanta–4 ml/kg.

Note: Surfactant therapy is a very costly therapy, it needs mechanical ventilation. It is available in certain specialized institutions.

Complications

- Pneumothorax
- Risk of Retinopathy of prematurity
- Bronchopulmonary dysplasia
- Respiratory insufficiency
- Death

Preventive Measures

- Prevention of premature delivery
- Avoid elective caesarean section, to expanding the alveoli and replacing the lung fluid with air.
- Amniocentesis and ultrasound are used to find out the maturity of foetus.
- Administration of corticosteroids is done to mothers for 24 hours to 7 days prior to delivery. It stimulates surfactant production in the foetus and decreases the incidence of hyaline membrane disease.

Nursing Intervention

- Expect the neonate to be on a ventilator or nasal CPAP to keep the alveoli open.
  - Administer oxygen as needed.
  - In neonates, mechanical ventilation is usually done in a pressure-limited mode rather than the volume-limited mode used in adults.

- Watch for signs of barotraumas
  - Increase in respiratory distress
  - Subcutaneous emphysema.
- Organize care to ensure minimal handling.
- Control the neonate's temperature to reduce stress and decrease additional energy use.
- Use aseptic technique to reduce the risk of infection.
- Administer I.V. fluids to ensure adequate hydration, but withhold oral food and fluid, if the neonate has a high respiratory rate; anticipate possible nasogastric tube feeding.
- Turn the neonate every 2 hours; raise the head of the bed; perform chest percussion before suctioning.
- Closely monitor blood gas as well as fluid intake and output.
  - If the neonate has an umbilical catheter, check for arterial hypertension or abnormal central venous pressure.
  - Watch for complication, such as infection, thrombosis, or decreased circulation to the legs.
  - If the neonate has a transcutaneous oxygen monitor, change the site of the lead placement every 2 to 4 hours to avoid burning the skin.
- Weigh the neonate once or twice daily
- To evaluate the neonate's progress, assess skin colour, rate and depth of respirations, severity of retractions, nasal flaring, frequency of expiratory grunting, frothing at the lips and restlessness.
- Teach the parents about their neonate's condition and let them participate in his care (using aseptic technique) to encourage normal parent neonate bonding.
- Advise parents that full recovery may take up to one year; when the prognosis is poor, prepare the parents for the neonates impending death and offer emotional support.

NEONATAL PNEUMONIA

Pneumonia is very common in the neonates. Pneumonia is an inflammation of the pulmonary parenchyma which occurs more frequently in infants. Such infection, be it bacterial or viral in origin, may be acquired before or at the time of birth or in the early postnatal period. The bacterial pneumonia carries a substantial mortality in the neonates.

Etiology

- Congenital bacterial pneumonia—acquired by transplacental route.
- Ascending infection from the genital tract before or during labour.
  - Prolonged rupture of membranes (exceeds 24 hours).
  - Bacteria may gain access to the foetus even with intact membrane.
  - Bacterial colonization of the infant always occurs during vaginal delivery.
  - Foetal asphyxia (gasping during delivery—the infant aspirates contaminated amniotic fluid).
- Nosocomial infection within the hospital environment.
- Pathogens like Group B streptococci are the major organisms that cause neonatal pneumonia, and
- Other organisms are:
  - *Escherichia*
  - *Klebsiella*
  - *Staphylococcus*
  - *Chlamydia trachomatis*
  - Group D streptococci
  - Listeria organisms and pneumococci
  - *Staphylococcus* and pseudomonas organisms,
  - Fungi.
- Viral pneumonia can be acquired by the foetus from transplacental passage of organisms—TORCH syndromes.

Clinical Manifestations

- Non-specific nature of the clinical signs.
- There are characteristics of neonatal sepsis in early diagnosis.
- In some cases it causes severe pneumonia.
- Other features include thermal instability, apneic spells, abdominal distension or jaundice.
- Tachypnea.
- Cyanosis or other signs of respiratory distress.

Investigation

- Chest roentgenogram—findings show unilateral or bilateral streaky densities.
- Blood and urine examination—for detection of Group B streptococcal antigen in urine and blood.

- Cerebrospinal fluid examination—for latex particle agglutination may facilitate the rapid diagnosis of group B streptococcal sepsis.
- Direct culture of blood, urine and nasopharyngeal or tracheobronchial secretions.
- Serological tests.
- Cord blood immunoglobulin to be measured—In intrauterine pneumonia, we can see elevated IgM levels.

Treatment

- Identification of organisms and its antibiotic sensitivities determined.
- Administration of antibiotics for 10 days or longer depend upon the infant condition.
- Chlamydial pneumonia—administration of oral erythromycin for 14 days course.
- Good supportive care is essential like fluid management, blood gas monitoring and ventilator assistance for the baby.

Complications

- Primary pulmonary hypertension.
- Decreased cardiac output.
- Pulmonary vascular injury.
- Death.

Nursing Management

- Maintain the airway pattern:
  - Administer oxygen as needed.
  - In neonates, mechanical ventilation is usually done in a pressure-limited mode rather than the volume-limited mode used in adults.
  - Watch for signs of barotraumas:
    - Increase in respiratory distress.
    - Subcutaneous emphysema.
- Organize care to ensure minimal handling.
- Control the neonate's temperature to reduce stress and decrease additional energy use.
- Use aseptic technique to reduce the risk of infection.
- Administer I.V. fluids to ensure adequate hydration, but withhold oral food and fluid, if the neonate has a high respiratory rate; anticipate possible nasogastric tube feeding.
- Turn the neonate every 2 hours; raise the head of the bed; perform chest percussion before suctioning.
- Closely monitor blood gas as well as fluid intake and output.
  - If the neonate has an umbilical catheter, check for arterial hypertension or abnormal central venous pressure.
  - Watch for complication, such as infection, thrombosis, or decreased circulation to the legs.
  - If the neonate has a transcutaneous oxygen monitor, change the site of the lead placement every 2 to 4 hours to avoid burning the skin.
- To evaluate the neonate's progress, assess skin colour, rate and depth of respirations, severity of retractions, nasal flaring, frequency of expiratory grunting, frothing at the lips and restlessness.
- Teach the parents about their neonates condition and let them participate in his care (using aseptic technique) to encourage normal parent neonate bonding.

NEONATAL HYPOGLYCAEMIA

Background and Pathophysiology

Glucose is the major energy source for foetus and neonate. The newborn brain depends upon glucose almost exclusively. Upto 90% of total glucose used is consumed by the brain. Alternate fuels (*e.g.*, ketones, lactate) are produced in very low quantities. The usual rate of glucose utilization is 4–8 mg/kg/minute. Glucose regulatory mechanisms are sluggish at birth. At birth the infant must rely on the glycogen stores deposited in the liver, heart and skeletal muscle during the last trimester of pregnancy for full time babies. It provides adequate source of energy for first 2 to 3 days of life. Thus, the infant is susceptible to hypoglycaemia when glucose demands are increased or when exogenous or endogenous glucose supply is limited. Severe or prolonged hypoglycaemia may result in long-term neurologic damage.

Definition

Hypoglycaemia in the first few days after birth is defined as blood glucose < 40 mg/dl. In preterm infants, repeated blood glucose levels below 50 mg/dl may be associated with neurodevelopmental delay.

Etiology

Conditions associated with an increased risk for neonatal hypoglycaemia include:

Decreased Substrate Availability

- Intrauterine growth retardation
- Inborn errors (*e.g.*, fructose intolerance)
- Prolonged fasting without IV glucose
- Glycogen storage diseases
- Prematurity/small for gestation age
- Postmature
- Prolong labour/difficult labour
- Mother did not receive supplementary glucose during pregnancy
- Infant of a pair of twins
- Infant born of toxaemic mother

Hyperinsulinemia

- Infant of diabetic mother
- Erythroblastosis foetalis
- Beckwith-Wiedemann Syndrome
- High umbilical arterial Catheter
- Exchange transfusion
- Abrupt cessation of IV glucose

Other Endocrine Abnormalities

- Pan-hypopituitarism
- Adrenal insufficiency
- Hypothyroidism

Increased Glucose Utilization

- Cold stress
- Sepsis
- Increased work of breathing
- Perinatal asphyxia

Miscellaneous Conditions

- Polycythemia
- CNS abnormalities
- Congenital heart diseases

Clinical Manifestations

Clinical signs and symptoms of hypoglycaemia are non-specific and include:

- Jitteriness, tremors
- Irritability, lethargy
- Weak or high–pitched cry
- Seizures
- Apnea, grunting and sweating (uncommon).
- Hypoglycaemic infants may not always be symptomatic.
- Other clinical features like cyanosis, irregular respiration, sweating, eye rolling and refusal to take feeds, the routine glucose monitoring for at-risk infants is mandatory.

Investigations

- Routine blood glucose monitoring is obtained from heel stick.

Management of Hypoglycaemia

- Take care to prevent hypothermia.
- Commence feed within 1 hour of birth and regularly 2–3 hours at breast or at least 80–90 ml/kg/day with EBM or formula milk.
- Measure blood glucose within 2 hours of birth if high risk, otherwise before the second feed.
- **Glucometer reading > 40 mg/dl** means infant is feeding normally. Follow the usual nursery protocol.
- **Glucometer reading 20–40 mg/dl**, infant is term and is able to feed:
  - Draw blood for stat blood glucose.
  - Give 5 ml/kg of D5W orally.
  - Repeat blood glucose or glucometer 20 min after feeding.
- Glucometer reading: If the reading is as given below treatment should be given as follows:

  (*a*) < 20 mg/dl or

  (*b*) < 40 mg/dl and NPO or preterm or

  (*c*) < 40 mg/dl after feeding or

  (*d*) < 40 mg/dl and symptomatic

Treatment

- Draw blood for stat glucose measurement.
- Give IV bolus of 2–3 ml/kg/minute.
- Begin continuous infusion of D10W at 4–6 mg/kg/minute.
- If infant is of diabetic mother, begin D10W at 8–10 mg/kg (100–125 ml/kg/dl).

Nursing Care

- Identification of problem of the baby, prepare the baby to feed immediately.
- Observe the signs and symptoms.
- Encourage the mother to feed the baby, educate the mother about correct position and good attachment (feeding technique).
- Secure the IV with aseptic manner and administer dextrose infusion.

ANAEMIA IN NEWBORN

Definition

The cord blood haemoglobin level of 14 gm% or lesser is considered to be anaemic.

Causes

1. Blood loss
2. Prematurity
3. Haemlytic disease of the newborn.
4. Delivery of the baby by caesarean section after cutting through the placenta in anterior placenta previa.
5. Unnoticed scalp injuries inflicted during caesarean section.
6. Ruptured vase previa.
7. Torn cord as in precipitated labour.
8. One baby is monozygotic twin (twin transfusion syndrome).
9. Excessive feto-maternal blood.

Anaemia Developing within First Week

- Slipping ligature (Improper ligature)
- Haemlytic disease.
- Hemorrhagic disease of the newborn.
- Secondary haemorrhage from the cord.
- Visceral trauma.
- Large cephlohaematoma.

Late Anaemia

Haemlytic disease

Increased RBC Destruction

Intrinsic Causes

Hereditary RBC disorders (rare) including

- **RBC** enzyme defect
- **RBC** membrane defects
- Hemoglobinopathies (*e.g.*, Meriitt syndrome)

Extrinsic Causes

- Haemlytic disease (Immune haemolysis)
  - Rh incompatibility
  - ABO incompatibility
  - Minor blood group incompatibility (*e.g.*, kell, duffy)
- Acquired haemolysis
  - Infection
  - Vitamin E deficiency (very rare)
  - Drugs.

Clinical Findings

Clinical features vary with the severity of anaemia and other associated conditions. There may be no signs with mild anaemia with more severe anaemia, findings includes:

- Pallor
- Tachypnea
- Tachycardia
- Apnea
- Poor feeding
- Lethargy
- Jaundice
- Hepatosplenomegaly
- Wide pulse pressure
- Hypotension
- Metabolic acidosis with severe anaemia.

History

- Family history: Anaemia, ethnicity
- Maternal and perinatal: Blood type and Rh; anaemia; complications of labour or delivery
- Neonatal: Age of onset; presence of other physical findings.

Laboratory Evaluation

- CBC with platelets, smear and reticulocyte count
- Blood glucose and type, direct antiglobulin test (Coomb's test)
- Bilirubin test (total and direct)
- Kleihauer-Betke test (to identify feto-maternal haemorrhage)

- Ultra sonogram for internal bleeding (head, abdomen)

Treatment

It will depend on cause and severity:

- **Prenatal** case diagnosis of significant fatal anaemia is usual except in haemolytic disease of the newborn and B-19 infection. Fetal transfusion may be needed for severe anaemia.
- **Postnatal**

  Anaemia of prematurity

The main methods of management are:

- Limit blood drawing for laboratory tests.
- In emergency transfusion of packed cell 10–15 ml/kg body weight should be given.
- Oral Iron in suspension may have to be continued for a longer period.

INJURIES OF THE NEWBORN (BIRTH INJURY)

The injuries are common in newborns during delivery, due to mismanagement during delivery. It causes injuries to infant's at birth. Various types of soft tissue injuries may be sustained during the process of birth, primarily in the forms of bruises and/or abrasions secondary to dystocia. Soft tissue injuries usually occur when there is some degree of disproposition between the presenting part and the maternal pelvis. Discolouration or abrasion occurs due to application of forceps. Petechiae or ecchymoses occurs due to pressure on the presenting part after a breech or brow delivery. Nerve injuries due to pulling the baby in breech delivery, even rarely, laceration occurs during caesarean section.

The injuries are described under two headings:

1. Injuries to the head
2. Other injuries.

Injuries to the Head

Cephalohaematoma

It is a collection of blood in-between the pericranium (periosteum) and the flat bone of the skull, usually unilateral and over a parietal bone.

Causes

- Forceps delivery.
- Ventose application.

Clinical Manifestations

- It is never present at birth but gradually develops after 12–24 hours.
- The swelling is limited by the suture lines.
- The blood is usually not significant.

Treatment

- No active treatment is necessary, the blood collection subsides itself within 2 weeks to 3 months.
- Do not aspirate the blood collection, it causes infection to infants.

Caput Succedaneum

The most commonly observed scalp lesion is Caput succedaneum, a vaguely outlined area of oedematous tissue situated over the portion of the scalp that presents in a vertex delivery.

Clinical Manifestations

- The swelling consists of serum or blood or both, accumulated in the tissues above the bone, and it often extends beyond the bone margins.
- The swelling may be associated with overlying petechiae or ecchymoses.

Treatment

- No specific treatment is needed, and the swelling subsides within a few days.

Subgaleal Haemorrhage

It subgaleal haemorrhage is bleeding into the subgaleal compartment. The subgaleal compartment is a potential space that contains loosely arranged connective tissues; it is located beneath the galea aponeurosis, the tendinous sheath that connects the fontal and occipital muscles and forms the inner surface of the scalp.

Causes

- Forceps delivery due to compression.
- Using vacuum extractor at birth.

Clinical Manifestations

- Increased head circumference.
- Increased oedema in the back of the neck and a firm mass.

Investigation

- Intranatal history-mode of delivery.
- Physical examination.
- X-ray.
- Computerized tomography or magnetic resonance image to conform the diagnosis.

- Check the haematocrit level.
- Serum bilirubin level—increase may be seen as a result of degradation of blood cells within the haematoma.

Management

- Monitoring the infant for changes in level of consciousness.
- Early identification of the problem and management.

Nursing Management

- Nurses should do the early assessment and observation for the common scalp injuries.
- Remain alert to the associated complication such as infection, rarely acute blood loss and hypovolemia.
- Assess the level of consciousness.
- Monitoring the vital signs constantly.
- Measuring the head circumference twice daily and recording.
- Reassure the parents.

Scalp Injuries

Causes

- Forceps delivery
- Caesarean section

Clinical Manifestations

- Abrasion of the scalp
- Incised wound in the scalp
- Swelling and tenderness
- Wound bleeding

Treatment

- Wound should be dressed with antiseptic solution 2% mercuro chrome.

Fracture of the Skull

Fracture of the vault of the skull (Frontal or Anterior part of the parietal bone) may be of fissure or depressed type.

Causes

- Difficult forceps delivery in disproportion or due to wrong application of forceps.
- Projected sacral promontory of the pelvis may produce depressed fracture.

Clinical Manifestations

- Fracture may be associated with cephalo-hematoma, infant with swelling and collection of blood in the scalp.
- Fracture may be associated with extradural or subdural haemorrhage—infants have convulsion, alteration in consciousness.
- If it is fissure fracture it is uncomplicated and is usually symptomless.
- Depressed fracture may occasionally cause pressure effect–increased intracranial pressure, convulsion, hypoxia-breathlessness, altered vital signs, pallor or cyanosis.
- Irritable cry
- Feeding difficulties, dehydration
- Fluid and electrolyte imbalance.

Investigation

- Intranatal history-mode of delivery
- Physical examination
- X-ray
- Computerized tomography or magnetic resonance image to conform the diagnosis
- Serum for electrolyte study
- Hematocrit.

Treatment

Principles of treatment

1. To control convulsions
2. To treat the underlying pathology
3. To maintain supportive therapy.

To Control Convulsions

- IV Phenobarbitone 10 mg/kg body weight slowly over a period of 3–5 minutes.
- A maintenance dose of 5 mg/kg/day IM for 4 weeks.
- If hypoglycemia is present administer 1 gm/kg of 10% dextrose IV stat.
- If hypocalcaemia—2 ml/kg of 10% calcium gluconate taken over 5 minutes followed by oral calcium chloride 250 mg with each feed for a month.
- If hypomagnesaemia—Administer 50% of magnesium sulphate 0.1 ml/kg.

Treat the Underlying Pathology

- Conservative treatment should be given for symptomless cases.
- In presence of symptoms, the depressed bone has to be deviated or subdural hematoma may have to be aspirated or excised surgically.

Maintain Supportive Therapy

- Nutrition—Exclusive breast feeding if infant can't suck the breast, expressed breast feeding to be encouraged.
- Infant is not conscious: Insert the nasogastric tube and feed the baby.
- Administration of oxygen.

Nursing Management

- Assessment of infant, identify at the level of consciousness and complications.
- Provide adequate nutrition by encouraging the mother to feed the baby.
- Depending on the infant's condition insert NG tube and start NG tube feeding.
- Assess the oxygen saturation level using pulse oxymeter and administer oxygen.
- Maintain thermoregulation by keeping the baby in warmer or in incubator.
- Maintain intake output chart for child.
- Assess for sign of complication.

Other Injuries

Skin and Subcutaneous Tissues

Bruises and lacerations on the face are usually caused by forceps blades. These are treated with application of 1% lotion mercurochrome. The healing is perfect without leaving behind any trace of the injury. The scalp may be oedematous and bruised, if allowed to remain on the perineum for a long period. Buttocks in breech presentation, or eyelids, lips or nose in face presentation, similarly become oedematous and congested, no treatment is required.

Muscles

Necrosis of the subcutaneous tissues may occur while the superficial skin remains intact. After a few days of birth, a small hard subcutaneous nodules appears. If it is the fat necrosis due to pressure and takes many weeks to disappear, no treatment is required.

Nerve Injuries

Facial Palsy

Due to direct pressure of the forceps blades cause haemorrhage and oedema around delivery.

Brachial Palsy

Either the nerve roots or trunk of the brachial plexus are involved due to nerve stretching or effusion or haemorrhage inside the sheath.

Causes

Traction applied on the neck while delivering mother with the shoulder dystocia or vaginal delivery with difficult labour.

Brachial palsy is of two types:

1. Erb's palsy
2. Klumpke's palsy.

Erb's palsy: This is the commonest type in which the 5th and 6th cervical nerve roots are involved. The resulting paralysis causes the arm to lie on the side with extension of the elbow, pronation of the forearm and flexion of the wrist.

Treatment is splint application in the hand.

Klumpke's palsy: It involves 7th and 8th cervical or even the first thoracic nerve roots, in this arm is flexed at the elbow, the wrist extended, the hand is flaccid and the fingers flexed.

Treatment: Splinting the arm with the forearm pronated and the fingers extended.

Bone Injury (Fractures)

Fractures are seen most often following breech delivery or infant with shoulder dystocia in large infants and occasionally in infants born by caesarean section.

Fracture of Clavicle

Fracture of Spines

Fracture of Long bones

Dislocation

The common sites of dislocations of joints are shoulder, hip, jaw and 5–6 cervical vertebrae.

Investigation

- X-ray.

Visceral Injuries

Liver, kidney, lungs are commonly injured mainly during breech delivery —Cause haemorrhage.

Treatment

1. To correct hypovolemia and anaemia
2. Specific management: Surgical treatment depends upon organ injury

Prevention

Prevention of injuries and intranatal care is the key to success in the reduction of birth injuries.

Antenatal Period

1. Screening out the high risk babies to avoid vaginal delivery—nurse should plan for elective caesarean section, it is important.

2. CP and CPD or pelvic malpresentation like breech and transverse lie to be identified posted or refer the case for caesarean section.

Intranatal Period

Normal, preterm labour, forceps, breech the management to prevent neonatal injuries.

1. *Normal Delivery*
   - Continuous foetal monitoring is desired to detect the early evidence of foetal distress.
   - Foetal blood sampling is done to identify the pH level to prevent traumatic cerebral anoxia.
   - Episiotomy should be carefully performed after placing two fingers in between the head and the stretched perineum to prevent injury to the scalp.
   - The neck should not be unduly stretched.
2. *Special Care in Preterm Labour*
   - To prevent anoxia
   - To avoid strong sedation
   - Liberal episiotomy and use of forceps to minimize intracranial compression
   - To administer vitamin K, 1 mg IM to prevent or minimize haemorrhage for the traumatized area.
3. *Forceps Delivery Management*
   - Majority of the severe injuries due to forceps.
   - Avoid forceps preference for caesarean section.
   - Never apply traction unless the application is a correct one.
4. *Vaginal Breech Delivery*
   - Care and gentleness is needed while conducting vaginal breech delivery, problems occur due to any fault in the technique during delivery.
5. *To Prevent Intracranial Injury*
   - Never be in hurry during delivery of the head which finds little time to mould.
   - Episiotomy should be done as a routine to minimize head compression.

HAEMOLYTIC DISEASE OF THE NEWBORN

Introduction and Definition

Haemolytic Disease of the Newborn (HDN), also known as erythroblastosis fetalis, isoimmunization, or blood group incompatibility, occurs when foetal red blood cells (RBCs), which possess an antigen that the mother lacks, cross the placenta into the maternal circulation, where they stimulate antibody production. The antibodies return to the foetal circulation and result in RBC destruction.

Differential Diagnosis

- Isoimmunization
- RBC enzyme disorders (*e.g.*, G6PD, pyruvate kinase deficiency)
- Haemoglobin synthesis disorders (*e.g.*, alpha-thalassemias)
- RBC membrane abnormalities (*e.g.*, hereditary spherocytosis, elliptocytosis)
- Hemangiomas (Kasabach-Merritt syndrome)
- Acquired conditions, such as sepsis, infections with TORCH or Parvovirus B 19 (anaemia due to RBC aplasia) and haemolysis secondary to drugs.

Isoimmunization

Rh Disease (Rh = Rhesus factor)

Genetics

Rh positive (+) denotes presence of D antigen. The number of antigenic sites on RBCs varies with genotype, Prevalence of genotype varies with the population, Rh negative (d/d) individuals comprise 15% of Caucasians, 55% of African-Americans, and < 1% of Asians. A sensitized Rh negative mother produces anti-Rh lgG antibodies that crosses the placenta. Risk factors for antibody production include 2nd (or later) pregnancies, maternal toxaemia, paternal zygosity (D/D rather than D/d), feto-maternal compatibility in ABO system and antigen load.

Clinical Presentation

Clinical presentation of Haemolytic Disease of the Newborn (HDN) varies from mild jaundice and anaemia to hydrops fetalis (with ascites, pleural and pericardial effusions). Because the placenta clears bilirubin, the chief risk to the foetus is anaemia. Extramedullary haematopoiesis (due to anaemia) results in hepato-splenomegaly. Risk during labour and delivery includes asphyxia and splenic rupture.

Postnatal problems include:

Asphyxia	Pulmonary hypertension
Pallor (due to anaemia)	Oedema (hydrops, due to low serum albumin)
Respiratory distress	Coagulopathies (platelets and clotting factors)
Jaundice	Kernicterus (from hyperbilirubinemia)

Hypoglycaemia (due to hyperinsulinemia from islet cell hyperplasia)

Laboratory findings

Laboratory findings vary with severity of HDN and include:

Anaemia	Hyperbilirubinemia
Reticulocytosis (6 to 40%)	↑nucleated RBC count (> 10/100 WBCs)
Thrombocytopenia	Leucopenia
+ve Direct Antiglobulin test	Hypoalbuminemia
Rh negative blood type	Smear Polychromasisa, anisocytosis No spherocytes

*HDN can occur in 1st pregnancy, but this is uncommon

↑Cord blood bilirubin > 4 mg/dl indicates severe isoimmunization

±With severe HDN, high quantities of antibody may block Rh antigen site resulting in Rh+ve infant typing as Rh –ve and having a negative direct antiglobulin test.

Treatment

Intrauterine Transfusion (IUT)

When iso-immunization is severe, IUTs are given to the foetus to prevent hydrops fetalis and foetal death. After multiple IUTs, most of the baby blood will be of Rh negative donor blood. Therefore, the direct antiglobulin test will be negative, but the indirect antiglobulin test will be positive. IUTs, the cord bilirubin are not an accurate indicator of rate of haemolysis of the likelihood of the need for post-natal exchange transfusion.

Minor Blood Group Incompatibility

It is uncommon. It occurs in 0.8% of pregnant women and usually with c, kell, Kidd or Duffy. Clinical presentation is similar to Rh disease. Anti-kell disease may be severe due to haemolysis or erythroid suppressor. Lewis antigen stimulates only lgM production, so maternal antibody screen may be positive, but foetus is not affected.

ABO Incompatibility

Genetics

With maternal blood types A and B, isoimmunization does not occur because the naturally occurring antibodies (anti–A and –B) are lgM, not lgG, In type O mothers, the antibodies are predominantly lgG, cross the placenta and can cause haemolysis in the foetus. The association of a type A or B foetus with a type O mother occurs in 15% of pregnancies. However HDN occurs in only 3%, is severe in only 1%, and < 1 : 1,000 require exchange transfusion. The disease is more common and more severe in African-American infants. Unlike Rh, ABO disease can occur in first pregnancies, because anti-A and anti-B antibodies are found early in life from exposure to A- or B-like antigens present in many foods and bacteria.

Clinical Presentation

Generally less severe than with Rh disease:

- Jaundice
- Anaemia
- Hepatospelenomegaly
- Hypovolmic shock

Laboratory Findings

Laboratory findings that differ from Rh disease:

- Smear, microspherocytosis.
- MCV < 95, microcytic for a newborn (normal for adults).
- Direct coombs test is often weakly +ve.

Management

Preparation Prior to Delivery

- Blood type O Rh negative packed RBCs, is cross-matched against the mother. For severe HDN, have blood in the resuscitation room to correct severe anaemia immediately after birth by partial exchange transfusion (ExTx). Anticipate need for later ExTx for hyperbilirubinemia and have additional blood for these.
- Surfactant therapy, if infant is preterm.
- Catheter (*e.g.*, angiocaths) for immediate drainage of hydropic fluid.

Resuscitation

At birth, the major problems are cardiopulmonary and relate to effects of severe anaemia, hydrops and prematurity, because of multiple problems, baby may need effective resuscitation.

- For investigation obtain cord blood for bilirubin, blood type and Rh, combs test, total count, and albumin.
- Infant is hydropic, immediately intubate the baby assisted by ventilation with oxygen, if ventilation is difficult, drain pleural and abdominal fluid, avoid complication like puncturing enlarged liver and spleen.
- Insert the umbilical catheters for checking BP and analysis for arterial blood gas, blood haematocrit.
- Correct the metabolic acidosis with alkali and by giving ventilation.
- Correct anaemia by blood transfusion of packed RBCs (*e.g.*, for Hct of 30%, push 10 ml/kg over 5 min, for Hct of 20%, push 10 ml/kg over 5 min, then repeat).
- Measure the blood sugar to correct hypoglycaemia.
- Follow platelet counts; consider platelet transfusion for count < 50,000.

Exchange Transfusion (ExTx)

- **Indications**

  Depending upon absolute serum concentration bilirubin, the rate of rise of bilirubin, gestational age, albumin concentration and acid base status.

  Exchange transfusion should be done at or soon after birth in baby born to Rh-Isoimmunized mother.

  - Hydrops fetalis
  - History of previous siblings requiring an exchange transfusion because of Rh-Isoimmunization.
  - Baby born with pallor, hepato-splenomegaly and positive direct Coombs test.
  - In general, perform ExTx for cord bilirubin > 5 mg/dl,
  - Cord TSB < 11 gm/dl
  - Rate of rise of TSB > 0.5 mg/dl
  - Any TSB > 12 mg/dl in the first 24 hours and TSB > 20 mg/dl in the neonatal period are also indications for exchange transfusion.
- Blood should be reconstituted (to Hct-40–50%) from fresh, 0 negative packed RBCs cross-matched against the mother and type-specific fresh frozen plasma.

Technique (procedure)

About 30 minutes before ExTx, give albumin 1 g/kg to increase the bilirubin bound to albumin in the circulation and make ExTx more effective. The blood should be warmed and the bag agitated every few minutes (to prevent settling of the RBCs).

Following equipment should be arranged for the ExTx:

- Exchange transfusion set
- One bottle of normal saline
- Three way stopcocks
- Disposable syringes 10 ml and 20 ml and needles (different size)
- Umbilical cannula number 6 and 9
- 10% calcium gluconate, sodium bicarbonate, distilled water, heparin.
- Blood transfusion set, intravenous set
- Resuscitation tray
  - Infant should be kept in the radiant warmer.
  - Exchange 2 × the blood volume (estimate blood volume at 85 ml/kg but is limited to no more than 500 ml).
  - A catheter is inserted into the umbilical vein and threaded into the inferior vena cava.
  - Depending on the infant's weight, 5 to 10 ml of blood is withdrawn within 15 to 20 seconds, and the same volume of donor blood is infused over 60 to 90 seconds.
  - If the blood has been citrated (addition of phosphate dextrose adenine to prevent coagulation).
  - Calcium gluconate may be given after the infusion of 100 ml of donor's blood to prevent hypocalcaemia.

Complications

- Hypocalcaemia
- Hypoglycaemia
- Thrombocytopenia especially with older units of blood
- Hypothermia
- Hyperkalemia

Nursing Management

- Initial nursing responsibility is to recognise the jaundice.

- If there is any possibility of haemolytic diseases, anticipate from the prenatal and perinatal history.
- Any prenatal evidence of incompatibility, do the investigation for coomb's test.
- If an exchanged blood transfusion is required, the nurse should prepare the infant and family and also assist the practitioner with the procedure.
- All emergency drugs and cardiopulmonary resuscitation equipment must be kept ready.
- The exchange transfusion is to be performed in a radiant warmer.
- Sterile equipment should be ready for the procedure. Aseptic procedure must be performed.
- Blood is also warmed before infusion.
- Maintain the documentation of blood volume exchanged, including the amount of blood withdrawn and infused, the time of each procedure and the cumulative record of the total volume exchanged.
- Monitor the vital signs electronically evaluated frequently and correlated with the removal and infusion of the blood (HR, RR, BP).
- If signs of cardiac or respiratory problems occur, the procedure is stopped temporarily and resumed once the infant's cardiopulmonary function stabilizes.
- The nurse also observes for signs of transfusion reaction which include tachycardia or bradycardia, respiratory distress, dramatic changes in blood pressure, temperature instability and rash.
- Maintain the thermoregulation throughout the procedure to prevent hypothermia and hyperthermia (hypothermia causes metabolic acidosis, hyperthermia causes damage donor erythrocytes, elevates free potassium, it predisposes to the infant's cardiac arrest).
- After the procedure is completed, the nurse inspects the umbilical site for evidence of bleeding, usually the catheter remains in place in case repeated exchange is required.
- Psychological support to prove to the parents.

HYPERBILIRUBINEMIA

Hyperbilirubinemia refers to increased bilirubin levels in the blood. Manifestation is yellowish discoloration of the skin and other organs (iterus). About 97% of healthy full term infants have biochemical hyperbilirubinemia (total serum bilirubin > 1.5 mg) and 65% are clinically jaundiced (TSB > 7 mg/dl). This is all known to be physiological jaundice in newborn babies. It appears between 24–72 hours of birth. The most important factors which contribute to the development of physiological hyperbilirubinemia in the newborn are:

- "Physiological polycythemia" and shorter life span of neonatal RBCs result in increased production of bilirubin.
- Hepatic uptake, conjugation and excretion of bilirubin are limited due to glucuronyl transferase enzyme in newborn, especially preterm babies.
- Due to paucity of bacterial flora in the gut of newborn babies and on the other hand the over activity of intestinal beta-glucuronidase enzyme, the conjugated bilirubin entering the duodenum is rapidly deconjugated and recirculated in the blood through entero-hepatic circulation.

Pathological Jaundice appears within 24 hours of birth with following characteristics of bilirubin level:

- Exceeds 6 mg/dl within the first 24 hours after delivery.
- Increases greater than 5 mg/day.
- Remains elevated more than 5 mg/dl/day.
- Remains elevated beyond 7 days in a full term neonate.
- Remains elevated for 10 days in a premature neonate.

Pathophysiology

Bilirubin is one of the breakdown products of haemoglobin as a result of the destruction of red blood cells. When red blood cells are destroyed their component substances are released into the circulation. Released haemoglobin splits into two fractions, heme and globin. The globin (protein) is used by the body, while the heme portion is converted to uncojugated bilirubin. An insoluble substance bound to albumin in the liver, the bilirubin is detached from the plasma protein and in the presence of the enzyme glucuronyl tranferase is conjugated with glucuronic acid to produce a highly soluble substance, bilirubin glucuronide, which is excreted in the bile.

In the newborn infant hyperbilirubinemia is usually the result of excess production of bilirubin, disturbed capacity to conjugate or bile duct obstruction. Excess production of bilirubin causes haemolytic diseases in newborn or infection. Reduced ability to conjugate bilirubin may be a complicating factor in haemolytic diseases. This is the so called physiologic jaundice in newborn. It causes serum bilirubin level to reach toxic levels that leads to Kernicterus, serious brain damage may result due to deposition of unconjugated bilirubin in brain cells.

Causes

- Haemolytic diseases of the newborn
- Rh incompatibility
- ABO incompatibility
- Isoimmune haemolytic diseases like erythroblastosis fetalis
- Hydrops fetalis
- Prematurity
- Polycythemia
- Pyloric stenosis
- Obstruction or atresia of the biliary duct
- Sepsis
- Hypoglycaemia
- Other perinatal predisposing factors like:
  - Hereditary
  - Diabetics of the infant
  - Intrauterine infection
  - Green negative bacilli infection
  - Drug ingestion—(sulfar, salicylates, and diazepam)

Clinical Manifestations

- Skin colour is pale or jaundice noticed in 1st 24–36 hours after birth
- Dark concentrated urine
- Changes in behaviour—lethargy, irritability—high pitched cry
- Hypoactive bowel sound
- Meconium passage may be delayed
- Neonate may have enlargement of spleen or liver
- Generalized oedema with pleural and pericardial effusion
- Seizures
- Decreased reflexes.

Diagnostic Test Findings

- Blood investigation: HB, Total serum bilirubin, packed cell volume (PCV), Complete blood count.
- Blood group of the baby with direct coomb's test.
- History: Neonatal history, Family history, Maternal Rh factors, Feeding method.
- Clinical examination or assessment: Gestational age at birth.
- Assessment of jaundice if there is no lab facilities:
  - Jaundice limited to face = 5–7 mg/dl.
  - Jaundice up to the level of the chest = 10 mg/dl.
  - Lower abdomen/thigh = 12 mg/dl.
  - Sole/palms stained yellow ≥ 15 mg/dl.

Medical Management

- Alleviating anaemia
- Exchange transfusion removing maternal antibodies and sensitized erythrocytes (if serum bilirubin level more than 20 mg/dl)
- Infusion of albumin
- Increasing serum albumin levels
- Reducing the levels of serum bilirubin
- Minimizing the consequences of hyperbilirubinemia
- Phototherapy
- Increased fluid intake
- Provide adequate feeding to the baby by breast feeding.

Complications

- Kernicterus
- Severe anaemia
- Oedema, ascitis
- Hydrothorax

Clinical Stages of Kernicterus

Stage I: Poor Moro reflex, decreased tone, lethargy, poor feeding, vomiting and high pitched cry.

Stage II: Opisthotinos, seizures, fever, rigidity, oclogyric crisis.

Stage III: Spasticity is decreased.

Stage IV: Late stage includes spasticity athetosis, deafness, mental retardation and paralysis of upward gaze.

Phototherapy

Phototherapy involves the use of intense fluorescent light on the infants exposed skin. Light promotes bilirubin excretion by **photoisomerization**, which alter the structure of bilirubin to a soluble form (lumirubin) for easier excretion. The studies indicate that blue fluorescent light is more effective in reducing bilirubin.

An alternative to traditional phototherapy "bililight" is the **fiberoptic blanket** or **panel**, which consists of a light generating illuminator, a bundle of plastic fibers affixed to a panel that distributes the energy, and soft, disposable, light permeable cover to protect the infant. The blanket delivers therapeutic light consistently and continuously to the infant and achieves the same photoismerization as conventional phototherapy. This fiberoptic blanket is portable and suitable for home phototheraphy, it permits more parent-infant interaction, there is no need for using eye pad and placing the baby in correct distance, it maintains the temperature, if very preterm babies it may cause dermal injury.

Indication

- Infant weight < 1500 g, serum bilirubin at the level of 5–8 mg/dl.
- Infant weight 1500 g – <2000 g, serum bilirubin at the level of 8–12 mg/dl.
- Infant weight 2000–2499 g, serum bilirubin at level of 11–14 mg/dl.

Contraindication

- Phototherapy is not recommended for conjugated hyperbilirubinemia, it may cause brooze discolouration of the skin in these babies.

Nursing Management

- Prevent neonatal jaundice –Encourage the mother to feed early.
- Identify infant at risk for hyperbilirubinemia and kernicterus.
  - Identify the evidence of jaundice.
- Assist in phototherapy
  - Keep the baby undressed (except for a diaper).
  - Shield the infant's eyes.
  - Cover the infant's head, testes to avoid exposure to the light, head is a large area evaporation occurs due to overheat, exposure of testes causes sterility.
  - Maintain the distance of light from the cot 45 cm.
  - Monitor the temperature every 4 hours.
  - Change the position frequently every 2 hours.
  - Maintain the nutritional status–encourage the mother to feed every 2 hours or as per infant's demands.
  - Check for any dehydration.
  - Monitor the serum bilirubin level everyday.
  - Change the diaper frequently after urination to prevent infection.
  - Strictly follow the instructions, duration of therapy is 6 to 8 hours per day.
  - Observe the skin for any heat rashes.
- Keep the neonate's anal area clean and dry, frequent greenish stools result from bilirubin excretion and can lead to skin irritation.
- Assist with an Exchange Transfusion
  - Inform the child's sickness and explain the procedure to the parents, get the consent form to be signed.
  - Check the infant blood group and Rh factors.
  - Keep infant Npo 3 to 4 hours before procedure.
  - Check donor blood with physician for correct blood group and Rh type.
  - Keep ready all the equipment needed for the procedure.
  - Ensure asepsis during procedure.
  - Keep accurate recordings of amount of blood infused and withdrawn.
  - Monitor the vital signs continuously.
  - Maintain the baby's body temperature during the procedure (cover the baby with blanket, keep the baby in radiant warmer).
  - Observe the signs of exchange transfusion reactions.
  - Keep ready the resuscitation equipment.
  - Apply the sterile dressing to catheter sit.
- Provide emotional support to parents:
  - Explain reason for jaundice.
  - Discontinue phototherapy during parents visits, remove infant's eye shields.

Complications

- Increased insensible water loss, therefore, these babies need extra fluid of 20 ml/kg/day.
- Retinal damage
- Erythematous skin rash
- Bronze baby syndrome.
- Dehydration
- Hyperthermia
- Burns.

INFECTION OF NEWBORN

Infection is still one of the leading causes of neonatal death in the developing countries. The neonates are more susceptible to infection. This is because they lack in natural immunity and take some time for the acquired immunity to develop. There is also deficiency in leucocytic response to infection.

Mode of Infection

- Antenatal
- Intranatal
- Postnatal

Antenatal

Transplacental: Maternal infection by syphilis, measles, toxoplasmosis, chicken pox, tuberculosis, poliomyelitis, etc., can affect the baby following aspiration or ingestion of infected amniotic fluid.

Intranatal

Provided the membranes are intact and there is no transplacental infection, the unborn baby is main in a bacteriological sterile environment.

The following are the modes of intranatal infection to the babies.

- Aspiration of infected liquor, which is inevitable in prolonged labour following early rupture of the membranes or repeated internal examination. This may lead to either congenital or neonatal pneumonia.
- While the foetus is passing the vagina contamination leads to Gonococci infection and this leads to Ophthalmic neonatorum.
- Oral thrush etc.
- Improper asepsis causes cord sepsis to the neonates.

Postnatal

- Transmission due to human contact—Infected mother, relatives, staff in the wards etc.
- Cross infection from an infected baby in the nursery.
- Infected utensils either used for feeding or bathing, clothing or airborne.

Common Organism that Cause Infection

In developing countries gram negative and gram positive organisms causes infection

- Group B Streptococci—*E. coli, Klebsiella*
- Group D
- Enterobacteria species

Prevention

- Proper antenatal care
- Asepsis care
- Clean the eyes
- Proper suctioning

Treatment

- Baby should be isolated.
- Control infection by adequate and appropriate antibiotics.
  - Ampicillin 100 mg/kg/day bid.
  - Gentamycin 2.5 mg/kg, Im/IV OD.
  - Ciprofloxacin 50 mg/kg/day every 24 hours.
  - Cefotataxime 100 mg/kg/day Bid.
- Maintain the general condition—if necessary by changing the feeding route.
- Adequate oxygenation.

NEONATAL SEPSIS

Definition

Neonatal sepsis or septicemia is a generalized acute bacterial infection in the blood stream, occurring in the first month of life with high mortality. It occurs in infants of any gestational age, with both innate and extrinsic reasons.

Risk Factors for Sepsis

- Perinatal infection.
- Prematurity.
- Infant with central lines/Indwelling catheter.

- Neutropenia (ANC ≤ 1000).
- Inadequate aseptic technique in general and hand washing in particular.
- Excessive and unplanned invasive procedures.
- Compromise on use of disposables.

Etiology

- Group B Streptococcus is the most common cause of sepsis
- *Escherichia coli*
- Group A Streptococcus
- *Streptococcus viridians*
- *Klebsiella pneumoniae*
- *Pseudomonous aeruginosa*

Pathophysiology

- Bacterial pathogens cause neonatal infection. It varies depending upon time of infection, presentation of sign and symptoms, neonatal infections are early and late sepsis.
- Immune defence mechanisms in neonates are immature.
- Posing the potential for rapid invasion spread and multiplication of infecting organisms the newborn is unable to locate the infection.

Early sepsis: Acute bacterial infection occurs during onset of first week of life after birth. All term babies, the likelihood of infection is greater among preterm infants. Gram-negative and gram-positive organism causes sepsis.

Late sepsis: Preterm and term infants with various medical and surgical conditions are at greater risk for late onset of sepsis. It is mostly due to horizontally transmitted nosocomial infection usually from invasive techniques. Lack of enteric feeding and exposure to broad spectrum antibiotics, which may alter normal flora and permit overgrowth and dissemination of fungal species and resistant bacteria.

Clinical Manifestations

- Infant generally "not doing well"
- Poor sucking and feeding
- Weak cry
- Lethargy
- Irritability,
- Fast breathing > 60/minute, followed by pallor, cyanosis or mottling, irregular respiration, severe lower chest indrawing, grunting
- Jaundice
- Decreased pain response
- Hypotension
- Tachycardia
- Dehydration
- Hyperthermia or hypothermia-temperature > 37.5°C or < 35.5°C.
- Gastrointestinal disturbances—diarrhoea/vomiting, abdominal distention
- Hepatomegaly, splenomegally
- Seizures
- Hypotonic
- Tremors
- Full fontanel
- Abnormal eye movement

Investigation

- Physical examination looking for potential sites of infection
- Blood culture—central line, peripheral site
- Urine culture
- Blood routine examination, CBC—shows sign of anaemia, leukocytosis or leucopenia, elevation or decreased total neutrophils, micro ESR
- Culture of any draining wounds
- Chest X-ray
- Lumbar puncture for sepsis.

Therapeutic Management

Early recognition and diagnosis are essential in order to increase the infant's chance for survival and reduce the likelihood of permanent neurologic damage.

- Antibiotic therapy is initiated before laboratory results are available to conform.

Specific therapy for less than 1 week of age

- Ampicillin 50 mg/kg 8 hourly,
- Gentamycin 2.5 mg/kg 12 hourly,
- Amikacin 15–25 mg/kg every 24 hours
- Treatment consists of circulatory support, respiratory support, aggressive administration of antibiotics and immunotherapy.
- Supportive therapy usually involves administration of oxygen, careful regulation of fluid and electrolytes, temporary discontinuation of oral feedings, blood transfusion if needed to correct anaemia, regulating thermal environment and monitoring the vital signs.

Nursing Management

- Nurses should observe and assess the infants with high risk and identify the problems of infants.
- Nurses should have knowledge of antibiotics and proper regulation and administration of the drug are vital to identify the side effects.
- Nurses must alert for evidence of complications. If infant has candida albicans, Nystatin oral suspension is swabbed on the buccal mucosa for prophylaxis against oral candidasis.
- Provide an optimum thermo regulated environment to keep the infant in warmer or in incubator.
- Provide adequate hydration by administrating IV fluids, maintain intake and output chart, avoid dehydration.
- Observe for hypoxia by pulse oximetery for oxygen saturation.
- Strictly follow the aseptic precaution to prevent infection (proper hand washing, using disposable equipments, disposal of excretions, etc.).
- Nurses should follow the standard precautions to prevent infection because they are most consistent caregivers.

NECROTIZING ENTEROCOLITIS (NEC)

Necrotizing enterocolitis is an acute inflammatory disease of the bowel with increased incidence in preterm and other high-risk infants; it is most common in infants who are preterm. Three factors appear to play an important role in the development of NEC: intestinal ischemia, colonization by pathogenic bacteria, and substrate (formula feeding) in the intestinal lumen.

Risk Factors

- Premature infants.
- Perinatal hypoxia.
- Hypertension, umblical sepsis.
- Feeding of cow's milk to babies.
- Asphyxia.
- Patent ductus arterioses.
- Bacterial infection.

Pathophysiology

The precise cause of NEC is still uncertain, but it appears to occur in infants whose gastrointestinal tract has suffered vascular compromise.

The damage to mucosal cells lining of the bowel wall is great. Diminished blood supply to these cells causes their death in large numbers; they stoop secreting protective, lubricating mucus; and the thin, unprotected bowel wall is attacked by proteolytic enzymes. Thus the bowel wall continues to swell and breaks down; it is unable to synthesize protective IgM, and the mucosa is permeable to macromolecules (*e.g.*, exotoxins), which further hamper intestinal defenses. Gas-forming bacteria invade the presence of air in the submucosal or subserosal surfaces of the bowel.

Clinical Manifestations

Early Symptoms

- Vomiting
- Temperature instability
- Lethargy
- Abdominal distension and tenderness
- Bradycardia
- Apnea
- Ileus and G.I. bleeding
- Decreased appetite
- Gross or occult blood in stool
- Bluish discolouration of abdominal wall

Later Stage

- Perforation
- Peritonitis
- Septic shock
- Death.

Investigation

- X-ray shows a sausage shaped dilation of the intestine
- Blood examination TBC, haematocrit
- Serum electrolytes
- Blood culture

Treatment

- Prevention of shock
- To correct electrolyte imbalance
- Nothing by oral for 24 to 48 hours
- NG Tube-aspiration
- Intravenous fluids to maintain fluid for correction of extra vascular volume
- Antibiotics intravenously

Nursing Care

- Early recognition of the problem by warning signs of NEC.
- Observe the abdomen frequently for distension.
- Measuring the abdominal girth and record every two hours.
- Insert the nasogastric tube for aspiration.
- Measuring residual gastric contents before feeding.
- Listening the bowel sound frequently.
- Maintain thermoregulation for the baby—keep the infant in warmer or in incubator.
- Administer the antibiotics on time.
- Observe for abnormal signs, if identified inform immediately.
- Maintain intake and output chart.
- Provide psychological support for the parents.

OPHTHALMIC NEONATORUM

It is an inflammation of conjunctiva during first three weeks of the life.

Causes

- Chlyamydian trachomatis
- Bacterial infection
- Chemical
- Rarely viral

Mode of Infection

- Occurs during delivery by contaminated vaginal discharge. It is more likely in face or breech delivery.

Clinical Manifestations

- Discharge may be watery from eyes
- Mucopurulent to frank purulent in one or both eyes
- Eyelids may be sticky or markedly swollen
- Cornea may be involved in severe cases

Prevention

- Any suspicious vaginal discharge during the antenatal period should be treated.
- Meticulous obstetric asepsis maintained at birth.
- Eyes should be cleaned when the head is delivered.
- Tetracycline ointment to be applied into each eye.

Treatment

- Isolation of baby
- Clean the eyes gently and wipe away the push.
- Apply Tetracycline ointment in both eyes 4–6 times/day.
- If gonococcal infection-tropical (1 : 10,000) penicillin drops should be applied.
- In severe cases, systemic benzyle penicillin 50,000 units/kg in 2 divided doses for 7 days.

ORAL THRUSH (ORAL CANDIDIASIS)

Infection of the buccal mucus membranes and the tongue by the fungus candidia albicans is not uncommon especially in bottlefed babies. Thrush present as white patch on the gums, palate and tongue, affects the skin around the mouth.

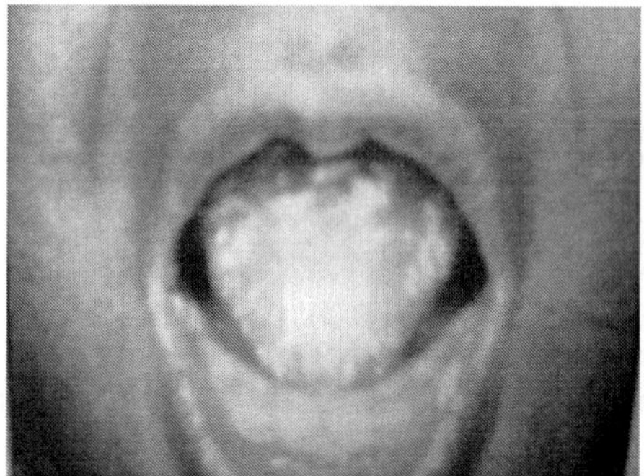

Fig. 3.6: Baby with oral candidiasis

Causes

- Contamination by the organisms occurs from the feeding bottles.
- Acquired during birth or from caregivers hands or feeding equipment.
- The fungus grows on the mucous membrane and produces milky white elevated patches resembling milk curd, which cannot be easily wiped off with gauze, rarely the fungal infection may spread down to involve the gastrointestinal or respiratory tract.

Clinical Manifestations

- It usually appears in the late first week or during the second week.
- Infant refuses to take feeding.
- White patches on the gums, palate and tongue and skin around the mouth.

- If spread to respiratory tract, the child has respiratory distress or difficulty in breathing.

Prevention

- Maternal fungal infection in the vagina is to be adequately treated before delivery (during antenatal period).
- Utensils including feeding bottles are cleaned well and steriled (boiled) before and after feed.
- After feeding, warm water to be given to clean the mouth.

Treatment

- Local application of 1% aqueous solution of gentian violet on the oral mucus membrane twice daily after feeding for 2–3 days is quite effective.
- Nystatin (mycostain) 100,000 units in 1 ml, oral suspension dropped under the tongue 4 times a day.
- Avoid feeding for 20 minutes after medication.
- Application of glycerine in the oral cavity, it gives soothing effect to the child.
- Advise the mother to wash breasts before and after feeds, if bottle fed advice change to spoon or cup.

NEONATAL SEIZURES

Seizures in the neonatal period are usually the clinical manifestation of serious underlying diseases. The most common causes of seizures in the neonatal period are hypoxic ischemic encephalopathy secondary to perinatal asphyxia. Seizures is a condition of medical emergency because they signal a disease process that may produce irreversible brain damage so recognize the seizures and identify the cause, treat the infant immediately.

Causes

- Hypoxic-ischemic injury
- Intracranial haemorrhage
- Electrolytes imbalance (sodium, calcium, magnesium)
- Hypoglycaemia
- Drug withdrawal
- Inborn error metabolism
- Intrauterine or perinatal infection
- CNS developmental defects (hydrocephalus)

Clinical Manifestations

The clinical manifestations of neonatal seizures are tabulated below:

TABLE 3.1: Classification of Neonatal Seizures

Type	Characteristics
Clonic	• Rhythmic jerking movements • Approximately 1 to 3 per second • May migrate randomly from one part of the body to another • Simultaneous involvement of separate areas • Movements may start at different times and at different rates
Tonic	• Extension of all four limbs (similar to decerebrate rigidity) • Upper limbs are maintained in a stiffly flexed position (resembles decorticate rigidity) appear more often in preterm infants commonly associated with IVH
Myoclonic	Single or multiple flexion jerks of limbs often indicate a metabolic etiology
Subtle	May develop in either full-term or preterm infants. Often overlooked by inexperienced observers. Signs: • Clonic horizontal eye deviation • Repetitive blinking or fluttering of the eyelids, starting • Twitching • Drooling, sucking, or other oral-buccal-lingual movements • Arm movements that resemble rowing or swimming • Leg movements described as pedalling or cycling • Apnea (Common) Signs may appear alone or in combination

Investigation

- History—Related to traumatic delivery, maternal infection, family history
- Clinical examination—look for birth injury, infection, congenital anomalies in addition to the seizures

- X-ray
- CT scan or ultrasound
- Blood for serum electrolytes
- Lumbar puncture
- Culture for urine, blood, CSF
- Total blood count/coagulation study (PT/PTT)
- Electro encephalogram
- Neuroimaging—MRI

Treatment

1. A/B/C's: Correct any abnormalities in oxygenation, ventilation, and perfusion, be ready to intubate if giving anticonvulsant therapy.
2. Anticonvulsant therapy.

   Phenobarbital—loading dose 20 mg/kg should be given IV over 10–15 min. If seizures persist for the baby, bolus amount should be increased to 5 mg/kg to achieve serum level > 40 mg/dl.

   Maintenance dose: 3–4 mg/kg/day initiate 12–24 hours after loading dose.

   Phosphenytoin—After continued, prolonged episodes of seizures activity on maximal Phenobarbital therapy

   Loading dose: 20 mg/kg bolus (no faster than 1 mg/kg/min)

   Maintenance dose: 5 mg/kg/day

   Benzodiazepines—For brief, episodic events,

   Lorazepam 0.1 mg/kg/dose or diazepam 0.5 mg/kg/dose
3. Correct all metabolic abnormality (IV glucose, electrolyte replacement, metabolic acidosis correction)
4. Antibiotics therapy
5. Surgical management (if indicated).

Nursing Management

- Nurses should observe the infant to recognize the seizure.
- If therapy regimen has started, observe the baby for response to the therapy.
- Inform to the parents their infant status. And provide psychological support.
- Maintain thermoregulation for infant.
- Encourage the parents to visit their baby and perform the parenting activities.
- Encourage mother to breastfeed the baby.
- Monitor the vital signs and recording, if any deviation of vital sign, inform to physician immediately.
- Observe for the sign of complication of the drugs (Myocardial and respiratory depression, cardiac arrhythmias, hypotension).

NEONATAL COAGULATION DISORDERS

Neonatal bleeding results from disorders of platelets, coagulation proteins, and disorders of vascular integrity, vitamin K deficiency. While healthy newborns have low levels of some coagulation proteins, this is normally balanced by the parallel decrease in fibrinolytic activity.

Platelet Disorders

1. **Thrombocytopenia** (Platelet count < 150×10^9/L) occurs in 1–4% of term newborns, 40–72% of sick preterms and 25% of NICU/NCCN admissions; of these, 75% occur before age 72 hours.

Causes

- Decreased platelet production occurs in congenital infections (*e.g.*, CMV, Rubella, HIV), certain syndromes (*e.g.*, Thrombocytopenia, absent radius, Fanconi), Sepsis and Haemolytic diseases of newborn.
- Increased platelet consumption, occurs in
  - Maternal autoimmune disease (*e.g.*, ITP, SLE)
  - Asphyxia/shock
  - Neonatal autoimmune thrombocytopenia
  - Maternal thiazide intake
  - IUGR with toxaemia of pregnancy
  - Neocrotizng enterocolitis
  - Thrombosis (due to catheters, hemangiomas)
  - Sepsis
  - Haemolytic disease of the newborn
  - Exchange transfusion
  - Heparin-induced thrombocytopenia
  - Polycythemia/hyperviscosity.

2. Impaired platelet function is rare in the newborn except for:
   - Decreased platelet adhesiveness associated with indomethacin therapy
   - Von Willebrand's disease

Coagulation Protein Disorders

1. Congenital factor deficiencies:
   - X-linked recessive: Haemophilia A (Factor VIII) and Haemophilia B (Factor IX)
   - Autosomal recessive (rare): Factors VII, X, XI, XII, XIII, afibrinogenemia
2. Acquired deficiencies: Most common is vitamin K deficiency.

Combined Platelet and Coagulation Factor Disorders

1. Disseminated intravascular coagulation (DIC) occurs secondary to inappropriate systemic activation of normal clotting mechanisms after endothelial injury. Infants have low platelet counts and fibrinogen levels, prolonged PT and PTT, and elevated fibrin degradation products.
2. Hepatic dysfunction due to several causes (*e.g.*, shock, infection, inherited conditions) most have prolonged PT and decreased factor and fibrinogen levels.

Disorders of Vascular Integrity

Haemangiomas or vascular malformations are in babies that may rupture and directly bleed, or sequester platelets and secondarily cause bleeding.

Clinical Features

- Magnitude of blood loss and underlying diseases
- Sign of abnormal bleeding tendency includes
  - Petechiae,
  - Excessive bruising,
  - Prolonged bleeding from puncture sites
  - Umbilical oozing
  - Gastrointestinal bleeding
  - Subgaleal haemorrhage and intracranial haemorrhage
  - Pulmonary haemorrhage
  - Haematuria
- When the blood loss is large, the infant may be present with signs of hypovolemia
  - Pallor
  - Tachycardia
  - Metabolic acidosis
  - Weak pulse
  - Hypotension

HAEMORRHAGIC DISEASE OF THE NEWBORN (HDN)

Vitamin K Deficiency

The most appropriate term for hemorrhagic disease in the newborn is vitamin K deficiency. Vitamin K is a fat soluble vitamin that can be absorbed from the GI tract in the presence of bile required for the production of coagulation factors II, VII, IX and X in the liver. A moderate decrease of factors II, VII, IX and X normally occurs in all newborn infants by 48–72 hours after birth, with a gradual return to birth levels by 7–10 days of age.

- This transient deficiency of vitamin K dependent factors probably is due to lack of free vitamin K in the mother.
- Immaturity of the infant's liver and absence of bacterial intestinal flora—normally responsible for synthesis of vitamin K.

Commonly Affected Babies

- Babies who did not receive vitamin K prophylaxis at birth
- Babies whose mothers have seizure disorder and taking anti-convulsant medications
- Babies whose mother is having tuberculosis and are on antituberculous medications
- Babies who are on antibiotic therapy for prolonged period of time
- Babies who are having persistent diarrhoea.

Clinical Manifestations

The clinical manifestation is classified as

Early HDN occurs within 24 hours of life, mainly due to maternal anticonvulsants, antituberculous drugs and salicylates.

Classical HDN occurs in newborns from 2–7 days of age. This is primarily due to low level of vitamin K in the newborns and low levels of vitamin K in breast milk.

Late HDN occurs, from one week to 12 weeks of life usually starts at 2 weeks of age. In this case the most important causes are prolonged antibiotic therapy and persistent diarrhoea.

The major clinical manifestations include; bleeding from the following sites:

- Bleeding from sero-mucous
- Bleeding or oozing from umbilicus
- Blood in the urine
- Blood in the stool

If any one of the clinical signs occur, in otherwise a relatively well baby, it is important to suspect HDN, and do coagulation profile and determine the levels of protein inducted by vitamin K antagonism or absence to confirm the diagnosis.

The findings suggestive of HDN are:

- Prolonged PT
- Prolonged PTT
- Platelets are normal
- Levels of PIVKAII increased.
- Plasma recalcification time prolonged
- Blood coagulation time prolonged.

Treatment

- Administration of 1 mg of vitamin K intramuscular injection at the time of birth.
- The disease may be effectively treated with an IV 5 mg of vitamin K.
- A Prothrobin time (PT) should be obtained on cord blood and the infant given 1-2 mg of vitamin K IV.
- If the PT is greatly prolonged and fails to improve, then 10 ml/kg of fresh frozen plasma should be given.

Diagnostic Evaluation of Abnormal Bleeding

History

- Family history of bleeding disorder or neonatal death
- Maternal history of bleeding disorders, medicine intake, autoimmune diseases.
- *Perinatal*: Toxemia of pregnancy, IUGR, antepartum bleeding
- *Neonatal*: History of asphyxia, birth injury, Administration of vitamin K.

Neonatal Physical Examination

- Signs of bleeding
- Signs of infection (hepatospleenomealy)
- Signs of hypovolemia
- Hemangiomas, vascular malformation
- Other malformations
- Other illness (*e.g.*, NEC, haemolytic disease)

Laboratory Investigations

- Blood examination—CBC, differential, smear
- Platelet count
- Prothrombin time (PTT)
- Fibrinogen

Note: Draw the blood from the infant non-heparinized source.

Management

For secondary bleeding disorders, treat underlying disease. Replacement of clotting factors is often necessary.

1. Severe, life threatening bleeding
   - Maintain adequate circulating blood volume
   - Send the blood for clotting study
   - If clotting defect is not known, consider to give following treatment
     - Vitamin K 1 mg IV slowly over 1 minute (Rapid infusion can cause cardiac dysarrhthmias)
     - Fresh Frozen plasma 10 ml/kg over 5–10 min
     - Transfusion of platelets one unit
     - Administration of cryoprecipate one unit
   - Send repeat blood sample for clotting studies in 4–6 hours
   - Obtain haematologist consultation needed if bleeding is not controlled quickly
2. Bleeding with known abnormal clotting screening tests:
   - Prolonged prothrombin time (PT) normal PTT, platelets and Fibrinogen
     - Give vitamin K 1 mg IV slowly over 1 minute. Repeat PT in 4 hours. If not improved, consult haematologist.
   - Prolonged PT and PTT
     - Give fresh frozen plasma 10 ml/kg and vitamin K 1 mg, send repeat clotting studies in 2 hours
   - Low fibrinogen
     - Give cryoprecipitate
   - Thrombocytopenia
     - Severe bleeding occurs in this condition of infants. Use platelet transfusion to maintain platelets $> 50 \times 10^9$ l.
3. For any bleeding problem that is not controlled adequately and quickly, refer the infant to haematologist consultation.
4. For significant bleeding from any cause, consider cranial ultrasound, especially in preterm infants.

CARE OF NEWBORN WITH COMMON CONGENITAL ANOMALIES

CONGENITAL ABNORMALITIES

Many congenital abnormalities can nowadays be treated surgically. A list of the more common types is of interest and some knowledge of them may lead to keener observation even in a maternity, neonatal ward or medical paediatric ward.

The Head: Microcephaly, hydrocephaly, Encephalocel, Craniosynostosis

The Eye: Congenital cataracts, strabismus microphthalmia

The Mouth: Cleft lip and cleft palate, microganthia (congenital smallness of the lower jaw)

Alimentary Tract: Pyloric stenosis, oesophageal atresia, trachea oesophageal fistula, hiatus hernia, Hirschsprung's diseases, ano-rectal anomalies.

Bones: DDH, Cleft foot, shortness of bone

Thorax: Diaphragmatic hernia, congenital heart disease

Abdomen: Umbilical hernia

Genito Urinary Tract: Hypospadias, epispadias, rectovaginal fistula, hydrocele.

Central Nervous System: Spina bifida, anenecephaly, microcephaly, hydrocephaly.

Extremities: Developmental displasia of the hip, cleft foot.

HEAD

Microcephaly

Microcephaly is a relatively uncommon congenital anomaly. Microcephaly is defined as an occipito frontal circumference (OFC) greater than 3 standard deviations below the mean (Vanucci, 1997).

Causes

- Autosomal—recessive disorder, a chromosome abnormality, or application of a toxic stimulus during the period of induction and major cell migration in prenatal development.
- Maternal infection (notably toxoplasmosis, rubella, or cytomegalovirus), or chemical agents.
- Secondary microcephaly can result from a variety of insults that occur during the third trimester of pregnancy, the perinatal period, or early infancy. Infection, trauma, metabolic disorders, and anoxia are all capable of causing decreased brain growth and early closure of cranial sutures.

Clinical Features

- Small skull
- Head circumference less than normal
- Severe mental retardation
- In both types the neurologic manifestations range from decerebration, complete unresponsiveness, and/or autistic behaviour to mild motor impairments, impairment, educable mental retardation, and/or mild hyperkinesis.

Treatment

No treatment.

Nursing Considerations

Nursing care is supportive and may be directed toward helping parents to adjust for rearing a child with cognitive impairment.

Hydrocephaly

Definition

Hydrocephaly is a condition characterized by an excess of cerebrospinal fluid within the ventricular and subarachnoid spaces of the cranial cavity.

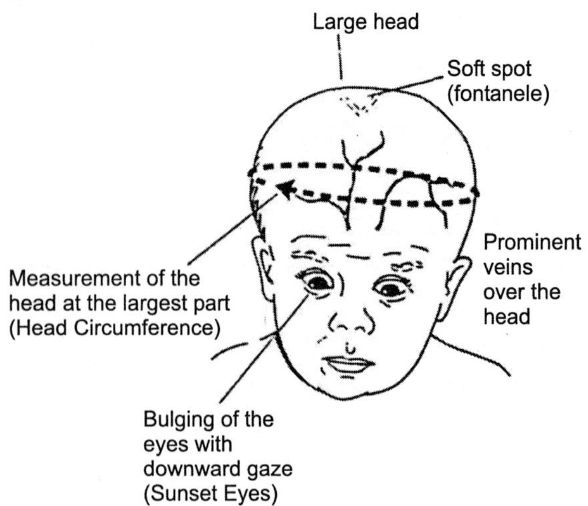

Fig. 4.1: Hydrocephaly (See Pl. 21)

Causes

1. **Non-communicating hydrocephaly** (due to developmental malformation), or **obstructive hydrocephaly**, is caused by a CSF-flow obstruction ultimately preventing CSF from flowing into the subarachnoid space (either due to external compression or intraventricular mass lesions).

- **Foramen of monro** obstruction may lead to dilation of one or, if large enough (*e.g.*, in colloid cyst), both lateral ventricles.
- **The aqueduct of sylvius**, normally narrow to begin with, may be obstructed by a number of genetically or acquired lesions (*e.g.*, atresia, ependymitis, haemorrhage, and tumour) and lead to dilation of both lateral ventricles as well as the third ventricle.
- **Fourth ventricle** obstruction will lead to dilatation of the aqueduct as well as the lateral and third ventricles.
- **The foramina of luschka and foramen of magendie** may be obstructed due to congenital failure of opening (*e.g.*, Dandy-Walker malformation).

2. **Communicating hydrocephaly**, also known as **non-obstructive hydrocephaly**

- It is caused by impaired cerebrospinal fluid resorption in the absence of any CSF-flow obstruction between the ventricles and subarachnoid space. It has been theorized that this is due to functional impairment of the arachnoid granulations, which are located along the **superior sagittal sinus** and is the site of cerebrospinal fluid resorption back into the venous system. Various neurologic conditions may result in communicating hydrocephalus, including subarachnoid/intraventricular haemorrhage, **meningitis, Chiari malformation,** and congenital absence of arachnoidal granulations (**Pacchioni's granulations**). Scarring and fibrosis of the **subarachnoid** space following infectious, inflammatory, or haemorrhagic events can also prevent resorption of CSF, causing diffuse ventricular dilatation.
- Surgery to repair a myelomeningocele.
- Adhesions between meninges at the base of the brain of meningeal haemorrhage.
- Rarely, a tumour in the choroids plexus that causes an overproduction of CSF.

Pathophysiology

CSF is formed by the choroid plexus mainly in the lateral ventricles. It is absorbed into the venous system through the arachnoid villi, CSF circulates within the ventricles and the subarachnoid space. (It is a colorless fluid, consisting of water with traces of protein, glucose and lymphocytes.) Any defect in this causes the problem.

Clinical Feature

Infancy—Head enlarges, suture line separate

- AF becomes tense and bulging.
- Setting sun eyes.
- Macewen sign (cracked pot sound).
- Fontal enlargement or bossing with depressed eyes.
- Infant reflexes persist.
- Failure in the development.
- Convulsion, nystagmus.
- Increased Cranial Pressure.
- Child has difficulty to turn the head or raising.
- Irritability to support the head when upright or lethargy.
- Vomiting not related to food intake.
- Distended scalp vein, thin, shiny and fragile looking scalp skin and weak muscles.
- High–pitched cry.

Investigation

- Physical examination and assessment findings of clinical features.
- Head circumference.
- Computerized axial tomography.
- Angiography.

- MRI.
- Light reflexion—Light reflects off the opposite side of the skull with skull transillumination.

Complications

- Physical injury
- Delayed growth and development
- Decreased intracranial adaptive capacity

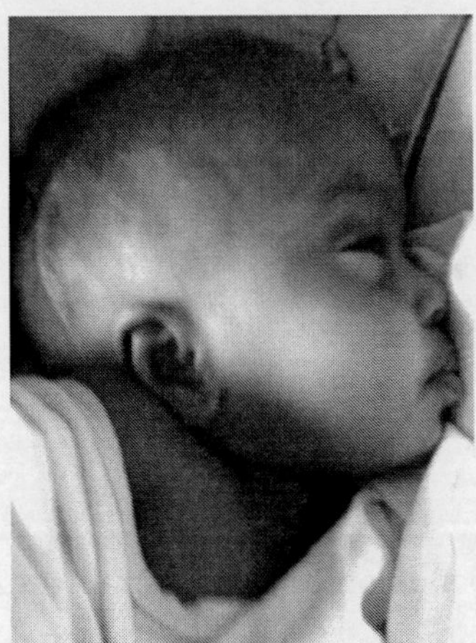

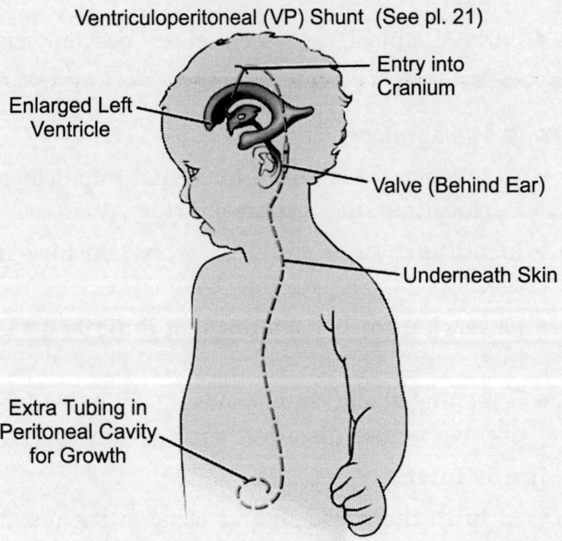

Fig. 4.2: Child with ventricular peritoneal shunt

Treatment

Medical therapy—towards reduction of production of CSF.

Surgical therapy

1. Remove the obstruction.
2. Ventricular bypass into a normal intracranial channel.
3. Drainage of fluid from a lateral ventricle into an extra cranial compartment (Right atrium or peritoneum) by the way of artificial passage or shunt.
   - Ventriculoatrial shunt
   - Ventriculo peritoneal shunt.

Mechanical Complication of Shunting

- Shunt malfunction, shunt failure
- Kinking of the tube
- Shunt infection
- Shunt block (clogged)
- Plugging or separation of the tubing and
- Bacterial infection
- Recurrent hydrocephaly due to failure of shunt
- Increased intracranial pressure.

Nursing Care

Preoperative Care

Preoperatively the infant should be observed carefully for the signs of increased intracranial pressure.

- Daily head circumference to be measured
- Fontanels and suture lines are gently palpated for size, signs of bulging, tenseness and separation
- Psychological aspect of care
- Adequate nutrition—small and frequent feeding
- Prevent pressure sores.

Postoperative Care

- Routine post operative care and observation.
- Assess the shunt function, if not functioning the cerebrospinal fluid will begin to accumulate again and a number of physical symptoms will develop (headaches, nausea, vomiting, photophobia/light sensitivity), some extremely serious, like seizures.
- Position the baby on unoperated side to prevent pressure on the shunt value.
- Observe the sign of increased intracranial pressure.
- Prevent infection—observe the sign of elevated vital signs, poor feeding, and vomiting, decreased response and seizure activity.
- Administration of antibiotics.
- Emotional support to the parents.
- Prevent post operative complications.
- Administer comfort measures.

Craniosynostosis

Premature closure of single or multiple sutures of cranial vault, face, and base of skull during the first 18 months of life. This condition occurs in upto 2000 births.

Causes

Unknown 15% have autosomal dominant inherited syndromes such as Crouzon syndrome.

Diagnosis

- Clinical appearance
- Palpitation of the skull reveals a bony ridge along a suture
- Skull X-ray
- CT scan
- MRI

Treatment

- Reconstructive surgery is performed to protect mental development and vision.

Nursing Care

Observe the child for symptoms of increased intracranial pressure like early signs and report immediately.

- Headache
- Visual disturbances, diplopia
- Nausea and vomiting
- Dizziness
- Slight change in vital signs
- Seizures
- Infant has the signs of bulging fontanels
- Wide sutures, increased HC
- Dilated scalp veins
- High piched, catlike cry.

THE EYE

Congenital Cataracts

Definition: Opacity of crystalline lens

Pathophysiology

Prevents light rays from entering eye and refracting them on retina.

Clinical Feature

- Gradually less able to see objects clearly
- May lose peripheral vision
- Gray opacities of lens
- Strabismus
- Absence of red reflex

Treatment

- Surgical treatment to remove cloudy lens and replace lens.
- Must be treated early to prevent blindness from amblyopia.

Strabismus

"Squint" or cross eye—malalignment of eyes.

Estropia—inward deviation of eye.

Exotropia—outward deviation of eye.

Pathophysiology

Strabismus results from muscle imbalance or paralysis, poor vision or congenital defect.

Treatment

Treatment depends on causes of strabismus

- May involve occlusion therapy (Patching stronger eye) or surgery to increase visual stimulation to weaker eye.
- Early diagnosis is essential to prevent vision loss.

Nursing Management

- Assessment of children for visual impairment is a critical nursing responsibility.
- Identifying those children whose history is at risk.
- Observing for behaviours that indicate a vision loss.
- Screening all children for visual acuity and signs of other ocular disorders such as strabismus.

If it is Infant

- At birth the nurse should observe the neonates response to visual stimuli like following a light or object and cessation of body movement.
- Lack of eye contact from the infant.
- Infancy of the child should be tested for strabismus.
- Lack of binocularity after 4 months of age is considered abnormal and must be treated to prevent amblyopia.

Note: Suspect blindness if the infant does not react to light and in any-age child if parents express concern.

MOUTH

Cleft Lip and Cleft Palate

Cleft lip with or without cleft palate is the most common craniofacial malformation. It occurs in 1 in 800 live births. Cleft palate occurs 1 in 2000 live births. Cleft lip results from failure of the bone and tissue of the upper jaw and palate to fuse completely at the midline.

Causes

- Congenital defects; in some cases inheritance plays a role.
- Part of another chromosomal abnormality.
- Prenatal exposure to teratogens or environmental factors.
- Maternal smoking.

Pathophysiology

- Development of the primary and secondary palates takes place at different times and involves different developmental processes.
- Primary palate of the maxillary process to fuse with the nasal elevation on the frontal prominence, which occurs normally during the sixth week of gestation.
- Merging of the upper lip at the midline is completed between the seventh and eighth weeks of gestations.
- Fusion of the secondary palate (hard and soft) takes place later in development, between the seventh and twelfth weeks of gestation.
- At the time the primary palate is completed, the two lateral palatine processes are situated in a vertical position at the side of the tongue.
- In the process of migrating to a horizontal position, they are, for a short time, separated by the tongue movement downwards, allowing the palatine process to fuse with each other and with the primary palate to form the roof of the mouth.
- If there is delay in this movement, or if the tongue fails to descent soon enough, the remainder of development proceeds but the palate never fuses.

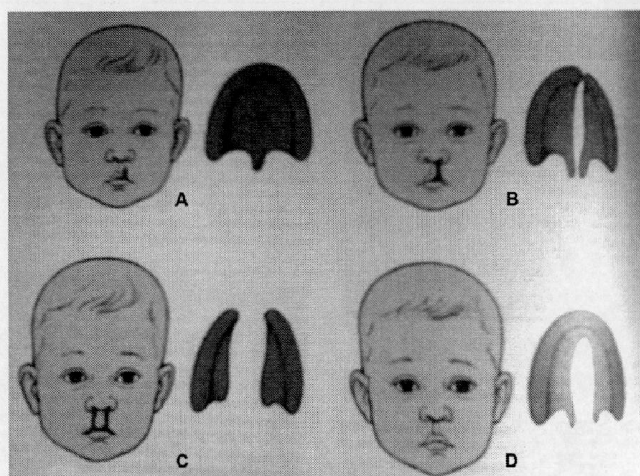

Fig. 4.3: Types of cleft lip and cleft palate

The above illustration shows the four variations of cleft lip and cleft palate.

A. Notch with vermilion border
B. Unilateral cleft lip and cleft palate
C. Bilateral cleft lip and palate
D. Cleft palate

Assessment Findings

- Abdominal distention from swallowed air
- Difficulty in swallowing
- If infant has cleft lip
  - Simple notch on the upper lip
  - Complete cleft from the lip edge to the floor of the nostril
  - On either side of the midline but rarely along the midline itself.
- If infant has cleft palate
  - Opening in the palate.
  - May be partial or complete.

Complications

- Speech defects.
- Dental and orthodontic problems.
- Nasal defects.
- Alterations in hearing.
- Shock, guilt and grief for the parents that may interfere with parent child bonding.
- Increased risk of aspiration, upper respiratory infection, and otitis media.

Management

Management of both defects is directed towards surgical closure of the cleft, prevention of complication and facilitation of normal growth and development of the child.

- Cheiloplasty (cleft lip repair surgery):
  - Performed between birth and age 3 years.
  - Unites the lip and gum edges:
    - Provides a route for adequate nutrition and sucking.
    - Performed in anticipation of tooth eruption.
- Staphylorrhaphy (cleft palate repair surgery):
  - Scheduled at about age 18 months:
    - Allow for palate growth.
    - Allow for surgery to be done before the infant develops speech patterns.
  - Infant must be free from ear and respiratory infection.
- Long-term, team-oriented care to address speech defects, dental and orthodontic problems, nasal defects, and possible alterations in hearing.
- If cleft lip is detected on sonogram while the infant is in utero, foetal repair may be possible.

Nursing Management

- Maintain the nutritional status of the infant:
  - To help determine an effective feeding method.
  - Assess the quality of the child's sucking by determining if the infant can form an airtight seal around a finger or nipple that's placed in his mouth.
  - Nurses should feed the infant with a specialized nipple used for cleft lip or palate infant.
  - Assess the infant's ability to swallow.
  - Secure the intravenous line, administer intravenous fluid to maintain the nutritional status.
- Assess infant for the complication:
  - Assess for abdominal distension from swallowed air.
  - Assess respiratory status to detect signs of aspiration (choking, respiratory distress, cyanosis, cough).
- Monitor vital signs (temperature, heart rate, respiration, BP).
- Maintain intake and output chart to determine fluid volume status.

Preoperative Nursing Care for Cheiloplasty

- Administer diet appropriate for age, provide adequate nutrition.
- Assist mother with breastfeeding if this is mother's preference, since the newborn with either defect can breast–feed.
- Position and stabilize nipple well back in oral cavity so that tongue action facilitates milk expression.
- Feed the infant slowly and in an upright position to decrease the risk of aspiration.
- Feed the infant using a commercially available cleft lip and cleft palate nipple.
- Position nipple between infant's tongue and existing palate to facilitate compression of the nipple.
- When using the device without nipple (*e.g.*, Breck feeder-syringe with rubber tube, Asepto syringe), deposit the formula on back of tongue to facilitate swallowing and adjust flow according to infant's swallowing to prevent aspiration.
- Burp often during feeding to eliminate swallowing air and decrease the risk of emesis.
- Use gavage feeding if oral feedings are unsuccessful.
- Administer a small amount of water after feeding to rinse the mouth to prevent accumulating the milk to form bacterial growth.
- Give small and frequent feeding to promote adequate nutrition and prevent tiring of the infant.
- Encourage the parents to begin feeding as soon as possible so that they become adopt in feeding technique before discharge.

Postoperative Nursing Care for Cheiloplasty

- Maintain a patent airway; edema or narrowing of a previously large airway may make the infant appear to be in distress.
- Observe for cyanosis as the infant begins to breathe through his nose to detect signs of respiratory compromise.
- Maintain an intact suture line; keep the infant's hands away from his mouth by using restraints or pinning his sleeves to his shirt.
- Anticipate the infant's needs to prevent crying; don't place him in the prone position.
- Give extra care and support because the infant's emotional needs can't be met by sucking.

- When feeding resumes, use a syringe with tubing to administer foods at the side of the mouth to prevent trauma to the suture line.
- Place the infant on his right side after feedings to prevent aspiration.
- Monitor for pain and administer pain medication as prescribed.

Preoperative Interventions for Staphylorrhaphy

- Position the child on his abdomen or side to maintain a patent airway.
- Assess for signs of altered oxygenation to promote good respiration.
- Keep hard or pointed objects (utensils, straws, frozen dessert sticks) away from the child's mouth to prevent trauma to the suture line.
- Use a cup to feed; do not use a nipple or pacifier, to prevent injury to the suture line.
- Use elbow restraints to keep the child's hands out of his mouth.
- Provide soft toys to prevent injury.
- Start the child on clear liquids and progress to a soft diet.
- Rinse the suture line by giving the child a sip of water after each feeding to prevent infection.
- Distract or hold the child to try to deep his tongue away from the roof of his mouth.

ESOPHAGEAL ATRESIA WITH TRACHEOESOPHAGEAL FISTULA

Congenital atresia of the oesophagus and tracheoesophageal fistula are rare malformations that represent a failure of the oesophagus to develop as a continuous passage.

Etiology

TA and TEF are not known

Incidence: 1 in 800 to 5000 live births

Predisposing facts—maternal polyhydramnios

Pathophysiology

During normal embryologic development, the gut and respiratory tract originate as a single tube. During 4 and 5 weeks of gestation, this tube lengthens and separates longitudinally. Two parallel tubes are formed both of which are joined at the pharynx. Atresia occurs because of the defective growth of ectodermal cells. When there is incomplete fusion of the lateral walls of the foregut, there is incomplete closure of the laryngotracheal tube and fistula is formed, generally it occurs at the level of tracheal bifurcation. If atresia there is a thin, non-canalized cord with an upper blind pouch connected to the pharynx and a lower pouch leading to the stomach.

- In fistulas commonly the cover pouch is connected through a fistulous tract with the trachea or a main stem bronchus.
- Less frequently a fistulous tract is present between the blind upper oesophageal pouch and the respiratory tree.

Types

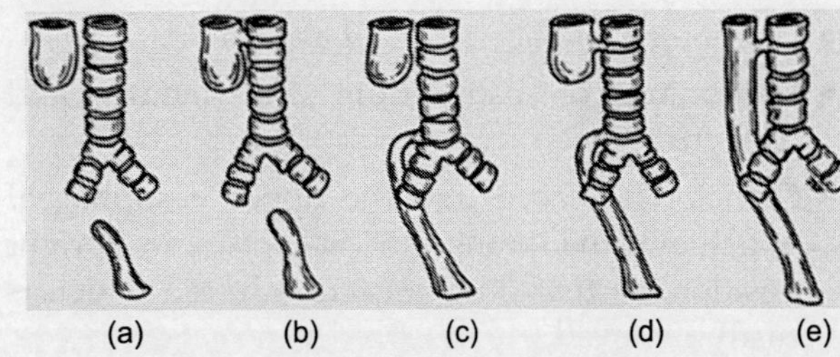

Fig. 4.4: Types of tracheoesophageal atresia and fistula

(*a*) Consists of a blind pouch at each end, widely separated and with no communication to the trachea.

(*b*) Involves a fistula from the trachea to the upper oesophageal segment.

(*c*) One in which the proximal oesophageal segment terminates in a blind pouch and the distal segment is connected to trachea or primary bronchus by a short fistula at or near.

(*d*) Extremely rare anomalies involve a fistula from the trachea to the upper oesophageal segment or to both the upper and lower segments.

(*e*) Less frequently normal trachea and oesophagus are connected by a common fistula.

Clinical Manifestations

Oesophageal atresia—Infant with excessive salivation and drooling accompanied by 3 Cs

- Choking, coughing, and cyanosis.
- Cyanotic, sneezing and may stop breathing in aspirated into the trachea or bronchus.
- Cyanosis—due to laryngospasm.
- Acute gastric distention.

Investigation

- To rule out oesophageal atresia a catheter is generally passed into the oesophagus and gets resistance if the lumen is blocked.

- Aspiration of stomach content or introduce the air to see patent oesophagus.
- Radio opaque fluid is carefully instilled in the oesophagus under fluoroscopy.
- Fistulas are not patent.

Treatment

- If oesophageal atresia and fistula need surgical repair of the anomaly.
- If fistula is suspected—the infant should be stopped oral intake, start only intravenous fluids.
- Positioning of baby to avoid aspiration.
- Suctioning of baby from the mouth and pharynx.
- Catheter is placed into the upper oesophageal pouch and the infant head is kept in an upright position, so that fluid collection in the pouch is easily removed.
- Gastrostomy is performed to decompress the stomach and prevent future aspiration of gastric contents by way of the fistula.
- Antibiotics therapy is administered.
- Surgical correction consists of a thoracotomy with division and ligation of the tracheophageal fistula and end to end anastomosis.
- For preterm babies with multiple anomalies and if condition is poor then it is preferred to involve palliative surgery like gastrostomy ligation of the oesophageal pouch.
- Oesophageal replacement is usually done when child is closed and the child is fed directly by gastrostomy, whereas the upper oesophageal segment is drained by means of a cervical esophageostomy.

Nursing Management

- Detection of malformation immediately after birth.
- Suction to be done to prevent aspiration.
- If there is cyanosis and excessive mucus secretion immediately inform the physician.
- Place the infant under a radiant warmer.
- O_2 is administered to help relieve respiratory distress.
- Observe the cyanosis—due to laryngospasm caused by overflow of saliva into the larynx.
- Positive pressure is contraindicated.

Preoperative Nursing Care

1. Maintain patent airway and lung expansion
   - Remove accumulated secretion from oropharynx.
   - Position for patent airway and prevent aspiration.
   - Observe for signs of respiratory distress.
2. Recognize the defect early
   - Be alert to danger signs.
   - Excess salivation.
   - Three Cs—coughing, choking and cyanosis.
   - Acute gastric distension.
3. Prevent aspiration pneumonia
   - Nothing Per Oral (NPO).
   - Positioning the infant in upright position.
   - Aspirate secretion through NG tube.

Postoperative Nursing Care

1. Maintain vital signs
   - Pulse rate and respiratory rate to be checked every 15 minutes.
   - Any alteration in vital signs, inform to physician.
2. Prevent infection at operative sites
   - Observe the signs of inflammation, bleeding and other drainage.
   - Clean dressing to be done.
3. Maintain fluid and electrolyte balance
   - Record intake output chart.
   - Maintain the IV fluid carefully.
   - Measure and record gastrostomy drainage.
   - Record weight daily.
4. Facilitate ventilation
   - Maintain patent airway.
   - Suction the secretions as needed.
   - Maintain care of chest tubes and drainage apparatus.
   - Position for optimum ventilation.
   - Administer O_2 as needed.
   - Prevent aspiration of feedings.
5. Control pneumonia
   - Administer antibiotics.
   - Administer O_2.
   - Suction out the secretion.
   - Position for optimum ventilation.

6. Administer comfort measures
   - Provide tactile stimulation.
   - Position comfortably.
   - Avoid restraints.
   - Administer mouth care.
   - Offer pacifier frequently.
7. Support parents (Psychological)
   - Encourage frequent visiting to ICU.
   - Encourage participation in infant's care.
   - Encourage expression of feelings.
8. Educate parents in home care
   - Teach parents about positioning.
   - Signs of respiratory distress.
   - Care of gastrostomy and esophagostomy.
   - Care of operative site anatomies, dressing change etc.
9. Administer oral feedings
   - Introduce foods at a time.
   - Begin with slightly liquid feedings and progress to more solid food.

HYPERTROPIC PYLORIC STENOSIS

Pyloric stenosis is the narrowing of part of the stomach (the pylorus) that leads into the small intestine. This narrowing occurs because the muscle around the pylorus has grown too large. Most babies with pyloric stenosis begin to vomit during the second to third week of life. Babies begin with "spitting up" that turns into forceful projectile vomiting.

Incidence: It is common in males than females

- Incidence: 5 in every 1000 males and 1 in every 1000 females.

Etiology

- Unknown
- Predisposing factor—Hereditary
- Monozygotic to dizygotic twins.

Pathophysiology

The circular muscle of the pylorus is grossly enlarged as a result of both hypertrophy and hyperplasia. These produces severe narrowing of the pyloric canal between the stomach and duodenum consequently the lumen at this point is partially obstructed, over a period of time inflammation and edema further reduce the size of the opening until the partial obstruction may progress to complete obstruction. The distal portions end abruptly and are externally distinct and easily palpated. The stomach is usually dilated.

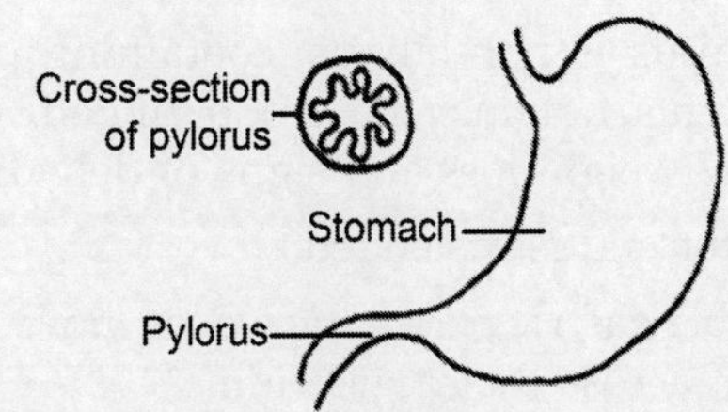

(a) Diagram of normal stomach and pylorus. Note the cross-section showing normal pyloric opening

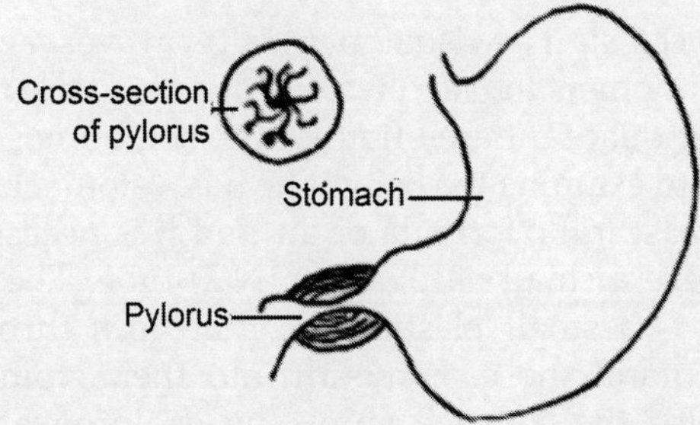

(b) Diagram of stomach with pyloric stenosis. Note the cross-section showing how the pyloric opening is narrowed

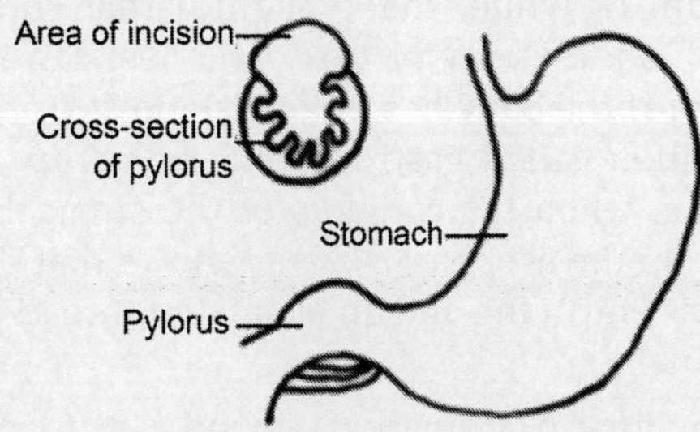

(c) Diagram of stomach after repair of pyloric stenosis. Note (in the cross-section) how an incision has been made in the muscle, enlarging the pylorus and relieving the obstruction

Fig. 4.5: Pyloric stenosis

Clinical Manifestations

Infants—1st week of life

- Initially there is only regurgitation or occasional non-projectile vomiting.
- 4 weeks after birth—Vomiting becomes projectile in nature then it may lead to complete obstruction by 4 to 6 weeks.
- Infant vomits may be ejected 3 to 4 feet from the child in a side lying position.
- Infant vomits 1 foot or more when the infant is lying on the back.
- Vomiting occurs most often shortly after a feed or several hours later.

- Vomitus is non-bilious, containing only gastric contents but may be blood tinged, infant may show weight loss and signs of dehydration.
- Upper end is distended.
- Visible gastric peristaltic waves move from left to right across the epigastrium.

Investigation

- History
- Physical signs—visual peristaltic waves across the abdomen and an olive-sized mass in the right upper quadrant are often found, sometimes it is hard to examine the baby if he has a stomach full of breast milk/formula or air and it is necessary to place a small nasogastric (NG) tube. The NG tube is a small plastic tube that goes through the infant's nose or mouth into their stomach. It helps the stomach empty by draining air or anything else that may be in it.
- One test is a barium study of upper GI. This test involves the baby drinking a small amount of barium (a white, chalky liquid) that shows up easily on an X-ray picture. This test can tell the doctor if the baby has pyloric stenosis or another condition called gastroesophageal reflux (GER). GER is when the contents of the stomach come back up the esophagus. X-ray shows that delayed gastric emptying and an elongated thread pyloric channel.
- Laboratory examination—blood serum electrolytes, sodium and potassium will be decreased.
- Haemoglobin level decreased or normal.
- Another test that may be done is an abdominal ultrasound. This test involves a metal wand that is moved over the baby's stomach. The metal wand is able to take pictures using sound waves. It is a common test used in pregnancy to look at the baby and does not harm the baby.

Treatment

Surgical Treatment

- Pyloromyotomy (Fredet—Ramstedt operation)

Nursing Management

Nursing assessment and intervention

- Observe the infant's abdomen for the presence of peristaltic waves
- Check for the bowel sound by auscultation
- Assess skin turgor, fontanels, mucus membranes and urine output for adequate hydration
- Check the serum electrolytes
- Observe the child for type of vomiting (nature), colour, content of vomitus
- Assess vital signs
- Assess for feeding disorder.

Intervention

- Maintain adequate hydration by meeting the fluid and electrolyte needs.
  - Oral feedings are withheld and administer intravenous fluids to correct fluid and electrolyte imbalance.
  - Monitor intake and output (including vomitus), diaper should be weighed to measure the output.
  - Check the urine specific gravity.
- Minimize weight loss
  - Monitor the weight daily, both preoperative and post operatively.
  - Small and frequent feedings consisting of clear liquids, are begun within 4 to 6 hours post operatively, if the child tolerates clear fluid, start with breast milk or formula feedings.
- Promote rest and comfort
  - Maintain warmth and provide comfort to the baby.
  - Encourage the parents to hold the baby.
  - Provide a pacifier to meet the infant's need to suck.
  - Post operation—instruct the parents to avoid pressure on the incision.
  - Change the diapers carefully and gently to avoid pain.
  - Use pacifier to relax the infant.
  - Acetaminophen or analgesics can be administered to relieve pain or discomfort.
- Prevent infection
  - Post operation the wound should be cleaned and dried, dressing to be done according to the instruction given.
  - Check the incision site for redness, swelling or discharge.
  - Monitor the infant's temperature every 4 hour.
  - Auscultate the lungs to listen for clear respiratory sounds.
- Provide supportive care

- Psychological support is imparted to the parents regarding preoperative and surgery, post operative care to relieve the anxiety.
- Encourage the parents to participate in the infant's care.
- Provide simple and clear explanation about the infant's condition and care.
- Advice the parents that occasional vomiting after surgery may occur.

- Educate the parents before discharge about regular medication, care of infants. Instruct the parents to observe the incision for redness, swelling if discharge and notify the physician immediately if temperature is above 38.5°C.
- Educate the parents to reduce the possibility of infection by proper hygienic conditions.

OBSTRUCTIVE DISORDERS

Obstruction in the GI tract occurs when the passage of nutrients and secretions is impeded by a constricted or occluded lumen, or when there is impaired motility (Paralyticileus). Obstructions may be congenital or acquired. Congenital obstructions, such as oesophageal or intestinal atresias and malrotation, usually appear in the neonatal period. Obstruction in the GI tract from many causes is characterized by similar signs and symptoms, although the progression may vary greatly.

Usually, acute intestinal obstruction is characterized by abdominal pain, nausea, vomiting, abdominal distension, and a change in stooling patterns.

Intestinal Obstruction

Causes

- Congenital
  - Atresia
  - Hernias
  - Intussusception
  - Imperforate anus
  - Meckel diverticulum
  - Hirschsprung
  - Stricture
  - Malrotation
  - Volvulus
  - Meconium plug
  - Meconium ileus

Diagnosis and Preoperative Management

Intestinal obstruction should be suspected with maternal history of polyhydramnios, large amount (> 20 ml) of gastric fluid at birth, bilious or non-bilious emesis, or progressive abdominal distention.

- Common causes include duodenal, jejunal, ileal, or colonic atresia, malrotation with mid gut volvulus, meconium ileus with associated cystic fibrosis, meconium plug, hirschsprung's disease, imperforate anus, and hypoplastic left colon.
- Infants with bowel atresia may pass meconium.
- The higher the obstruction, the more prominent is the vomiting. The lower the obstruction, the more prominent is the distention.
- Make infant NPO, start IV, and monitor electrolytes, urine output and hypoplastic left colon.
- Place nasogastric tube to continuous suction and measure output.
- Obtain X-ray of abdomen looking for:
  - "Double bubble" sign of duodenal atresia. If present, no further GI workup is needed and patient should go to surgery when stable.
  - Multiple dilated loops of bowel indicating a more distal obstruction.
  - Intraperitoneal calcifications suggestive of perforation with meconium ileus.
  - Air throughout bowel to the rectum gives suspicion for Hirschsprung's disease.

    Bubbly-appearing stool filling the bowel is suggestive of meconium ileus and cystic fibrosis.
- Upper GI contrast study may be required to assess for malrotation and possible volvulus.
- Contrast enema using GastrograffinTM or dilute hypaque TM may be done to identify an area of obstruction or to relieve meconium plug or meconium ileus.
- Suspect acute volvulus secondary to malrotation if the baby has signs of shock, metabolic acidosis or peritonitis. If there are signs suggesting volvulus, emergency operation is indicated since gut viability may be threatened.
- Suspect Hirschsprung's disease with repeated episodes of abdominal distension or much delayed passage of meconium. Diagnosis can be

made with suction rectal biopsy. If no ganglion cells are seen, a surgical biopsy will confirm the diagnosis.

- Infants with Hirschsprung's disease are at risk for development of fatal toxic megacolon until the bowel has been decompressed by corrective with rectal irrigation. This is different from simple enemas.
- Imperforate anus may be the sole abnormality or may be part of the urethral or perineal fistula. Ultrasound may help determine if the defect is low (and easily repaired) or high (requiring colostomy drainage). These patients will need eventual workup for tethered spinal cord and urinary tract anomalies.

HIRSCHSPRUNG'S DISEASE (CONGENITAL AGANGLIONIC MEGACOLON)

Hirschsprung's disease is a congenital absence of normal ganglionic cells in the mesenteric plexus of the bowel, resulting in abnormal peristalsis. It may cause delayed passage of meconium (after 24 hours of birth), or the infant may have enterocolitis. In older children, they may have chronic constipation. It may be mechanical obstruction caused by inadequate motility in part of the intestine. It is more common in male children than in female children.

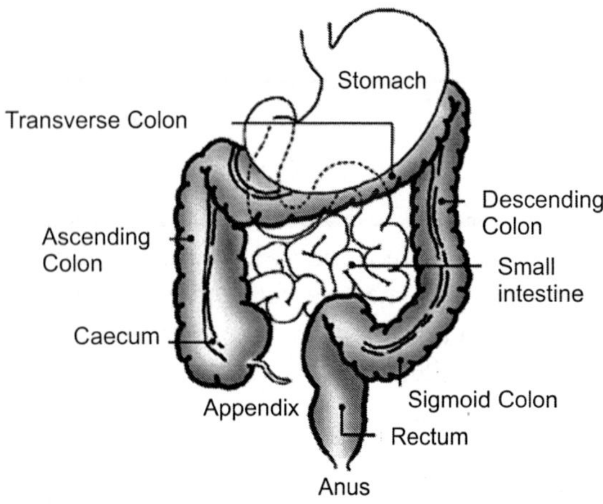

Fig. 4.6: Diagram of the colon and rectum

Causes

- Congenital
- Common in Down syndrome

Pathophysiology

The primary absence defect is para sympathetic ganglion cells in one segment of colon. The functional defect as a results of lack of innervation is absence of propulsive movement (Peristalsis) causing accumulation of intestinal contents and distention of the bowel proximal to the defect, hence the term 'mega colon' or large colon. In addition there is failure of the internal rectal sphincter to relax. This adds to the clinical manifestations because it prevents evacuation of solids, liquids and gas.

Clinical Manifestation

During Infancy

- Failure to pass meconium within 2–8 hrs after birth.
- Refuses to suck
- Reluctance to ingest fluids
- Bile–Strain vomit,
- Abdominal distension
- Child does not thrive and has constipation
- Episodes of diarrhoea and vomiting
- Watery diarrhoea, fever and severe prostration are ominous because these often signify the presence of enterocolitis, which greatly increases the risk of fatality.

During Childhood

- Choric and include constipation
- Passage ribbon like stools
- Foul smelling stools
- Abdominal distention and visible peristalsis
- Fecal masses are easily palpable,
- Child is usually poorly nourished, anaemic and has hypoproteinemia from malabsorption of nutrition.

Investigation

- Clinical sign of intestinal obstruction
- Failure to pass meconium
- Barium enema
- Anorectal manometric examination
- Rectal biopsy demonstrates absence of ganglia

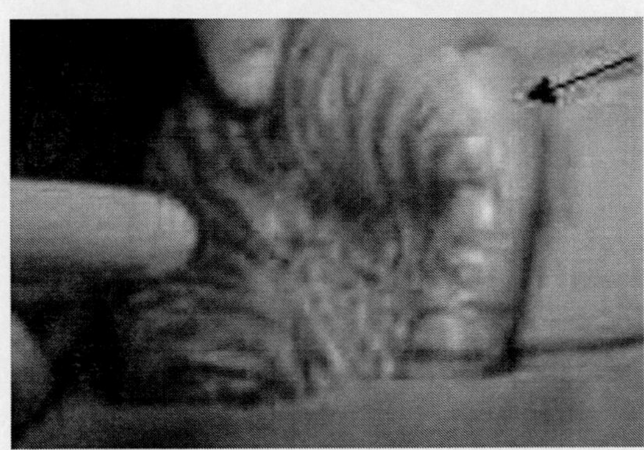

Fig. 4.7: Sigmoid colon showing a transition zone. The big, enlarged colon is normal while the smaller colon has the Hirschsprung's disease. The arrow points to the transition zone

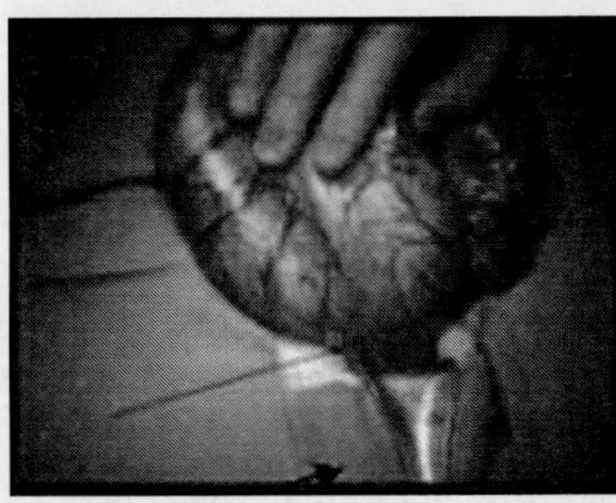

Fig. 4.8: A huge "megacolon" consisting of sigmoid colon in an older child with Hirschsprung's disease. There is a transition zone in the last part of the sigmoid colon (arrow) which has a "funnel". A colostomy was formed to allow the colon to get smaller before a pullthrough was performed

Treatment

Symptomatic Treatment

- Saline enemas
- Stool softeners
- Low residue diet (bread, grains, dairy products, meat, vegetable, fruits) not to be given.

Corrective Therapy (surgical treatment)

The removal of the aganglionic bowel and improve functioning of the internal sphincter. In severe cases or in ill infants, a temporary colostomy is created. Closure of the colostomy and reanastomosis are performed at a later point.

Nursing Management

- Nursing assessment at birth, when child has not passed stool within 24 hours
- Preoperative nursing care
  - Routine preoperative care.
  - Maintain temperature of infant by keeping the baby in warmer atmosphere.
  - Monitor the vital signs and record to prevent sepsis and enterocolitis.
  - Carefully maintain the fluid and electrolyte balance and nutrition to prevent dehydration and shock.
  - Rectal washout using 10 ml/kg of 0.9% normal saline solution is necessary to promote adequate elimination and prevent obstruction.
  - Teach the parents to give the rectal irrigation and teach them how to prevent skin breakdown in the rectal area by cleaning the area and applying protective ointment. Change the diaper frequently.
- Post operative care after colostomy or ileostomy
  - Monitor the vital signs every 15 minutes.
  - Monitor fluid intake and output.
  - Keep the area around the stoma clean and dry; use the gauze pad to collect the drainage.
  - Monitor for return of bowel sounds to begin diet.
  - Meticulous skin care and stoma care after corrective surgery
  - NG Tube aspiration for abdominal decompress.
  - Keep the wound clean and dry to prevent infection.

ANORECTAL MALFORMATION

These malformations are common congenital malformations caused by abnormal development. Incidence one in 5000 live births. Anorectal malformation includes several forms of imperforate anus which are often associated with anomalies of the genitourinary and pelvic organs.

Imperforate anus is a malformation without an obvious anal opening.

Fistula is abnormal connection from the distal rectum to the perineum or genitourinary system.

Anorectal malformation may occur as a part of the **VACTERL** or **VATER** syndrome.

Cloaca is a complex anorectal malformation in which the rectum, vagina and urethra drain into a common channel that opens onto the perineum via the visual urethral site.

Cloacal exstrophy is a rare condition, it is a severe defect in which there is externalization of the bladder and bowel through the abdominal wall. Anorectal anomalies are classified according to sex and abnormal anatomic features including genitourinary and associated pelvic anomalies.

TABLE 4.1: Classification of Anorectal Malformation

Level	Male	Female
High	Anorectal agenesis With rectoprostate-urethral fistula Without fistula Rectal atresia	Anorectal agenesis With rectovaginal fistula Without fistula Rectal atresia
Intermediate	Recto-bulbar Urethral fistula Agenesis without fistula	Rectovestibular fistula Rectovaginal fistula Agenesis without fistula
Low	Anocutaneous fistula Anal stenosis Imperforate anus	Anovestibular fistula Anocutaneous fistula Anal stenosis Cloaca Imperforate anus

Investigation

- Check for patency of the anus and rectum is a routine part of the newborn assessment.
- Observe the passage of meconium.
- Inspection of the perineal area for normal or absence of anal opening.
- Check for fistulas may not be apparent at birth but may become obvious as peristalsis gradually forces the meconium through the fistula.
- Rectourinary fistulas should be suspected if there is meconium in the urine.
- Anal stenosis may not be identified until the child is older and parents observe a history of difficulty in defecation, abdominal distention and passing a ribbon like stool.
- Abdominal ultrasound is performed for further evaluation of anatomic malformation.
- Intravenous pyelogram (IVP).
- Cystourethrogram is used for a high malformation to identify associated anomalies of the urinary tract.
- Further examination is done if a syndrome is suspected.

Treatment

- Malformation of the lower rectum often can be corrected in the neonatal period by simple dilation or minor perineal procedure.
- *For Anal stenosis*: Manual dilations of anus.
- *Imperforate Anus*: Anal membrane is excised and followed by daily anal dilations.
- Infant with high anomalies requires a temporary colostomy in the newborn period.
- Final correction of higher defects is usually for a year, when a pull-through procedure with anorectoplasty is performed.

Nursing Management

- It is nurse's responsibility to identify the anorectal malformation after birth by neonatal assessment.
- Observe the newborn for poorly developed anal dimple, a genitourinary fistula or vertebral abnormalities.
- Monitor the newborn when it passes stool within 24 hours of birth, if not passed, infant requires further assessment.
- Observe the meconium, if it is not passed in appropriate orifice, it is reported immediately.
- Maintain the temperature of the infant.

Preoperative Care

- NG tube insertion and decompression of the stomach content.
- Secure the IV and administer the intravenous fluids.
- Take preoperative consent from the parents.
- Explain about the child's condition and about the surgery or any minor procedure.

Postoperative Care (Anorectoplasty)

- Routine postoperative care.
- Prevention of infection.
- Care for the operative site, sterile dressing, or stoma care is important to prevent infection.
- Prevent complication.

- Meticulous skin care or stoma care.
- Prevent skin irritation, protective ointment such as zinc oxide to be applied in anal area.
- Keep the anal area as clean as possible with scrupulous perineal care because a temporary dressing and drain may be placed initially to manage the continuous passage of stool.
- Preferred position is a side lying prone position with the hips elevated or a supine position with the legs suspected at a 90 degree angle to the trunk to prevent pressure on perineal sutures.
- Maintain the nutritional status of the infant slowly and frequently by feeding breast milk or formula. If peristalsis movement is noticed, in the mean time, there may be a nasogastric tube for abdominal decompression and intravenous fluids to be continued.
- Special care for infant with colostomy involves frequent dressing changes; a gauze dressing may be applied over the stoma and water to absorb stomal drainage.
- Educate the parents on discharge for home care.
- Teach the parents regarding procedure done for her child, toilet training is delayed, sphincter control takes 2 to 3 years.
- Prevention of constipation is important, breast feeding is encouraged, if a cow's milk-based formula is used, a laxative may be given.
- Bowel habits training, diet modification and administration of stool softeners are important aspects of bowel management.
- Psychological support and reassurance is important to the parents and children regarding the slow progression to normal function.
- Parents are instructed in perineal and wound care or care of the colostomy.
- Parents are advised to observe stool patterns and signs of anal stricture or complication should be notified to the physician or child must be brought to the hospital.

HERNIAS

Definition

A hernia is a protrusion of portion of an organ or organs through an abnormal opening. The herniations of concern are those that protrude through the inguinal canal.

Diaphragmatic Hernia

In diaphragmatic hernia, abdominal contents protrude into the thoracic cavity through an opening in the diaphragm. Sites of herniation include the substernal space, posterolateral region and the oesophageal hiatus. The cause is a delay or failure in closure of the pleuroperitoneal musculature. The overall incidence is 1 in 5000 live births and associated anomalies, particularly cardiac defects occur in some infants. Diaphragmatic hernia is a life–threatening condition, it needs immediate attention.

Symptoms

- Mild to severe respiratory distress within few hours after birth; tachypnea, cynosis, dyspnea, absent breath sound in affected area.
- Difficulty in respiration, nasal flaring, chest retraction.
- Pressure is more in left side organ shifted to right side, heart sound is displaced to right side.
- Difficulty in feeding.
- Bowel sound may be heard in thoracic cavity, because abdominal organs extend into the thoracic cavity.
- Barrel shape chest and sunken abdomen.
- Rapid labored respiration and cyanosis are present on 1st day.
- Breathing becomes increasingly difficult.
- Possible symptoms of shock, severe acidosis.

Investigation

- Some cases of congenital hernia are diagnosed in utero by ultrasound before birth.
- After birth chest X-rays to be done to diagnose the baby.

Treatment

- Positioning of the newborn—keep the baby's affected side to take advantage of gravity.
- Ventilation support is necessary to manage the respiratory compromise.
- Administration of O_2 to the baby.
- NG tube suctions for decompression of the stomach.
- Prevent crying—Reduce the thoracic pressure, it leads to gravity.
- Extracorporeal membrane oxygenation.
- Prophylactic antibiotic administration.

Surgical Treatment

- Abdominal viscera are replaced in the abdominal and the defect repaired.

Nursing Care

Preoperative Care

- Reduce stimulation—environmental/care activities.
- Prompt recognition; resuscitation and stabilization.
- O_2 administration.
- **NG** tube aspiration.
- Keep the baby in high semi Fowler's position.
- Turn to affected side to allow unaffected lung expansion.
- Aspirate and irrigate tube with air or sterile water.

Postoperative Care

- Routine postoperative care and observation.
- Relieve pain and provide comfort.
- Support family because this is a critical illness.

Abdominal Hernias

Omphalocele: This is rare anomaly existing at birth. Some of the abdominal contents protrude through into the root of the umbilical cord and form a sac lying on the abdomen. This sac may be large and contain much of the intestines and the liver, the sac is covered with peritoneal membrane instead of skin.

Symptoms

- Obvious on inspection
- Observe for other malformation

Treatment

Surgical repair of the defect

- Prophylactic antibiotics administration.

Nursing Care for Non-operative Omphalocoele

- Keep the baby in warmer.
- Monitor the vital signs.
- Prevent infection, aseptic procedure should follow.
- Swab the omphalocoele 4 hourly with 70% ethanol alcohol or as per the surgeon's instructions.
- Observe the scab (Eschar) formation which then peels off, leaving granulation tissue forming over the defect.
- Observe for any signs of infection.
- Administration of antibiotics as prescribed.
- Ensure that comfort of the baby is maintained, use minimal handling, carefully support omphalocoele with folded up napkins when baby is lying on other side.

Umbilical Hernia

Normally the ring that encircles the foetal end of the umbilical cord closes gradually and spontaneously after birth. When this closure is incomplete or there is weakness of the umbilical rings, portion of the intestine protrudes through the opening. It is more common in preterm and black infants. It will close spontaneously by age of 3, if not closed surgery can be performed later.

Symptoms

- Noted by inspection and palpation of abdomen, hernia appears as a soft swelling covered by skin.
- The herniated area protrudes with coughing, crying or straining during a bowel movement. It is easily reduced by pushing the bowel back through the fibrous ring.

Treatment

- No treatment is required of small defect
- Operative repair if persists to age 4–6 years or if defect is > 1.5–2.0 cm by age 2
- Strangulation requires immediate attention

Nursing Care

- Reassure the parents.
- Discourage the parents to use home remedy.

Inguinal Hernia

Inguinal hernia is common in preterm infants. When the small sac of peritoneum surrounding of the testes (vaginalis) fails to close off after the testes descend from the abdominal sac into the scrotum. This allows intestine to slip into the inguinal canal as a result infants get hernia. It is most common in males (90%) and 15% of infants will have bilateral hernia. A palpable hernia in a female could represent an ovary.

Signs and Symptoms

- Swelling
- Mass at the inguinal ring which can be reduced.
- Sac contains bowel.
- Intestine becomes trapped.
- And the circulation to the trapper intestine (Strangulated).
- Intestinal obstruction and gangrene of the bowel.

Treatment

Surgical treatment herniotomy.

Nursing Care

- Newborn assessment is important to identify earlier.
- Nurses should be trained to differentiate between hernia and a hydrocele. In a hernia bowel enters the inguinal canal. There is a mass at the inguinal ring which can be reduced. Hydrocele are collections of fluid within the processus vaginalis and scrotum. If you can palpate above them, they transiluminate, and are irreducible.
- Positioning the child with legs elevated little to reduce the hernia.
- Observe for the complication.
- Prepare the baby for surgery if the infant is planned for surgery.

Postoperative Care

- Routine postoperative care.
- Observe the wound for signs of bleeding, excess bleeding is reported to the doctor.
- Prevent from infection- minimal handling of the infant, administration of antibiotics, aseptic care.

NEURAL TUBE DEFECT

It is a congenital malformation that produces skull and spinal column defects, Neural tube defects (NTDs) result from the failure of the neural tube to close during embryonic development at approximately 28 days after conception.

Neural tube defects include:

- Spina bifida
- Encephalocele
- Ancephaly

Causes

- Exposure to a teratogen
- Isolated birth defects
- Multiple malformation—chromosomal abnormalities such as trisomy 18 or 13 syndrome
- Lack of folic acid in the maternal diet around the time of conception

Spina Bifida (SB)/Myelodysplasia

Myelodysplasia refers broadly to a malformation of the spinal canal and cord. It is a neural tube defect. Midline defects involving failure of the osseous (bony) spine to close are called spina bifida, through which the spinal meninges and spinal cord may protrude.

SB is categorized into **two types**:

1. Spina bifida occulta and
2. Spina bifida cystica.

Spina bifida occulta refers to a defect that is not visible externally. It occurs most commonly in the lumbosacral area, it occurs with a bony defect without soft tissue involvment.

Clinical Features

- In most cases it is asymptomatic and presents no problems.
- Superficial cutaneous indications include a skin depression or dimple (Which may also mark the outlet of a dermal sinus tract that extends to the subarachnoid space).
- Port wine angiomatous nevi.
- Dark tufts of hair, and soft.
- Subcutaneous lipomas. These signs may be absent, appear singly, or be present in combination.
- Occasionally foot weakness.
- Occasionally, bowel and bladder disturbances.

Investigation

- Plain radiography or X-ray is employed to disclose the precise bony defect in the symptomatic lesion and to establish the diagnosis in the suspected disorder.
- Magnetic resonance imaging (MRI) is the most sensitive tool for evaluating the defect, like no symptomatic occult variety.
- Computed tomography (CT) scan.
- Ultrasound and myelography are also used to differentiate between SB occulta and other spinal disorders.

Spina bifida cystica refers to a visible defect with an external saclike protrusion.

The two major forms of SB cystica are

- *Meningocele* which contains meninges and spinal fluid, but no neural elements.
- *Myelomeningocele or meningomyelocele* which contains meninges, and spinal fluid, and a portion of the spinal cord or nerves roots.

Myelomeningocele (Meningomyelocele)

Myelomeningocele develops during the first 28 days of pregnancy when the neural tube fails to close and fuse at some point along its length. It may be detected prenatally or at birth, accounts for 90% of spinal cord lesions, and may be located at any point along the spinal column.

Usually the sac is encased in a fine membrane that is prone to tears through which cerebrospinal fluid leaks. In other instance the sac may be covered by dura, meninges, or skin, in which instances there is rapid and spontaneous epithelialization.

The largest number of myelomeningoceles is found in the lumbar or lumbosacral area. The location and magnitude of the defect determine the nature and extent of neurologic impairment.

When the defect is located below the second lumbar vertebra, the nerves of the caudal equina are involved, giving rise to symptoms such as flaccid, are flexic partial paralysis of the lower extremities and varying degrees of sensory deficit. Unlike a spinal cord injury, the degree of deficit is not necessarily uniform on both sides.

The anomaly most frequently associated with myelomenigocele is hydrocephalus; 90% to 95% of children with SB have hydrocephalus.

Pathophysiology

The pathophysiology of SB is best understood when related to the normal formative stages of the nervous system. At approximately 20 days of gestation, a decided depression, the neural groove, appears in the dorsal ectoderm of the embryo. During the fourth week of gestation the groove deepens rapidly, and its elevated margins develop laterally and fuse dorsally to and from the neural tube.

The primary defect in neural tube malformations is believed by most authorities to be a failure of neural tube closure. However, there is evidence to indicate that the defects are a result of splitting of the already-closed neural tube as a result of an abnormal increase in cerebrospinal fluid pressure during the first trimester.

Clinical Manifestations

- Manifestation of spinabifida varies according to the degree of defect of the spinal defect.
- The degree of neurologic dysfunction is directly related to the anatomic level of the defect and thus the nerves involved.
- The infant will respond to the sensory stimulus with limb movement, arousal, and crying.
- Defective nerve supply to the bladder affects both dribbling of urine or produces overflow in continence in childhood.
- Frequently there is poor anal sphincter tone and poor anal skin reflex, which result in lack of bowel control and sometimes rectum prolapse.
- Sometimes the innervation to the muscles of the lower extremities will produce joint deformities in utero. These are primarily flexion or extension contractures, talipes valgus or varus contractures, kyphosis, lumbosacral scoliosis, and hip dislocations.

Investigation

- On the basis of clinical manifestations and examination of the meningeal sac, the diagnosis is made.
- MRI, and ultrasound.
- CT scan and, myelography is done as diagnostic measures used to evaluate the brain and spinal cord.
- Laboratory examinations like urinalysis, culture, and evaluation of blood urea nitrogen (BUN) and creatinine clearance.

Therapeutic Management

Management of the child who has a myelomeningocele requires a multidisciplinary approach involving the specialties of neurology, neurosurgery, paediatrics, urology, orthopaedics, rehabilitation, physical therapy, occupational therapy, and social service, as well as intensive nursing care in a variety of specialty areas.

The collaborative efforts of these specialists are focused on

1. The myelomeningocele and the problems associated with the defect-hydrocephalus,

paralysis, orthopaedic deformities, and genitourinary abnormalities;

2. Possible acquired problems that may or may not be associated, such as meningitis, hypoxia, and haemorrhage; and
3. Other abnormalities, such as cardiac or gastrointestinal malformations.

Surgical repair of a myelomeningocel cannot be expected to decrease the neurological disability

- To improve the future function.
- If leaking sac cells for immediate repair to prevent meningitis.
- Primary objective is to close the defect, with replacement of neural elements with the vertebral canal, whenever possible.
- Nerve roots that can be freed are replaced in the canal, the sac amputated at its base or turned inward and plastic surgery employed for covering the site of the defect.

Immediate Care of the Newborn

- Care of the newborn involves prevention of infection.
- Neurologic assessment, including observation for associated anomalies; and dealing with the impact of the anomaly on the family.
- Most authorities believe that early closure, within the first 24 to 72 hours is desired.
- Early closure, preferably in the first 12 to 18 hours, not only prevents local infection and trauma to the exposed tissues, and also avoids stretching of other nerve roots, thus preventing further motor impairment.
- A variety of neurosurgical and plastic surgical procedures are employed for skin closure without disturbing the neural elements or removing any portion of the sac.

Complication

- Meningitis
- Paralysis

Encephalocele

It is a sac like portion of the menginges and brain protrudes through a defective opening in the skull, usually in the occipital area but may occur in the parietal, nasopharyngeal or frontal area.

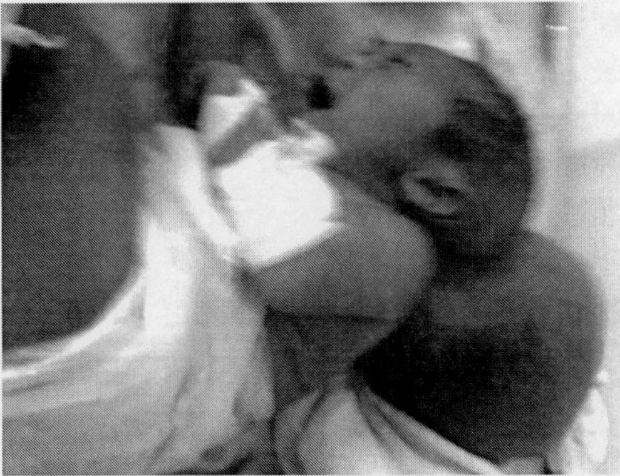

Fig. 4.9: Baby with encephalocele (See Pl. 20)

Anencephaly

It is a closure defect that occurs at the cranial end of the neuroaxis and as a result, part of or the entire top of the skull is missing, severely damaging the brain. Portion of the brain stem and spinal cord may also be missing. This defect is invariably fatal.

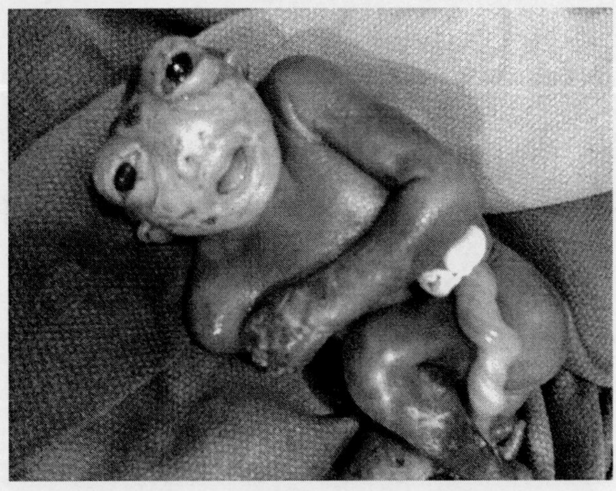

Fig. 4.10: Baby with anencephaly

Nursing Intervention

Prenatal Care

- Identify the problems from the couples, refer them to genetic counselling.
- Encourage all the pregnant mothers to take folic acid supplement to prevent the risk of neural tube defect.
- Provide psychological support to the parents to help them accept the diagnosis and preoperative and postoperative care.

Preoperative Care

- Keep the baby in the warmer to maintain the temperature.

- Sac should be covered to prevent skin irritation, sac should be clean and dry and cover it with saline-soaked sterile dressing, and pressure should be avoided.
- Child should be positioned on his abdomen or side position.
- Rolled towel or blanket should be kept under ankles or legs to prevent pressure on his toes.
- Nutritional need should be met by encouraging the mother to give breast feeding.
- Educate the mother how to handle the baby without pressing the sac.
- Avoid contamination from urine or foecal material to prevent infection.
- Any leakage of spinal fluid must be reported immediately.
- Assess for signs and symptoms of CNS infection.
- Measure the head circumference to establish baseline data.
- Assess bowel and bladder function and pattern, monitor intake and output.
- Provide emotional support to parents, be aware that surgery usually occurs 24 to 48 hours after birth.

Postoperative Nursing Care

- Provide routine post operative care.
- *Positioning*: Provide prone or knee chest position.
  - Should not be moved unnecessarily until the operative site is completely healed.
  - Even feeding and bathing should be carried out in this position.
- *Prevention of infection*: Prevent operative site from infection by keeping the observed site clean and dry with catheter care.
- *Skin care* is very important to prevent infection if child has paralysis.
- *Provide nutrition*: Provide adequate nutrition if breast feeding is not possible.
- Direct breast feeding or give bottle feeding (expressed breast milk).
- *Prevent complication*: Observe for the sign of any infection and sign of meningitis or paralysis.
- Prevent constipation.
- Provide psychological support to parents.

CLEFT FOOT

Definition

A congenital disorder in which the foot and ankle are twisted and can't be manipulated into the correct position, also known as talipes. It may be unilateral clubfoot which is more common than bilateral.

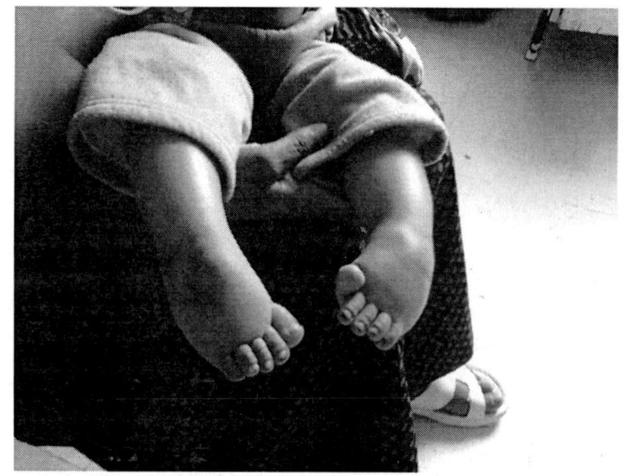

Fig. 4.11: Baby with Talipes Equinovarus

Causes

- Arrested development during the 9th and 10th weeks of embryonic life, when the feet are formed.
- Deformed talus and shortened Achilles tendon.
- Possible genetic predisposition.

Pathophysiology

- Abnormal development of the foot during foetal growth leads to abnormal muscles and joints and contracture of soft tissue.
- Apparent clubfoot
  - Results when a foetus maintains a position that gives his feet a clubfoot appearance at birth; it can usually be corrected manually.
  - Another form of apparent clubfoot is inversion of the feet, resulting from the denervation type of progressive muscular atrophy and progressive muscular dystrophy.

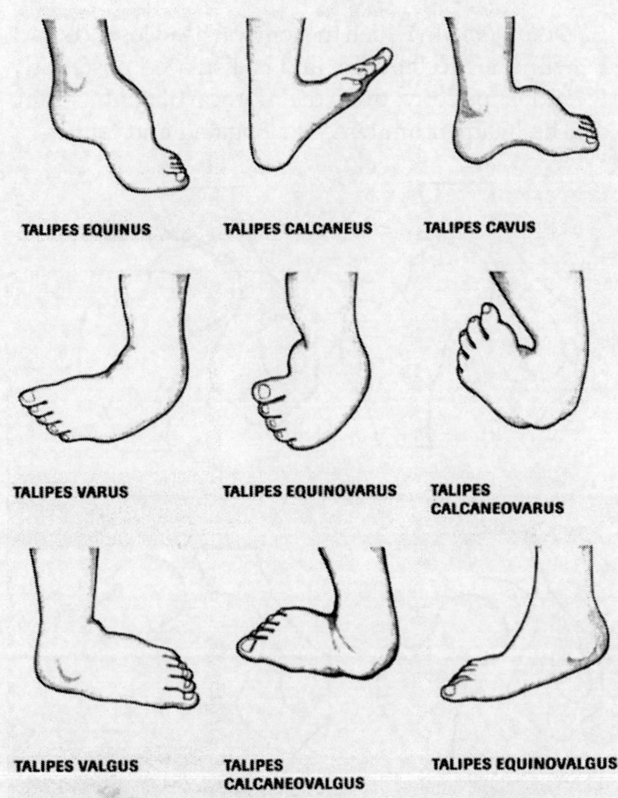

Fig. 4.12: Types of various deformity of foot

Clinical Feature

- Clubfoot involves three areas of deformity,
  - The midfoot is directed downwards (equinus).
  - The hindfoot turns inwards (varus).
  - The food curls towards the heel (adduction) and upward in partial supination.
- Deformity is usually obvious at birth (depends on involvement of ankle and foot.)
- Depends in involvement of ankle and foot.
- The foot is small with a shortened Achilles tendon.
- Muscles in the lower leg are atrophied but leg lengths are generally normal.

Investigation

- Assessment on birth on the basis of visual inspection.
- X-rays show superimposition of the talus and calcaneus and a ladder like appearance of the metatarsals.

Complications

- Delayed growth and development.
- Impaired mobility.
- Physical injury.

Medical Management

- Correcting the deformity.
- Early treatment is essential to achieve successful correction and reduce the chance of complication by application of cast.
  - After birth a series of casts to gradually stretch and realign the angle of the foot and, after cast removal, application of Denis Browne splint at night until age one.
- Surgical correction
  - Can improve clubfoot with good function but can't correct it.
  - The affected calf muscle will remain slightly underdeveloped.
  - Correction usually occurs in sequential order (correcting all three deformities at once results in a misshapen, rocker-bottomed foot).
    - Fore foot adduction.
    - Varus (inversion)
    - Equinus (Plantar flexion)
- Maintaining the correction until the foot gains normal muscle balance.
- Observing the foot closely for several years is required to prevent the deformity from recurring.

Nursing Interventions

- For the patient with a cast
  - Assess neurovascular status to ensure circulation to the foot.
  - Use a blow-dryer on a cool setting to provide relief of itching.
  - Discuss the importance of placing nothing inside the cast.
- Ensure that shoes fit correctly to promote comfort and prevent skin breakdown.
- Prepare the patient for surgery, if necessary, to maintain and promote healing process and decrease anxiety.
- Keep corrective devices on the patient as much as possible.
- Encourage the patient to walk as exercise after surgical repair.
- Perform passive range-of-motion (ROM) exercises; don't use excessive force when trying to manipulate the foot.

DEVELOPMENTAL DYSPLASIA OF THE HIP

The broad term developmental dysplasia of the hip describes a group of disorders related to abnormal development of the hip. DDH more properly reflects a variety of hip abnormalities in which there is a shallow acetabulum, subluxation, or dislocation.

The incidence of hip instability of some kind is approximately 10 per 1000 live births. The incidence of frank dislocation or a dislocatable hip is 1 in 1000. The left hip defect is involved in 60% of cases, the right hip defect in 20% and both hips in 20%. Sixty percent of the patients are girls. White children have a higher incidence than other groups.

Causes

- Prenatal factors:
  - Maternal hormone secretion.
- Mechanical factors of intrauterine posture:
  - High incidence of hip deformity with breech presentation and caesarean section (due to abnormal intrauterine position).
  - Legs in frank breech position (with the hips acutely flexed and knees extended).
- Other factors related to infant handling due to cultural practice.
- Twinning and large infant size.

Pathophysiology

There are three degrees of DDH that can be identified:

1. *Acetabulardysplasia or preluxation*: The mildest form, where there is neither subluxation nor dislocation. The dysplasia reflects an apparent delay in acetabular development evidenced by osseous hypoplasia of the acetabular roof that is oblique and shallow, although the cartilaginous roof is comparatively intact. The femoral head remains in the acetabulum.
2. *Subluxation*: Accounts for the largest percentage of congenital hip dysplasia. Subluxation implies incomplete dislocation of the hip and is sometimes regarded as an intermediate state in the development from primary dysplasia to complete dislocation. The femoral head remains in contact with the acetabulum, but a stretched capsule and ligamentum teres causes the head of the femur to be partially displaced. Pressure on the cartilaginous roof inhibits ossification and produces a flattening of the socket.
3. *Dislocation*: In which the femoral head loses contact with the accetabulum and is displaced posteriorly and superiorly over the fibrocartilaginous rim. The ligamentum teres is elongated and taut.

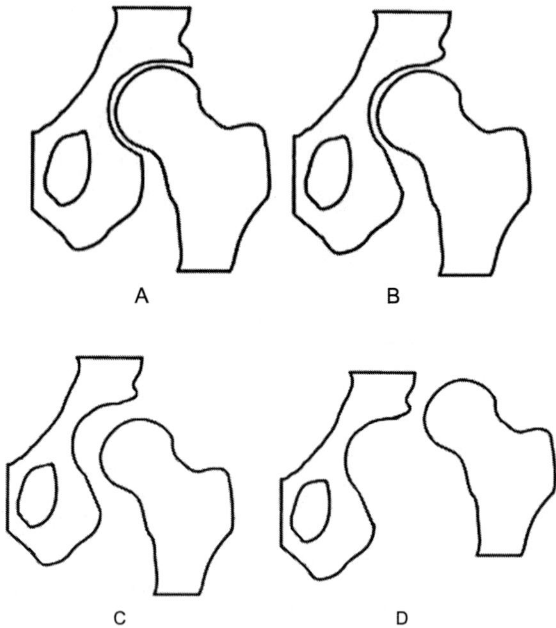

Fig. 4.13: Degree of developmental dysplasia A. Normal B. Dysplasia C. Subluxation or Sublocation D. Dislocation

Complications

- Delayed growth and development
- Impaired mobility
- Impaired skin integrity
- If corrective treatment isn't begun until age 2
- Degenerative hip changes
- Abnormal acetabular development
- Lordosis (abnormally increased concave curvature of the lumbar and cervical spine)
- Joint malformation
- A vascular necrosis of the femoral head

Clinical Features and Assessment Findings

- Asymmetry of gluteal and high fat fold and telescoping or pistoning of the thigh.
- On the affected side, an increased number of folds on the posterior thigh when the child is in a supine position with knees bent.
- Appearance of a shortened limb on the affected side.
- Restricted abduction of the hips.

- Barlow's sign:
  - A click is felt when the infant is placed supine with abducted hips flexed 90 degrees, knees fully flexed, and the hip adducted to midline.
  - Ortolani's click:
    - The infant is placed on his back, with hip flexed and in adduction the hip is then abducted while the examiner presses the femur downward to dislocate the hip.
    - A click or jerk (produced by the femoral head moving over the acetabulum rim) indicates subluxation in a neonate younger than 1 month; the sign indicates subluxation or complete dislocation in an older infant.
  - Positive Trendelenburg's test:
    - When the child stands on the affected leg, the opposite pelvis dips to maintain erect posture.

Investigations

- Sonography and MRI may be used to assess reduction.
- Ultrasonography shows the involved cartilage and acetabulum.
- X–rays show the location of the femur head and shallow acetabulum. It can also be used to monitor progression of the disorder.

Medical Management

- Infants younger than age 3 months:
  - Gentle manipulation to reduce the dislocation, followed by splintbrace or harness to hold the hips in a flexed and abducted position to maintain the reduction.
  - Splint brace or harness worn continuously for 2 to 3 months, then a night splint for another month to tighten and stabilize the joint capsule in correct alignment.
- Infants older than age 3 months:
  - Bilateral skin traction (in infants) or skeletal traction (in children who have started walking).
  - Bryant's traction or divarication traction (both extremities placed in traction, even if only one is affected, to help maintain immobilization) for children younger than 3 years and weighing less than 35 lb (16 kg) for 2 to 3 weeks.

    Gentle closed reduction under general anesthesia, followed by a spica cast (the legs are abducted with a bar between them) for 3 months if traction fails.
  - If hip is not reducible, open reduction and pelvic or femoral osteotomy to correct bony deformity, followed by immobilization in a spica cast for 6 to 8 weeks.
- In children ages 2 to 5:
  - Treatment is difficult; if begun after age 5, rarely restores satisfactory hip function.
  - Skeletal traction and subcutaneous adductor tenotomy (Surgical cutting of the tendon).

Nursing Interventions

- Assess circulation before application of cast or traction. After application, have the child wiggle toes to detect signs of impaired circulation. The nurse should be able to place one finger between the child's skin and cast.
- Give reassurance that early, prompt treatment will probably result in complete correction to decrease anxiety.
- Assure the parents that the child will adjust to restricted movement and return to normal sleeping, eating, and play in a few days.
- Inspect the skin and provide skin care, especially around bony prominences, to detect cast complications and prevent skin breakdown.
- Be aware that the goal of treatment is to enlarge and deepen the socket by pressure.

DEFECTS OF GENITOURINARY TRACT

External defects of the genitourinary tract are usually obvious at birth. Several, such as hypospadias, epispadias and undescended testes do not necessitate immediate repair but may require one or more stages of repair during early childhood.

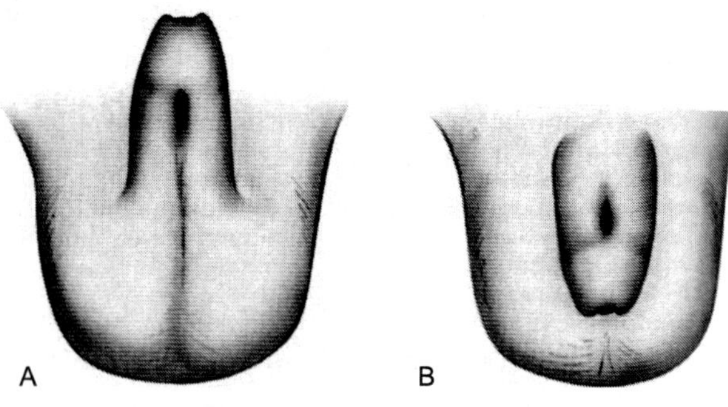

Fig. 4.14: Congenital defect in urethral opening
A. Hypospadias
B. Epispadias

Hypospadias

Refers to a condition in which the urethral opening is located behind the glans penis or anywhere along the ventral surface of the penile shaft.

- In mild cases the meatus is just off center from the tip of the penis.
- In the most severe malformation the meatus is located on the perineum between the two halves of the scrotum.

Treatment

Surgical correction is done as a urethroplasty.

The surgery is usually performed at about 3 years of age. When the phallus is of sufficient size and child has not yet developed mutilation anxiety and is not yet attending school.

Epispadias

In this congenital anomaly the urethra is located on the dorsal surface of the penis.

- In the mildest cases the meatus is located in front of the glans penis.
- In the most severe instance epispadias extends to exstrophy of the bladder.

Phimosis

Phimosis is an abnormal narrowing or stenosis of the preputial opening of the foreskin over the glans penis.

Pathophysiology

Phimosis can occur as a congenital anomaly or more commonly as a result of poor hygiene. In the later case smegma accumulates between the prepuce and penis. Infections occur, adhesions form and prevents the easy retraction of the foreskin.

Clinical Feature

- In an uncircumcised child the foreskin cannot be retracted over the penis.
- The narrowing obstructs the flow of urine resulting on a dribbling stream rather than a steady flow of urine during voiding.
- Tight band of skin constricts the blood vessels causing oedema, blush discoloration, pain dysuria causes necrosis.

Treatment

- Circumcision is done to treat phimosis.
- Treatment of mild cases includes manual retraction of foreskin and proper cleansing of the area.
- Retraction is best accomplished during the child's bath.

Nursing Management

- Cold compress to the area.
- Analgesics to reduce the pain.

Undescended Testis (Cryptorchidism)

Cryptochidism is failure of one or both testes is to descend in the scrotal sac, because the testes normally descend during the seventh to ninth month of gestation, infants born prematurely are likely to have cryptorchidism

Etiology

- Cause is not known, but congenital.
- Preterm babies have increased chance of finding an upper urinary tract anomaly on the same side as the undescended testis.

There are **two types** of cryptorchidism.

In true—undescended testis the organ has never been in the scrotal sac, but ties somewhere along the path of descent above the inguinal ring.

In ectopic testes—The organ has passed down the inguinal canal through the external rings but is fixed in an upward direction such as in the perineum or proximal scrotum, congenital hydrocele or inguinal hernias frequently accompany the defect.

Treatment

Hormonal therapy—in the form of human chorionic gonadotropin may be initiated to help enlarge the scrotum or testes. Testes that blow the external ring may descend by hormonal treatment.

If lodged inside the inguinal canal or fixed in an abnormal position surgery is desired.

Surgical Treatment—The surgery orchiopexy is done at the age 5 years.

- Rubber band to retraction suture in the scrotum and securing the other end to the inner thigh with adhesive tape for about 5–7 days.
- Positioning
- Prevention of infection—by careful cleaning of stool and urine.
- If surgery is done after the child's toilet training, prevention of contamination is simplified.

DOWN'S SYNDROME

Definition

Down's syndrome is a common chromosomal abnormality, occurs in 1.66 per 1000 live births. This condition is characterized by mental retardation in varying degrees and multiple associated defects. It occurs in all socioeconomic classes and both sexes

Causes

- Trisomy 21
- Genetic non dysfunction, with three chromosomes on the 21st pair (total of 47 chromosomes).
- Unbalanced translocation of chromosome 15 and 21 or 21. This type of genetic aberration is usually hereditary and not associated with advanced parental age.
- Risk factor is parental age; maternal age—the women age 35 (80%), especially in men 55 years of age or older (5%).
- Mosaicism (1–2%) which refers to cells with both normal and abnormal chromosomes.

Pathophysiology

A chromosomal aberration characterized by:

- Mental retardation
- Dysmorphic facial features
- Other distinctive physical abnormalities
- Commonly associated with congenital heart defects (in approximately 60% of patients; up to 44% of these patients die before age 1) and other abnormalities.

Complications

- Impaired growth and development
- Physical injury
- Aspiration
- Death

Clinical Features

Head

- Hair is dry and coarse
- Round and small head(brachycephaly) with slow brain growth
- Flat occiput
- Enlarged anterior fontanel
- Flat, broad forehead

Face

- Face is round

Eyes

- Palpebral fissures are narrow
- Upward slanting eyes with increased epicanthic fold,
- Strabismus
- Short, sparse eyelashes
- Brushfield's spots (marbling and speckling of the iris)

Nose

- Short,
- Flat bridge of nose (depressed)

Ear

- Small
- Short pinna
- Overlapping upper helices
- Narrow canals

Mouth and Teeth

- Thick and fissured, protruding tongue (due to small oral cavity)
- High arched palate
- Mouth kept open
- Hypoplastic mandible
- Small teeth (microdontia)
- Delayed eruption
- Alignment abnormality of teeth

Chest

- Shortness of rib cage
- Twelfth rib anomalies

Neck

- Short and broad

Abdomen

- Protruding
- Umbilical hernia

Genitalia

- Small penis
- Cryptorchidism
- Bulbous Vulva

Hands

- Hands are short with an incurved fifth finger, (clinodactyly).
- Single palmar crease (Simian crease).
- Stubby fingers.

Feet

- Wide space between first and second toes.
- Planter crease between big and second toes.

Musculoskeleton

- Hypotonic
- Hyperflexibility
- Muscle weakness
- Mild to moderate retardation

Skin

- Dry, cracked and frequent fissuring
- Mottling

Other congenital abnormalities like intestinal atresia, imperforate anus, heart disorder.

Diagnostic Test Findings

- Amniocentesis allows prenatal diagnosis.
  - Recommended for women older than age 34, regardless of a negative family history.
  - Recommended for women of any age if she or the father carries a translocated chromosome.
- Karyotype shows the specific chromosomal abnormality.
- Fetal ultrasound may reveal varying degrees of abnormalities, but many fetuses have few detectable defects.

Medical Management

- According to the IQ (Intelligence Quotient) level. Anti convulsant therapy to be given.
- Provide gavage feedings, if necessary, because the infant's sucking reflex may be poor.
- Treat coexisting conditions. Congenital heart problems, vision defects, hypothyroidism.
- Skeletal, immunologic, metabolic, biochemical, and oncologic problems treated according to specific problem.
- Rehabilitation therapy and Occupation therapy given later on.

Nursing Interventions

- Provide activities and toys appropriate for the child to support optimal development.
- Set realistic, reachable goals; break tasks into small steps to make them easier to accomplish.
- Use behaviour modification, if applicable, to promote safety and prevent injury to the child and others.
- Provide stimulation and communicate at a level appropriate to the child's mental age rather than the chronological age to promote a healthy emotional environment.
- Provide a safe environment to prevent injury.
- Mainstream daily routines to promote normalcy.
- Encourage parents to care for, bond with, and hold their child.
- Teach parents to perform all of the above interventions because care will mostly be provided at home by the parents.
- Refer the parents of the affected child for genetic counselling to explore the cause of the disorder and discuss the risk of recurrence in a future pregnancy.
- Refer the parents to a social worker or grief counsellor for additional support, if needed.

Altered Respiratory Conditions

RESPIRATORY INFECTION

Respiratory tract infection is very common in the children. Respiratory infections account for the majority of acute illnesses in children. Infections of the respiratory tract are described according to the areas of involvement. It is classified into two.

1. The upper respiratory infection
2. The lower respiratory infection

Upper respiratory tract infections (URTI) are:

- Common cold
- Pharyngitis
- Laryngitis

Lower respiratory tract infections (LRTI) are:

- Bronchitis
- Bronchiolitis
- Bronchiectasis
- Atelectasis
- Pneumonia
- Pneumothorax
- Asthma
- CROUP syndrome

Etiology

The etiology and cause of this infection are influenced by the age of the child, season, living conditions, and pre-existing medical problems.

Causative organisms are many, the most common organism are

- Virus particularly respiratory syncytial virus (RSV)
- Other agents are B-haemolytic streptococci
- *Staphylococci*
- *Haemophilius influenzae*
- *Chlamydia trachomatis*
- Mycoplasma
- *Pneumococci*

Age

- Infants age 3–6 months have increased infection rate.
- Viral infection rate continues to remain high during toddler and preschool age.
- Group A β–haemolytic streptococci infection increases in school age children.

Size

- Anatomic difference influences the response to respiratory tract infection.
- The diameter of the airways is smaller in young children and becomes narrow due to oedematous of mucus membranes and increased production of secretion.
- The structure of the respiratory tract is shorter so infants get an infection rapidly.
- The relatively short and open Eustachian tube in infants and young children allows organisms to easily access to the middle ear and cause otitis media.

Resistance

- Deficiency of immune system places the child at risk for infection.
- Other conditions cause decreased resistance in the children leading to disorders like malnutrition, anaemia, fatigue, chillness of the body.

Seasonal Conditions

- Winter and spring seasons are common for respiratory infection.
- Cold weather conditions.

Clinical Manifestations

- Fever
- Anorexia
- Vomiting
- Abdominal pain

- Nasal blockage
- Nasal discharge
- Cough
- Respiratory sounds associated with respiratory diseases like Grunting, stridor, wheezing, crackles.
- Sore throat

COMMON UPPER RESPIRATORY TRACT INFECTIONS (URTI)

Acute Viral Nasopharyngitis

Acute viral nasopharyngitis or common cold is caused by a number of viruses.

Causes

- Rhinovirus
- Respiratory syncytial virus (RSV)
- Adenovirus
- Influenza virus or Parainfluenza virus

Clinical Manifestations

- Fever is very common
- In older children low grade fever
- Dryness and irritation of nasal passage
- Sneezing
- Chilly sensation
- Nasal discharge
- Irritability
- Restlessness
- Decreased appetite
- Decreased activity
- Mouth breathing due to nasal obstruction

Complication

- Nasal inflammation leads to obstruction
- Otitis media
- Pneumonia

Treatment

- Children having nasopharyngitis are managed at home, no specific treatment.
- Antipyretics (paracetamol) are usually given for the child who has mild fever.
- Advise the child to take rest.
- Decongestants may be prescribed for the children as nasal drops.
- Cough suppressants should be given, it contains dextromethorphan if the children have cough.
- Antihistamines are largely ineffective in treatment of nasopharyngitis.
- Encourage the mothers to give more hot fluids and fruit juices.

Prevention

- Children should be made to protect from exposure to the causes.

Nursing Management

- Explain the illness to parents, most discomfort in this condition is due to nasal obstruction.
- Elevating the head of the bed or crib mattress assists with drainage of secretions.
- Suctioning and vaporization may also help to provide relief to the child.
- Administer saline nasal drops and gentle suction with a bulb syringe before feeding.
- Maintaining adequate fluid intake is essential during any infection process.
- Encourage the child to take frequent and more fluid diet to prevent dehydration, and also the child who has poor appetite and refuses to take solid foods.
- Isolate the children from infected person.
- Minimize the visitors or other persons' contact.
- Encourage them to carefully dispose of tissues, not sharing the towels with others, eating utensils, covering the mouth and nose with tissue or handkerchief when coughing or sneezing and washing the hands thoroughly after nose blowing or sneezing.
- Children should be taught to wash their hands thoroughly before putting them near their nose, mouth or eyes.
- Educate the parents to notify the health professionals if any of the following symptoms (respiratory complications) are present:
    - Evidence of earache
    - Fast respiration
    - Fever
    - Increased irritability with or without fever
    - Persistent cough
    - Wheezing
    - Crying
    - Refuses to eat
    - Restlessness and poor sleeping pattern.

Tonsillitis

Tonsillitis is an inflammation of the tonsils that is also included in upper respiratory tract infections.

Etiology

- Mostly viral and bacterial.
- Group a beta-haemolytic streptococcus is the most common and the most important bacterial agent after 2 year of age.
- Oral anaerobes.

Pathophysiology

- The tonsils are involved in immunity and antibody production. Because of their location, tonsils are exposed to pathogens on a regular basis. This can lead to micro abscesses with chronic or recurring infections.
- Waldeyer's tonsillar ring—a mass of lymphoid tissues around the nasal and oral pharynx that consists of three pairs of tonsils.
- Palatine tonsils, also known as faucial tonsils:
  - Located on both sides of the oropharynx, behind and below the opening of the mouth.
  - Surface is visible on oral examination.
  - Removed during tonsillectomy.
- Pharyngeal tonsils, also known as the adenoids:
  - Located on the back wall of the nasopharynx above the palatine tonsils.
  - Close to the nares and eustachian tubes, which causes problems when they become inflamed.
- Lingual at the base of the tongue:
  - Located at the base of the tongue.
  - Rarely removed.

Complications

- Obstruction from tonsillar hypertrophy.
- Complications include the following supportive: Otitis media, Retropharyngeal and Peritonsillar abscess.
- Non-supportive—Acute glomerulonephritis, Rheumatic fever.

Clinical Manifestations

Acute Tonsillitis

- Mild to severe sore throat.
- Decreased food intake.
- Dysphagia.
- Abdominal pain.
- Vomiting.
- High grade fever.
- Headache.
- Other signs of URTI (runny nose, sneezing, coryza, etc.).
- Tenderness in the lymphglands in the submandibular area.
- Muscular and joint pain.
- Chills, Malaise.
- Pain that commonly refers to ears.
- Excess secretions that cause a constant urge to swallow.
- A feeling of constriction in the back of the throat.

Chronic Tonsillitis

- Recurrent sore throat.
- Purulent drainage in the tonsillar crypts.
- Diffuse redness and exudates, petechiae over palates, and, tender cervical lympho adenopathy.

Investigation

- Throat culture may be positive for streptococcal organisms
- Serum analysis reveals leukocytosis

Medical Management

- Treatment of viral tonsillitis consists of supportive care such as, salt water gargles.
- Antibiotics for bacterial infections:
  - Benzathine penicillin or another broad-spectrum antibiotics are the drugs of choice for a group A beta-haemolytic streptococcus infection.
  - Most oral anaerobes also respond to penicillin.
  - Antipyretics—syrup or tablet paracetamol.
  - Analgesics to relieve pain and inflammation.
  - To prevent complication, antibiotic therapy should continue for 10 to 14 days.
  - Chronic tonsillitis or the development of complications may require tonsillectomy; but only after the patient has been free from tonsillar or respiratory tract infection for 3 to 4 weeks.

- Lozenges, analgesics, and antipyretics may be used to maintain comfort.

Surgical Management

Tonsillectomy or adenoidectomy, or both, may be indicated in chronic enlargement that interferes with swallowing or breathing, or in recurrent streptococcal infections, peritosillar abscess, or retropharyngeal abscess.

Nursing Management

- *Preoperative Care*
  - Explain why the child is coming to the hospital.
  - Encourage the parents to stay with the child until surgery.
  - Prepare the child for the sights and sounds of surgery; explain that the child will be sleeping during surgery.
  - Allow the child to play with the equipment.
  - Provide reassurance that the child will never be alone and won't feel the procedure.
  - Put a transitional object in the recovery room for the child.
  - Prepare the child for throat surgery.
  - Maintain a soft to liquid diet.
  - The child may breathe through his mouth; a vaporizer (cool mist) may help to keep mucous membranes from drying out.
- *Postoperative Care*
  - Place the child in a prone or side-lying position to facilitate drainage.
  - Don't do suction except to remove an obstruction; this will prevent trauma to the site.
  - Check for signs of haemorrhage, which require immediate attention:
    - Frequent swallowing
    - Restlessness
    - Fast, thready pulse
    - Vomiting bright red blood; however, be aware that vomiting dried blood is common.
  - Provide an ice collar for comfort and for reducing edema.

CROUP SYNDROME

Croup is a term applied to a broad classification of upper airway illness that results from swelling of the epiglottis and larynx. The swelling usually extends into the trachea and bronchi; it causes severe inflammation and obstruction of the upper airway.

Causes

- Viral-induced edema around the larynx.
  - Parainfluenza viruses (two-thirds of the infections)
  - Adenoviruses
  - RSV
  - Influenza
  - Measles virus
- Bacterial
  - Pertussis
  - Diphtheria
  - Mycoplasma.

Pathophysiology

In croup, inflammatory swelling and spasm constrict the larynx, thereby reducing air flow. Inflammatory changes almost completely obstruct the larynx and significantly narrow the trachea.

- Spasmodic laryngitis—typically involves paroxysmal attacks of laryngeal obstruction generally occurring at night.
- Acute obstructive laryngitis—a sudden narrowing of the upper airway results from vocal cord edema.
- Acute laryngotracheobronchitis—inflammation of the mucosal lining of the larynx and trachea results in a constricted airway.
- A childhood disease that affects boys more than girls, usually between ages 3 months and 5 years, in the winter.

Complications

- Respiratory insufficiency

Clinical Manifestations

- Barking cough or hoarseness, sometimes described as a "Seal bark" cough.
- Usually begins with cold like symptoms for 1 to 2 days.
- Worse at night and can last 5 to 6 days.

- Crackles and decreased breath sounds (indicates condition has progressed to bronchi).
- Increased dyspnoea and chest retraction.
- Inspiratory stridor with varying degrees of respiratory distress.
- Sudden or gradual onset.
- Muffled vocal sounds.
- Inability to swallow.

Investigations

- Throat cultures may identify the organism and its sensitivity to antibiotics as well as rule out diphtheria.
- Laryngoscopy may reveal inflammation and obstruction in epiglottal and laryngeal areas.

Neck X-ray shows areas of upper airway narrowing and edema in subglottic fold and rules out the possibility of foreign body obstruction as well as masses and cysts.

Table 5.1: Scale to Identify the Severity of Croup

Signs	Severity Score			
	0	1	2	3
Stridor	None	Mild	Moderate at rest	Severe, on inspiration
Retractions	None	Mild	Suprasternal, intercostals	Severe, may see sternal retractions
Colour	Normal	–	–	Dusky or cyanotic
Breath	Normal sound	Mild decreased	Moderately decreased	Markedly decreased
Level of consciousness	Normal	Restless when disturbed	Anxious	Lethargic

Scoring: To quantify the severity of croup, add the individual scores for each of the sign categories. A score between 0 and 15 is possible. The rating of mild, moderate, and severe is as follows: 4–5 is mild, 6–8 is moderate, >8 or any sign in the severe category is severe.

Source: Adapted from Davis, H.W., Gartner, J.C., Galvis, A.G., Michaels, R.H., and Mestal P.H. (1981). Acute upper airway obstruction: Croup and epiglottitis; *Pediatric Clinics of North America*, **28**(4): 859–880.

Medical Management

- Cool humidification during sleep with a cool mist tent or room humidifier.
- Exposure of child to cool air.
- Oxygen administration, if necessary.
- Medications
  - Antipyretics such as acetaminophen (Tylenol or paracetamol).
  - Beta-agonist and beta-adrenergics (*e.g.*, albuterol, racemic epinephrine (Asthma Nefrin) aerosolized through face mask. It is a rapid acting bronchodilator; it relieves bronchial spasm and decreases the secretion.
- Corticosteroids (*e.g.*, dexamethasone); IM, PO, Nebulized budeonide—It is an anti-inflammatory, it reduces the oedema.
  - Antibiotics if the infection is bacterial.
- Administration of intravenous fluids to prevent dehydration.
- Tracheostomy or ET intubation for impending airway failure in very severe cases.

Nursing Management

- Keep the child calm to ease respiratory effort and conserve energy.
- Take the child into the bathroom, close the door, turn on the shower's hot-water spigot full-force, and sit with the child as the room fills with steam; this should decrease laryngeal spasm.
- Take the child outside into cool air.
- Use a cool-mist vaporizer near the child's bed after an acute episode (after a crisis, mucus production increases, and the child may vomit in large amounts; this vomiting doesn't require medical treatment).

- Encourage clear fluid intake to promote liquification of secretions and provide calories for energy.
- Provide steam tent bed to reduce the edema and lubricate the secretion in the throat.
- Anticipate that the child may need hospitalization for tracheotomy, oxygen, or mist if the crisis doesn't resolve.
- Assess respiratory and cardiovascular status to detect any indication that the obstruction is becoming worse.
- Monitor vital signs and pulse oximetry to detect early signs of respiratory compromise.
- Administer medications, as ordered, and note effectiveness to maintain or improve the child's condition.
- Provide emotional support for the parents to decrease anxiety.
- Monitor for rebound obstruction when administering racemic epinephrine; the drug's effects are short-term and may result in rebound obstruction.

LOWER RESPIRATORY TRACT INFECTIONS (LRTI)

Bronchitis

Bronchitis is inflammation of the trachea and bronchi, which is frequently associated with a URTI.

Causes

- Virus is primary cause.
- Mycoplasma pneumonia is common in children less than 6 years of age.

Clinical Manifestations

- Fever
- Dry coarse, hacking and productive cough that is worse at night.
- Sleep disturbance
- Irritable
- Weak
- Pain in the abdomen and chest, ribs due to deep and frequent cough.
- Wheezing sound heard even without stethoscope in some children.

Investigation

- Physical examination
- Blood examination
- X-ray.

Treatment

- Need symptomatic treatment that includes:
  - Antipyretic
  - Analgesic
  - Humidifier steam inhalation
  - Cough suppressants, it helps the children for rest but can interfere with clearance of the secretions.

Nursing Management

- Provide supporting respiratory function through.
  - Adequate rest
  - Humidification—oxygen administration.
  - positioning the child—Fowler's position to facilitate for easy breathing.
  - Maintain hydration to the child by giving adequate fluids.
  - Administration of medication as prescribed.
  - Psychological support to the child and family.

Broncholitis

Brocholitis is an acute viral infection with maximum effect at the bronchiolar level. The infection occurs in winter and springs seasons. It commonly occurrs in less than two years children; it can be a serious condition, the children need to be admitted in the hospital for treatment.

Causes

- Viral, bacterial, and mycoplasmal organisms may cause broncholitis.
- Adenovirus and parainfluenza viruses.
- Respiratory syncytial virus is a 50% most common organism.
- Winter and springs seasons.
- In tropical regions.
- Rainy seasons.

Pathophysiology

- RSV is transmitted by direct or close contact with an infected person.

- Virus acting as a parasite is able to invade the mucosal cells that line the small bronchi and bronchioles.
- Invaded cells die when the virus bursts from inside the cell to invade adjacent cells.
- Results in cells debris clogs and obstructs the bronchioles and irritates the airway.
- In response the bronchiole swells, produces excessive mucus.

  Mucus and lumina are subsequently filled with mucus and exudates.
- The walls of the bronchi and bronchioles are infiltrated with inflammatory cells, and peribronchiolar interstitial pneumonia is usually present.
- In response, the airway lining swells and produces excessive mucus.
- Despite this protective effort by the bronchioles, the actual effect is partial airway obstruction and bronchospasms.
- The cycle is repeated throughout in both lungs, the partially obstructed airways allow air in, but the mucus and airway swelling blocks expulsion of the air, and this creates wheezing and crackles in the airway.
- Air trapped below the obstruction also interferes with normal gas exchange.
- So child will get a risk of respiratory failure, as the oxygen level decreases and carbon dioxide level increases.
- Apnoea and pulmonary oedema may occur, air flow continues to decrease, and breath sound diminishes.

Clinical Manifestations

- Possible air trapping and atelectasis
- Sternal retractions
- Nasal flaring
- Tachypnea
- Thick mucus
- Wheezes and crackles
- Cough.

Complications

- Respiratory insufficiency
- Obstructed airway.

Investigation

- Bronchial mucus culture shows RSV
- Chest X-ray.

Medical Management

- Cardio respiratory monitor and pulse oximetry–to follow the treatment and there is need for specific therapies.
- Administration of humidified oxygen via hood or face mask, tent or nasal cannula.
- Administration of I.V. fluids or oral fluids.
- Isolation to prevent healthcare-associated infection.
- Administration of systemic medication includes antipyretics (acetaminophen or paracetamol preferred, no antibiotics are given unless the evidence of secondary bacterial infection such as otitis media is present).
- Medication for children at risk for chronic disease or severely affected infants.
  - Children may be intubated and ventilation for apnoea or respiratory failure.
  - Epinephrine may improve airway resistance in some cases; should only be continued if improvements appear.
  - Palivizumab (synagis) IM, Respigm IV may prevent RSV in high-risk infants.

Nursing Management

Maintain Respiratory Function

- Monitor vital signs and pulse oximetry to determine oxygenation needs and to detect deterioration or improvement in the child's condition.
- Administer humidified oxygen therapy to liquify secretions and reduce bronchial oedema.
- Assess respiratory and cardiovascular status; tachycardia may result from hypoxia or effects of bronchodilator use.
- Administer chest physiotherapy after oedema has abated; it helps loosen mucus that may be blocking small airways.

Prevent Infection

- Use gloves, gowns, and aseptic hand washing as secretion precautions to prevent spread of infection.

Maintain Hydration

- Administer and maintain I.V. therapy to promote hydration and replace electrolytes.
- Administer fluids by mouth after acute crisis.

Support Physiological Functions

- Administration of medication to control the temperature and promote comfort to the children.
- Provide rest.
- Provide position to improve the breathing pattern.

Reduce the Anxiety

- An important part of nursing care is anticipating, recognizing and acting to decrease the child's and parents' anxiety.
- Provide the parents with thorough explanation and daily updates and encourage their participation in the children care.
- Encourage and involve the parents in children care, it may reduce the anxiety to the child.

Asthma

Asthma is a condition in which laboured breathing is accompanied by wheezing, which is caused by a spasm of bronchial tubes or swelling of their mucous membranes. Asthma is a reversable form of airway obstruction.

Incidence

It is the most common chronic disease in children, 5%–10% fall children – 4000 deaths annually occur.

Causes

- Extrinsic factors.
- Polluted dust, mole feathers, animal dander.
- Food—eg gs, milk, nuts, grains
- Parainfluenza virus, rhinovirus, influenza virus.
- Stress or emotional changes.
- Air pollution, smoke.
- Changes in climate, excessive exercise.
- Some medications.
- Hyper responsiveness of the lower airway.
- May be idiopathic or intrinsic; may be caused by a hyper responsive reaction to an allergen, exercise, or environmental change.

Pathophysiology

- The obstructive symptoms of asthma are caused by three mechanisms.
    - Inflammation of the mucous membranes.
    - Smooth muscle broncheospasm.
    - Increased mucus secretion, leading to airway obstruction and air trapping bronchial smooth muscle spasm.
    - Inflammation and oedema of bronchial mucosa and production and retention of thick, tenacious pulmonary secretion.
    - Due to this increased airway resistance premature closure of the airway.
    - Hyper inflation, increased work of breathing and impaired gas exchange.
    - Normally during inspiration, the negative pressure within the thorax pulls the airway, allowing air to enter.
    - On expiration the lung contracts and air moves out of the lungs.
    - In asthma the airways are swollen and mucus filled.
    - Air moves into the lungs and becomes trapped because of the obstruction.
    - The lungs become hyper inflated. In addition spasm of the bronchial smooth muscles contributes to this over inflation

      The child expends increased energy to breath and experiences hypoxemia and hypercapnia.

Complications

- Respiratory insufficiency.
- Death.

Clinical Manifestations

- Alteration in chest contour from chronic air trapping; barrel chest.
- Tachycardia with prolonged respiration.
- Altered cerebral function.
- Exercise intolerance.
- Fatigue and apprehension.
- Prolonged expiration with an expiratory wheeze; in severe distress, possible inspiratory wheeze.
- Unequal or decreased breath sounds.
- Use of accessory muscles (intercostals retractions and nasal flaring).
- Cough.
- Increased capillary refill time.

- Cyanosis.
- Child complains of abdominal pain.

Investigation

- Pulse oximetry may show decreased oxygen saturation.
- ABG measurements may show increased $PaCO_2$ from respiratory acidosis.
- Skin test identifies the source of the allergy.
- Sputum analysis rules out respiratory infection.
- Chest X–ray shows hyper expansion of airways.
- PFTS indicates air trapping and decreased expiratory flow.

Medical Management

- Chest physiotherapy (after oedema has abated).
- Hyposensitization through the use of allergy shots, if appropriate.
- Parenteral fluids to thin mucus secretions.
- Oxygen therapy as tolerated.

Medication

Bronchodilator

- Beta-adrenergic blockers, bronchodilators (Short-acting) Epinephrine – 0.01 mg/kg – 0.5 mg.
- Bronchodilator – albuterol (Proventil), Salmeterol (Serevent).

Aminophylline

- Albutemol sulfate (Ventoline) Inhalation about 12 yrs.
- Oral-2–6 yrs—0.1 mg/kg qid.
- 6–14 yrs old—0.1 mg/kg.
- Steroids Prednisone—0.15 mg/kg/day or 4–5 mg.
- Mast cell stabilizer—Cromolyn (Intal) to prevent the release of mast cell products after an antigen–antibody union has taken place.
- Anticholenergic—Ipratropium (Atrovent) to inhibit broncho-vasoconstriction.
- Inhaled corticosteroids to decrease oedema of the mucous membranes (for chronic asthma, daily doses to control chronic inflammation); also oral and I.V. steroids are used in severe cases.
  - Leukotriene modifiers or leukotriene receptor antagonists-zileuton (Zyflo), montelukast (Singulair), Zafirlukast. (Accolate) to inhibit bronchoconstriction and inflammation.

Nursing Management

Assessment

- Assess respiratory and cardiovascular status; tachycardia, tachypnea, and quiet breath sounds signal worsening respiratory status.
- Monitor vital signs to detect changes and prevent complications.
- Assess the nature of the child's cough (hacking, unproductive progressing to productive), especially at night in the absence of infection; early detection and treatment lessens respiratory distress.

Provide Proper Ventilation

- Oxygen administration to the child.
- Fowler's positioning improves the child's ventilation.
- Chest physiotherapy and suctioning to remove the secretion.
- Administration of nebulizer to relax the bronchial muscle for air entry.

Administer Medication

- Modify the environment to avoid an allergic reaction:
  - Remove the offending allergen.
  - Allergens can trigger an asthma attack.
- Rinse the child's mouth after he inhales medication to promote comfort and prevent irritation to the oral mucosa.
- For exercise – induced asthma, give prophylactic treatments of beta-adrenergic blockers or cromolyn 10 to 15 minutes before the child exercises; premedication before exercise may prevent an asthma attack.
- Forbid smoking in the child's environment; second hand smoke can trigger an asthma attack.
- During an acute attack:
  - Allow the child to sit upright to promote chest expansion and ease breathing; provide moist oxygen, if necessary, to promote mobilization of secretions.
  - Monitor for alterations in vital signs (especially cardiac stimulation and hypotension) to detect signs of impending respiratory arrest and cardiac decompensation.

- Administer medications through a metered dose inhaler (MDI) or a nebulizer:
  - A child as young as age 4 can use an MDI if a spacer (Chamber) is attached.
  - The child puffs the medication into the spacer and then inhales, avoiding the problem of trying to coordinate the activities of pressing the MDI and inhaling slowly.
  - Monitor peak flow rates, which indicate the degree of lung impairment (baseline values need to be established when the child is healthy to set comparison rates).

Position the Child

- Provide semi upright or sit upright position to promote chest expansion and ease breathing.
- Maintain a calm environment; provide emotional support and reassurance to decrease anxiety and oxygen demands.
- Monitor effectiveness of drug therapy; failure to respond to drugs during an acute attack can result in status asthmaticus, a potentially fatal complication that arises when impaired gas exchange and heightened airway resistance increase the work of breathing.

Provide Adequate Nutrition

- Encourage the child to take small and frequent diet.
- Encourage fluid diet first then slowly change to semisolid diet.
- Encourage to take the dinner earlier so that it reduces the breathing difficulty and sleep disturbance to the child (increases the chest expansion).

Pneumonia

Pneumonia is an inflammation of the bronchioles and alveolar spaces of the lungs (Pulmonary parenchyma), it occurs most often in infants and young children.

- Pneumonia is classified according to etiology: Bacterial, viral.
- Pneumonia may also be classified according to location and extent of pulmonary involvement.
  - **Lobar** involves a large segment of one or more lobes.
  - **Broncho pneumonia** begins in terminal bronchioles and involves the nearby lobes.
  - **Interstitial** confined to the alveolar walls and bronchial and interlobular tissues.

Causes

- Bacteria (Pneumococcal, streptococcal, staphylococcal).
- Viral cause adenovirus, myxovirus syncytial virus.
- Aspiration of (lipid or hydrocarbon) substances.

Pathophysiology

Entry of the organism to the lungs through inhalation or from the bloodstream

↓

As the disorder progresses, parenchyma inflammation occurs

↓

Infiltration of exudates into the alveoli (consolidation)

↓

RBC and exudates serum are invading the alveoli

↓

Alveoli full of fibrin, leukocytes, and organism

↓

While coughing-blood-tinged sputum and thick purulent material comes

↓

Bacterial pneumonia most often causes lobular involvement and sometimes consolidation; viral pneumonia usually causes inflammation of interstitial tissue.

Clinical Manifestations

- Cough and cold
- High fever
- Nasal flaring, retraction
- Chest pain
- Chills and dyspnoea, cyanosis
- If high fever—leads to febrile convulsion
- Tachypnea or fast breathing
- Respiratory rales (due to fluids) on auscultation
- Percussion—reveals that there is dullness over a lobe (due to consolidation)
- Diminished breath sounds.

TABLE 5.2: Cut off for Fast Breathing According to IMNCI Guidelines–2009

Age Group	Cut off for Fast Breathing
2 months up to 12 months	50 breaths per minute or more
12 months up to 5 years	40 breaths per minute or more

Note: The child who is exactly 12 months old has fast breathing if you count 40 breaths per minute or more.

Investigation

- Physical assessment
- Chest X-ray shows an abnormal density of tissue, such as lobar consolidation, pleural effusion, atelectasis, or abscess formation.
- Blood exam—ESR, total count.

Medical Management

Symptomatic Treatment

- Antipyretic drugs—Paracetamol
- Analgesic drugs
- Anti-inflammatory drugs

Supportive Treatment

- Airway management—oxygen administration, positioning.
- Administration of fluid by oral or intravenously depends upon the child's conditions.
- Provide adequate rest.

Specific Treatment

Antibiotics

- Children with pneumonia are treated at outpatient level with cotrimoxazole or amoxicillin orally for 5 days.
- Children with severe pneumonia are given intravenous antibiotics—crystalline penicillin as first line drug.
- Anti congestant.
- Steam inhalation.
- Chest physiotherapy.

Nursing Management

- Nursing care incorporates supportive measures and medical therapies as appropriate.
- Nursing measures used to manage the child with bronchiolitis are generally applicable to the child with pneumonia.
- Administration of oxygen to the child by mask or mist tent, with cool humidification moistening the airway and providing an atmosphere that assists in temperature reduction.
- Provide positioning for adequate ventilation.
- Provide hydration, fluids are frequently administrated intravenously in acute phase, oral fluids are given carefully to avoid aspiration to the child.
- Provide rest to the child; involve the parents in daily care.
- In addition to ongoing respiratory assessment and supportive therapies (Pulmonary care, antibiotics, hydration), the child may need relief from pain when coughing and deep breathing.
- Pain medication (acetaminophen or ibuprofen) can provide the added benefits of temperature control and may aid in sleep.
- The goal of nursing care is to restore optimal respiratory function.
- Discharge planning should be addressed early in the hospital stay. Medications, especially antibiotics must be taken at prescribed intervals and for the full course.
- Parents should be taught the proper administration of drugs and any side effects.
- Follow-up may include a chest X-ray to see if the lungs are clear. Symptoms of pneumonia usually disappear long before the lungs are completely healed.

Otitis Media

Middle ear infection is one of the most common early childhood diseases particularly as a complication of upper respiratory infection respiratory allergy, adenoiditis, or unrepaired cleft palate.

It is classified as:

1. **Acute or chronic supportive otitis media**—in which bacterial or viral agents cause a purulent exudates to accumulate behind the eardrum in the space of the middle ear.
2. **Serous otitis media**—in which a nonpurulent sterile mucoid effusion collects as a result of blocked – Eustachian tubes.

Etiology

Acute supportive otitis media caused by the *Hemophilus influenza,* pneumococci, or streptococci, chronic supportive otitis media caused by inadequately treated the acute otitis media, the recurrent adenoiditis or unrepaired cleft palate.

- Allergic rhinitis or hypertrophic adenoids

Pathophysiology

Dysfunctioning of Eustachian tubes—the Eustachian tube connects the middle ear to the nasopharynx. Normally it is closed and flat, preventing organisms from the pharyngeal cavity from entering the middle ear, it opens to allow drainage if secretions are produced by the middle ear mucosa and to equalize air pressure between the middle ear and outside environment.

If the tube is blocked

↓

Alter in protective function

↓

Drainage impaired and the normal secretions are retained type

↓

Air cannot escape blocked tube so is absorbed through the vascular circulation

↓

Causing a negative pressure within the middle ear

↓

If the tube opens—bacteria enter to the middle chamber

↓

Organism proliferates and invades the mucosa (suppurative type)

Clinical Manifestations

- Pain

  Infant becomes irritable and feels discomfort by
  - holding or pulling their ears.
  - rolling their head from side to side.

  Young children—Complain of the pain.
- Temperature 40°C is common.
- Cervical or post auricular lymph gland enlargement.
- Rhinorrhea.
- Vomiting and diarrhoea.
- Anorexia is common.
- Sucking or chewing—child has pain.
- Tympanic membrane may rupture. It relieves pain, decreases temperature, there is purulent discharge in the external auditory canal.
- Severe pain or fever is usually absent in serous otitis media.
- Feeling fullness in the ear.
- If chronic serous otitis media, conductive hearing loss in young children.

Investigation

- Otoscopy—shows redness, inflammation or bulging of the tympanic membrane is usually present.
- Audiometry.
- Tympanometry.

Treatment

- Suppuration otitis media—Administration of antibiotics especially ampicillin for 10–14 days.
- Myringotomy—drainage of the middle ear with insertion of tympanic membrane.
- Tympanostomy tube—pressure-equalizing tubes may be inserted to drain fluid from the middle ear.
- Decongestant.
- Analgesic and antipyretic drugs.
- Ear drops to promote comfort and relieve pain.

Nursing Management

1. *Recognize Present Signs and Symptom*
   - Older child
   - Assess for evidence of discomfort
   - Crying – complaining pain
   - Irritability
   - Lethargy
   - Anorexia

   Infant
   - Crying
   - Restless, irritable
   - Tendency to rub, hold the ear
   - Inspect external auditory canal (drainage)
   - Assess for learning impairment

2. *Eliminate Infective Agent*
   - Administration of antibiotics.
   - Emphasize the patient importance of regular administration of medication.
3. *Reduce Inflammation*
   - Administration of decongestants as prescribed.
   - Apply cold compress.
4. *Promote Comfort*
   - Positioning and comfort.
   - Instil soothing substance into internal ear.
   - Administration of analgesic.
   - Apply external heat or cool compresses.
   - Avoid chewing by offering liquid or soft food.
5. *Reduce Fever*
   - Administration of Antipyretic drugs.
   - Provide tepid sponge bath.
6. *Facilitate Drainage when Appropriate*
   - Position with affected ear.
7. *Prevent Skin Breakdown*
   - Keep skin around ear and pinna clean and dry.
   - Change the cotton when soiled with drainage.
8. *Prevent Complication*
   - Continue the medicine and ask the mother to come for follow up.
   - Avoid injuring ear or eardrum.
9. *Educate Parents*
   - Teach correct administration of medication.
   - Teach to recognize signs of hearing impairment in the infant or child.
   - Avoid water in the ear.

Chapter 6 ALTERED CARDIOVASCULAR FUNCTIONS

ANATOMY AND PHYSIOLOGY OF PAEDIATRIC DIFFERENCES

Transition from Fetal to Pulmonary Circulation

After the umbilical cord has been cut, the newborn must quickly adapt to receive oxygen from the lungs. The transition from foetal to pulmonary circulation occurs in just a few hours. During foetal circulation, the constricted pulmonary vessels limit blood flow to the lungs (high pulmonary vascular resistance). Blood, however, flows easily to the extremities because systemic vascular resistance is low. The foramen ovule, an opening between the atria in the foetal heart, allows blood to flow from the right to the left atrium. Systemic vascular resistance increases after the umbilical cord is cut, causing a backup of blood flow. The pressure in the left side of the heart increases stimulating closure of the foramen ovule. Once breathing has been initiated, the lungs expand and pulmonary vascular resistance falls. Blood that was previously shunted through the ductus arteriosus to the aorta flows to the lungs.

The ductus arteriosus, responding to higher oxygen saturation normally constricts and closes within 10 to 15 hours after birth, permanent closure occurs by 10 to 21 days after birth, unless oxygen saturation remains low. Fetal tissues are accustomed to low oxygen saturation. This may explain why newborns with cyanotic heart disease appear relatively comfortable even when the arterial partial pressure of oxygen (PaO_2) is 20 to 25 mm Hg. Older children and adults would rapidly develop acidosis and cerebral anoxia with such a low PaO_2.

The ventricles are equal in size at birth, but by 2 months of age the left ventricle is twice as large as the right ventricle. The higher systemic vascular pressures force the left ventricle to develop quickly.

Infants have a greater risk of heart failure than older children because the immature heart is more sensitive to volume or pressure overload. During infancy the muscle fibres of the heart are less developed and less organized, resulting in limited functional capacity. Less compliance (amount of distention or expansion the ventricles can achieve to increase stroke volume) of the heart muscle means that stroke volume cannot increase substantially. The heart muscle fibers develop during early childhood and by 9 years of age, the weight of the heart has increased by 6 times.

Normal Anatomy of Heart

- Completely normal diagram (all septa intact)
- Situs solitus
- Levocardia
- Normal atrioventricular connections
- Normal connected great arteries

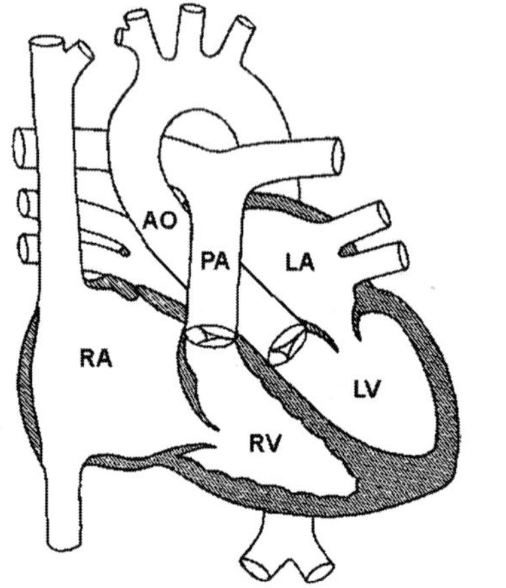

Fig. 6.1: Normal heart features

CONGENITAL HEART DISEASES

Congenital heart disease refers to a defect in the heart or great vessels or persistence of a foetal structure after birth. Congenital heart defects are estimated to occur in 1% of live births (American Heart Association).

Most congenital heart defects develop during the first 8 weeks of gestation.

They are usually the result of a combined or interactive effect of generic and environmental factors as follows:

- Foetal exposure to drugs such as phenytoin and lithium.
- Maternal viral infections such as rubella.

- Maternal metabolic disorders such as phenylketonuria and diabetes mellitus.
- Maternal complications of pregnancy such as increased age and antenatal bleeding.
- Genetic factors (family recurrence patterns).
- Chromosomal abnormalities such as Turner's syndrome, Noonan syndrome, Marfan syndrome, Downs syndrome and Trisomy syndromes 13, 15, 18 and 21.

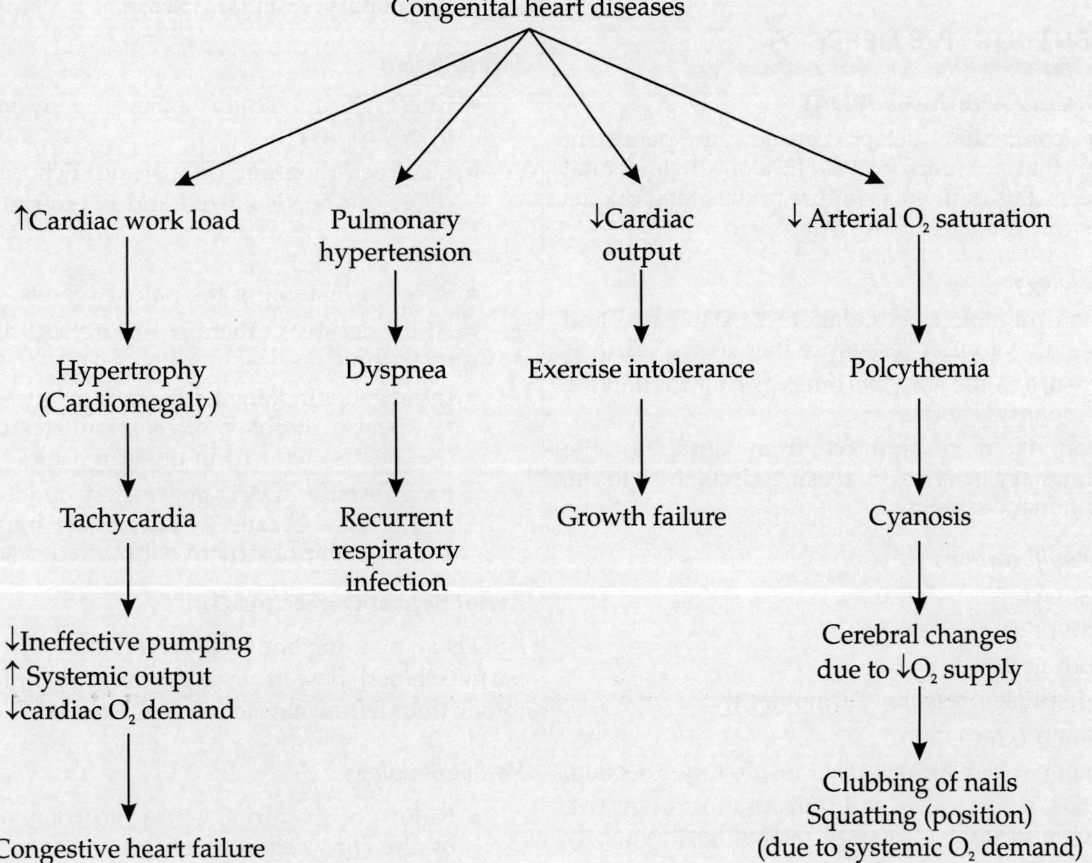

Pathophysiology (Compensatory Mechanism)

Children often have more than one defect at the same time. Depending on the type of the defect, signs and symptoms may be present at birth or develop later.

Congenital heart defects are generally divided into two categories,

1. Acyanotic (in which there is no mixing of unoxygenated blood in the systemic circulation).
2. Cyanotic (in which unoxygenated blood enters to the systemic circulation).

Clinical Manifestation

- Growth retardation
- Cardiac murmur
- ↓Exercise tolerance
- Recurrent respiratory infection
- Dyspnoea, tachypnea
- Tachycardia
- Cyanosis and tissue hypoxia
- Syncope
- Mental confusion
- Seizure

ACYANOTIC DEFECTS

The majority of children with congenital heart defects have acyanotic conditions. There are two types of acyanotic defects:

- Non-obstructive lesions which do not interfere with the flow of blood.
- Obstructive lesions which block the outflow of blood from the heart.

1. Non-obstructive defects include:

- Patent ductus arteriosus (PDA)
- Atrial septal defect (ASD)
- Ventricular septal defect (VSD)

- Atrioventricular (AV) canal defect (endocardial cushion defect)

2. Obstructive defects include:

- Pulmonic stenosis (PS)
- Aortic stenosis (AS)
- Coarctation of the aorta

NON-OBSTRUCTIVE DEFECTS

Patent Ductus Arteriosus (PDA)

Common congenital defect caused by persistent circulation that accounts for 9%–12% of all congenital heart defects. It is defined as failure of the foetal ductus arteriosus to completely close after birth.

Pathophysiology

- When pulmonary circulation is established and systemic vascular resistance increases at birth.
- Pressure in the aorta becomes greater than in the pulmonary arteries.
- Blood is then shunted from aorta to the pulmonary arteries, increasing circulation to the pulmonary system.

Clinical Manifestations

- Dyspnea
- Tachypnea
- Bonding pulse
- Wide pulse pressure, Cardiomegaly.
- Growth retardation.
- Infancy is risk for recurrent respiratory infection.
- If PDA is large size, child may go for congestive heart failure, intercostals retraction, hepatomegaly and growth failure.
- Continuous systolic murmur (machinery) is auscultated in mid and upper sternal border and thrill may be palpated in the pulmonary area.

Complications

- Congestive heart failure.
- Recurrent pneumonia.
- Bacterial endocarditis.
- Pulmonary hypertension.
- Pulmonary vascular disease.

Investigation

- Chest X-ray study (shows left ventricular hypertrophy).
- Electrocardiogram (ECG) and Echocardiogram (PDA can be visualized and left-to-right shunt).

Treatment

- Surgical ligation of the patent vessels.
- Anticongestive therapy—diuretics and fluid restriction.
- Intravenous indomethacin (Indocin) prostaglandin synthetase inhibitor often stimulates closure of the ductus ateriosus in preterm babies.

  Prognosis: If PDA is not treated, child's life span is shortened because of pulmonary hypertension and vascular obstructive disease develops.

Atrial Septal Defect (ASD)

ASD is an opening between the left and right atria and permits blood flow from left atrium to right atrium, rather than left atrium to left ventricle.

Pathophysiology

- Failure of the atrial septum to completely close by the 7th week of gestation.
- Blood shunts from the left atrium to the right atrium because left atrial pressure is normally slightly higher than right atrial pressure.

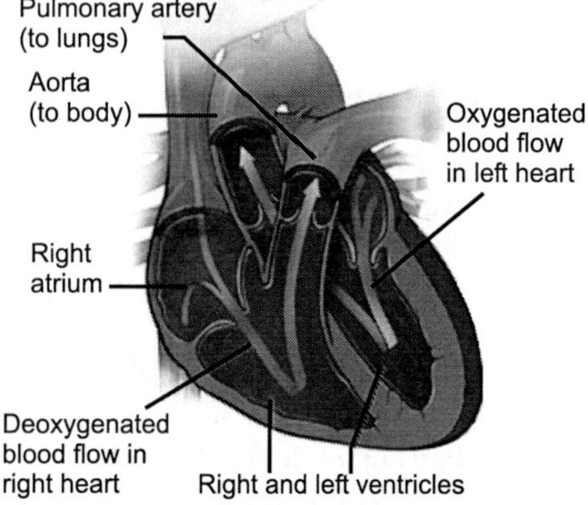

(A)

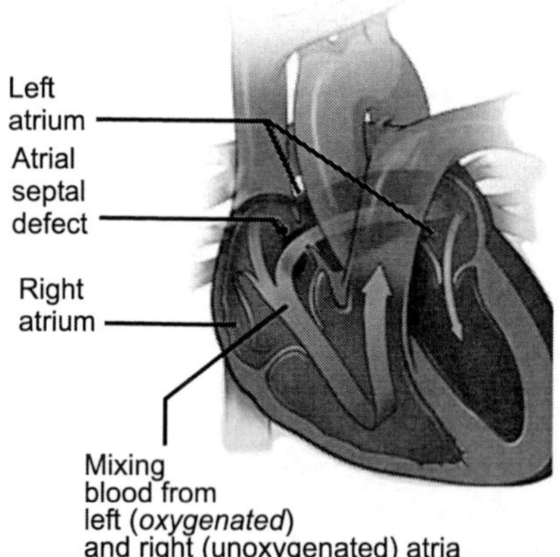

(B)

Fig. 6.2: (A) Normal heart (B) Heart with atrial septal defect

Clinical Manifestations

- Infants and young children usually have no symptoms.
- Children get easily tired (fatigue).
- Retarded growth with large size of ASD.
- Systolic ejection murmur ascultated to left sternal border in the pulmonic area with wide splitting of S_2.
- Dyspnea and fatigue on exertion.
- Clubbing of nails and cyanosis, if right-to-left shunt develops.

Investigation

- Chest X-ray (shows enlargement of right atrium and ventricle).
- Electrocardiogram (ECG).
- Echocardiography (determines the location and size of the defect, visualization of the shunt, RT ventricular enlargement).

Complications

- Heart failure
- Pulmonary hypertension
- Pulmonary vascular disease
- Bacterial endocarditis
- Atrial arrhythmias
- Stroke (rare)

Treatment

Surgical Closure

- Direct closure of the defect if small defect, purse string closure or large defect found with Dacron patch closure.
- Procedure is performed under cardiopulmonary bypass through an atrial approach.

Placement of an atrial occluder (done in the cardiac catheterization laboratory) is emerging as a prominent medical intervention for ASD closure.

Medication

- Digoxin (Lanoxin) and diuretics if signs and symptoms of heart failure are present.

Prognosis: Many persons uncorrected with small and moderate size ASDs have lived to middle age without symptoms; atrial arrythmias are common late complications.

Ventricular Septal Defect (VSD)

VSD is an opening in the septum between the ventricles that allows blood to shunt between the left and right ventricle.

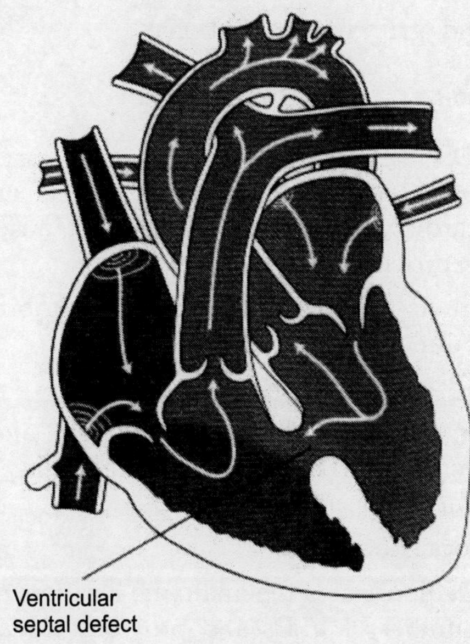

Fig. 6.3: Ventricular septal defect

Pathophysiology

- Delay in closure of the ventricle septum after the 7th week of gestation.
- As the pulmonary vasculature gradually relaxes (between 4 and 8 weeks after birth), right ventricular pressure decreases, allowing blood to shunt from the left to the right ventricle.
- Initially, large VSD shunts cause left atrial and left ventricle hypertrophy.
- Later, an uncorrected VSD causes right ventricle hypertrophy due to increasing pulmonary resistance; eventually biventricular heart failure occurs.

Clinical Manifestations

- Weight loss or absence of weight gain.
- Drop in height and head circumference percentile.
- Loud, harsh systolic murmur (along the left sternal border at third or fourth intercostals space), palpable thrill.
- Loud, widely split pulmonic component of S_2.
- Displacement to left of point of maximal impulse.
- Prominent anterior chest.

- Liver, heart and spleen enlargement.
- Diaphoresis.
- Tachycardia.
- Rapid, grunting respirations.

Investigation

- Chest X-ray
  - May be normal for small defects or shows cardiomegaly with a large left atrium and ventricle.
  - In a large defect, it may show prominent pulmonary vasculature.
- ECG
  - In a large defect shows left and right ventricular hypertrophy, suggesting pulmonary hypertension.
- Echocardiography
  - Demonstrates the anatomic location, size and number of VSDs and provides visualization of the shunt.
- Cardiac catheterization
  - Helps determine the size and number of the VSD.
  - Helps determine the degree of shunting.

Complications

- Bacterial endocarditis.
- Heart failure or pulmonary hypertension.
- Acquired left ventricular outflow tract obstruction.
- Aneurysm of the ventricular septum.
- Failure to thrive.
- Arrhythmia.
- Aortic insufficiency.
- Pulmonary stenosis.

Treatment

- Digoxin and diuretics if signs and symptoms of heart failure develop.
- Prophylactic antibiotics to prevent bacterial endocarditis.
- Oral iron therapy if anaemia develops.

Surgical Closure

- Direct closure of the defect with a patch or stitch closure.
- Performed under cardiopulmonary bypass or deep hypothermia, preferably through an atrial approach.

Prognosis: Pulmonic stenosis does not typically increase in severity, lifelong infective endocarditis prophylaxis is necessary.

Atrioventricular Canal Defect

A defect occurs when the endocardial cushions fail to fuse completely. The defect includes a low ASD continuous with a high VSD with clefts in the mitral and tricuspid valves (creating a common AV valve).

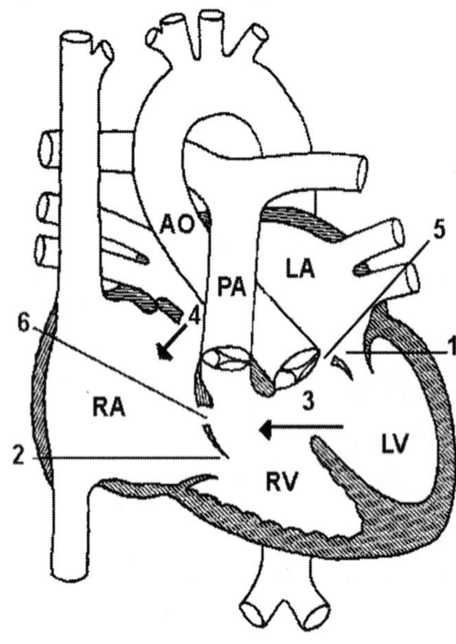

Fig. 6.4: Atrioventricular canal defect. 1. Left atrioventricular valve 2. Right atrioventricular valve 3. Inflow VSD (type III) 4. Ostium primum ASD 5. Cleft left atrioventricular valve 6. Cleft right atrioventricular valve

Pathophysiology

- Results from incomplete fusion of the endocardial cushions.
- Generally, blood is shunted from left to right once pulmonary vascular resistance drops; however, depending on the extent of the defect, blood may flow between all four heart chambers.

Clinical Manifestations

- Weight loss or absence of weight loss.
- Drop in height or head circumference percentile
- Signs of heart failure (usually present 6 to 8 weeks after birth due to the fall in pulmonary vascular resistance that normally occurs).

- Tachycardia.
- Tachypnea.
- Systolic regurgitant murmur heard at the left lower sternal border due to mitral insufficiency.
- Repeated respiratory failure.

Investigation

- Chest X-ray
  - Cardiomegaly.
  - Increased pulmonary vascular markings and prominent pulmonary artery segment.
- ECG
  - Shows right ventricular hypertrophy or right bundle branch block.
- Echocardiography
  - Determines the anatomy and functional significance of the atrioventricular canal defect and provides visualization of shunting and any regurgitation.

Treatment

- Frequent feedings of high-calorie formula, orally or through a nasogastric tube, to help reverse growth failure.
- Medications.
- Digoxin and diuretics if signs of heart failure develop.
- Prophylactic antibiotics to prevent bacterial endocarditis.
  - Surgical repair is indicated for all children with an AV canal defect.
  - Patch closure of the ASD and VSD, with reconstruction of the valves.
  - Procedure is performed under cardio-pulmonary bypass or deep hypothermia.

Nursing Management

- Explain the heart defect to the child and parents and answer any questions to prepare the child for cardiac catheterization or surgery.
- Monitor vital signs, pulse oximetry and intake and output to assess renal function and detect changes.
- Assess cardiovascular and respiratory status to detect early signs of decompensation.
- Monitor fluid status, enforcing fluid restriction as appropriate to prevent fluid overload.
- Weigh the child daily to determine fluid overload or deficit.
- Weigh soiled diapers to monitor fluid output.
- Organize physical care and anticipate the need to reduce the child's oxygen demands.
- Give the child high-calorie foods that are easy to ingest and digest.
- Raise the head of the bed to ease respiratory system.
- Take the child's apical pulse for 1 minute before giving digoxin.
- Withhold the drug to prevent toxicity if the child's heart rate is below 100 beats/minute.

OBSTRUCTIVE DEFECTS

Defects that obstruct the flow of blood out of the heart, including coarctation of the aorta, aortic stenosis and pulmonic stenosis.

Pulmonic Stenosis

Stenosis (narrowing of valve or valve area) can be above valve, below valve, or at valve. Stenosis obstructs blood flow into the pulmonary artery, which increases preload and results in right ventricular hypertrophy. Pulmonic stenosis is the second most frequent congenital heart defect, accounting for 8%–12% of all cases.

Causes

- Congenital
- Rheumatic fever

Pathophysiology

- Obstructed right ventricular outflow causes right ventricular hypertrophy, resulting in right-sided heart failure.

Complications

- Cyanosis
- Bacterial endocarditis
- Congestive heart

Clinical Manifestations

- May be asymptomatic
- Cyanosis
- Signs of heart failure
- Systolic ejection murmur heard loudest at 2nd left intracostal space of the upper left sternal border, split S_2.

Investigation

- Chest X-ray, ECG and echocardiography may show evidence of right ventricular hypertrophy.
- Cardiac catheterization demonstrates the degree of the stenosis.

Medical and Surgical Management

- Medications
  - Digoxin and diuretics for signs of heart failure.
  - Anticoagulant therapy to prevent bacterial endocarditis.
- Surgical repair
  - Balloon angioplasty is being used widely to relieve pulmonic stenosis.
  - Pulmonary valvulotomy may be necessary.

Nursing Interventions

- Explain the heart defect to the child and parents and answer any questions to prepare the child for cardiac catheterization or surgery.
- Monitor vital signs, pulse oximetry, and intake and output to assess renal function and detect changes.
- Assess cardiovascular and respiratory status to detect early signs of decompensation.
- Take the child's apical pulse for 1 minute before giving digoxin and withhold the drug to prevent toxicity if the child's heart rate is below 100 beats/minute.
- Monitor fluid status, enforcing fluid restrictions as appropriate to prevent fluid overload.
- Weigh the child daily to determine fluid overload or deficit.
- Weigh soiled diapers to monitor fluid output.
- Organize physical care and anticipate the need to reduce the child's oxygen demands.
- Give the child high calorie foods that are easy to ingest and digest.
- Raise the head of the bed to ease respiratory status.

Aortic Stenosis

Narrowing or fusion of the aortic valve obstructs blood flow to systemic circulation. Aortic stenosis accounts for 3%–6% of all cases of congenital heart defects. This defect is often associated with bicuspid rather than normal tricuspid valve. Stenosis is usually progressive during childhood.

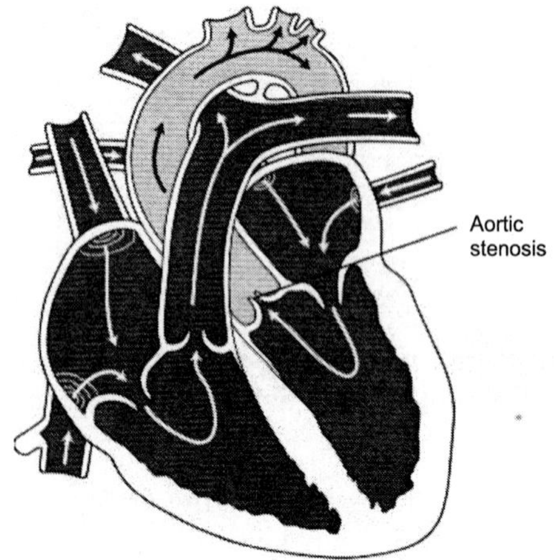

Fig. 6.5: Aortic stenosis of the heart

Causes

- Unknown
- Rheumatic fever

Pathophysiology

- Left ventricular pressure rises to overcome the resistance of narrowed valvular opening.
- The added workload increases the demand for oxygen and diminished cardiac output causes poor coronary artery perfusion, ischemia of the left ventricle and left-sided heart failure.

Complications

- Bacterial endocarditis
- Pulmonary edema
- Coronary insufficiency
- Ventricular failure
- Heart failure
- Sudden death due to myocardial ischemia.

Clinical Manifestations

- Rough, systolic murmur heard loudest at the second intercostals space
- Decreased cardiac output
- Exercise intolerance
- Diminished carotid pulses
- Systolic thrill
- Syncope
- Hypotension
- Poor feeding
- Angina—like chest pain on activity.

Investigation

- X-rays show
  - Left ventricular hypertrophy.
  - Prominent pulmonary vasculature.
- ECG shows left ventricular hypertrophy.
- Echocardiography
  - Thickened left ventricular wall.
  - Cardiac catheterization demonstrates the degree of the stenosis.

Medical Management

- Digoxin and diuretics for signs of heart failure.
- Anticoagulant therapy to prevent thrombus formation around the stenotic or replaced valve.
- Prophylactic antibiotics to prevent bacterial endocarditis.

Surgical Repair

- Aortic valvulotomy or prosthetic valve replacement (Commissurotomy).
- Balloon angioplasty may be used to dilate the stenotic valve.

Coarctation of the Aorta

Narrowing or constriction in the descending aorta, often near the ductus arterious, obstructs systemic blood flow. This defect is common, occurring in 5%–8% of all children with congenital heart disease.

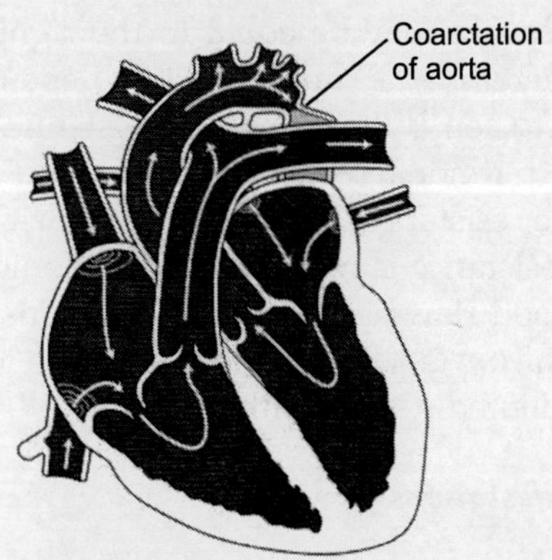

Fig. 6.6: Coarctation of aorta

Pathophysiology

- Obstruction causes hypertension in the aortic branches before the constriction and diminished pressure in the vessel after the constriction.

Clinical Manifestations

- High blood pressure.
- Blood pressure greater in upper extremities than in lower extremities.
- Pink upper extremities and cyanotic lower extremities.
- Absent or diminished femoral pulses.
- Continuous mid systolic murmur.
- Lower extremities cooler than upper extremities.
- Muscle cramps.
- Dizziness, headache, fainting and epistaxis.

Complications

- Rupture of the aorta.
- Systemic hypertension.
- Stroke and Intracranial haemorrhage.
- Congestive heart failure or shock in infancy.
- Left ventricular failure.
- Infective endocarditis.

Investigation

- Chest X-ray shows:
  - Left ventricular hypertrophy.
  - Pulmonary edema.
  - Wide ascending and descending aorta.
  - Rib notching from collateral circulation.
- Electrocardiogram shows:
  - Right ventricular hypertrophy or right bundle branch block in infant.
  - Left ventricular hypertrophy in children with long-standing coarctation of the aorta.
- Echocardiography shows:
  - Demonstrates the location, size and extent of the coarctation.
  - Increased left ventricular muscle thickness.
  - Coexisting aortic valve abnormalities.
- MRI
  - Reveals location of the coarctation of the aorta and determines whether other vessels are affected.

Management

Medical Management

- Prostaglandin E infusion to reopen or maintain a patent ductus arteriosus.

- Inotropic agents: dopamine, dobutamine.
- Prophylactic antibiotics to prevent bacterial endocarditis.

Surgical Management

- Performed without bypass through a left posterolateral thoracotomy.
- Types of repair:
  - *End-to-end anastomosis*: the area of coarctation is resected and the distal and proximal aorta are anastomosed end to end.
  - *Patch aortoplasty*: the area of coarctation is incised and an elliptical dacron patch is sutured in place to widen the diameter.
  - Subclavian flap aortoplasty the proximal portion of this vessel is used to expand the coarcted area.
  - Bypass graft repair is performed by inserting a graft between the ascending and descending portion of the aorta.
  - The ductus arteriosus is always ligated with each of these surgical techniques.
  - Balloon angioplasty may be performed if recoarctation occurs.

Nursing Interventions

- Explain the heart defect to the child and parents and answer any questions to prepare the child for surgery.
- Monitor vital signs, pulse oximetry and intake and output to assess renal function and detect changes.
- Assess cardiovascular and respiratory status to detect early signs of decompensation.
- Monitor fluid status, enforcing fluid restrictions as appropriate to prevent fluid overload.
- Weigh soiled diapers to monitor fluid output.
- Organize physical care and anticipate the need to reduce the child's oxygen demands.
- Give the child high-calorie foods that are easy to ingest and digest.
- Raise the head of the bed to ease respiratory status.

CYANOTIC HEART DEFECTS

Cyanotic heart defects are the most common heart defects in the children. These defects cause mixed blood flow, the oxygenated and deoxygenated blood mix in the heart or great vessels. The most common malformations of cyanotic heart disease are tetralogy of fallot, transposition of the great vessels and truncus arteriosus.

Tetralogy of Fallot

Tetralogy of fallot classic form includes four defects:

1. Ventricular septal defect
2. Pulmonic stenosis
3. Hypertrophy of right ventricule
4. Overriding aorta

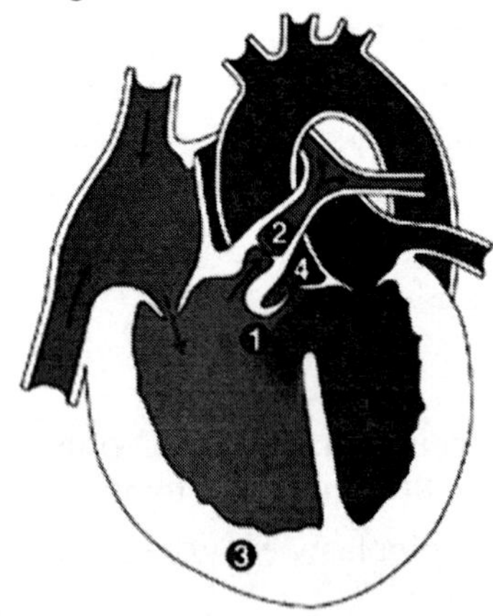

Fig. 6.7: Heart defect with Tetralogy of fallot

Pathophysiology

The altered haemodynamics varies widely, depending primarily on the degree of pulmonary stenosis, but also on the size of the VSD and the pulmonary and systemic resistance to flow. Because the VSD is large, the pressure may be equal to the right and left ventricles. Therefore the shunt direction depends on the difference between pulmonary and systemic vascular resistance. If pulmonary vascular resistance is higher than systemic resistance, the shunt is from right to left. If systemic resistance is higher than pulmonic stenosis decreases, blood flows to the lungs and, consequently, the amount of oxygenated blood from both ventricles may be distributed systemically.

Clinical Manifestations

Infants

- Cyanosis and hypoxia often called "blue spells."
- Anoxic spell occurs when the infants' oxygen requirement exceed the blood supply, usually during crying or often feeding.
- Infant may assume a knee chest position.

Children

- Delayed physical growth and development.

- Cyanosis.
- Diminished exercise intolerance and increased dyspnoea on exertion.
- Clubbing of the fingers.
- Squatting to relieve the chronic hypoxia.
- Difficulty in eating.
- Fainting and mental slowness in chronic hypoxia to the brain.
- Seizures.
- Pan systolic murmur heard at mid or lower left sternal border.

Investigation

- Chest X-ray-studies reveal a "boot shaped" due to the large RT ventricle with decreased pulmonary vascular markings.
- Electrocardiogram shows right ventricular hypertrophy.
- Echocardiography demonstrates VSD, obstruction of pulmonary outflow, and overriding aorta.
- Cardiac catheterization required before surgery to completely identify the location of all anatomic structures and any additional defects.

Complications

- Polycythemias, thrombophlebitis, embolism.
- Cerebrovascular diseases, brain abscess.
- Hyperpnoea with severe cyanosis leads to unconsciousness and death.

Surgical Management

Palliative Shunt

- In infants who cannot undergo primary repair, a palliative procedure to increase pulmonary blood flow and increase oxygen saturation may be performed.
- In the procedure an artificial opening is created between aorta and pulmonary artery to increase the pulmonary blood flow (Waterston–Cooley shunt), a side to side anastomosis of the ascending aorta to the right pulmonary artery in neonates.
- The preferred procedure is the Blalock-Taussing or modified Blalock-Taussing shunt, which provides blood flow to the pulmonary arteries from the left or right subclavian artery. (Blalock Taussing operation—a subclavian artery and pulmonary artery anastomosis in older infants and children.)
- In general, however, shunts are avoided because they may result in pulmonary artery distortion.

Complete Repair

- Elective repair is usually performed in the first year of life.
- Indications for repair include:
  - Increasing cyanosis and the development of hyper cyanotic spells.
  - Complete and the development of hyper cyanotic spells.
- Complete repair involves closure of the VSD and resection of the infundibular stenosis, with a pericardial patch to enlarge the right ventricular outflow tract. The procedure requires a median sternotomy and the use of cardiopulmonary bypass. (That is closure of the ventricular septal defect, pulmonic valvotomy as well as correction of the overriding aorta (3–4 yrs optimal age).

Prognosis: The operative mortality for total correction of TOF is less than 5% with improved surgical techniques, there is a lower incidence of arrhythmias and right ventricular dysfunction may be residual problems, surgical heart block is rare. CHF may occur postoperatively. Lifelong infective endocarditis prophylaxis is required.

Transposition of the Great Vessels

The pulmonary artery from left ventricle and the aorta exist from the right ventricle with no communication between systemic and pulmonary circulations.

Pathophysiology and Associated Defect

- The transposed pulmonary artery carries oxygenated blood back to the lungs, rather than to the left side of the heart.
- The transposed aorta returns unoxygenated blood to the systemic circulation rather than to the lungs.
- Communication between the pulmonary and systemic circulation is necessary for survival; the presence of other congenital defects, such as ASD or VSD, is necessary to sustain life.

Associated defects such as septal defects or patent ductus arteriosus must be present to permit blood to enter the systemic circulation and/or the pulmonary circulation mixing of unoxygenated and oxygenated blood. The most common defect associated with TGA is a Patent foramen ovale, PDA, VSD, presence of these defects increases the risk of congestive heart failure.

Clinical Manifestations

Clinical manifestations occur depending on the type and size of the associated defects.

- Child with minimal communication are severely cyanotic and depressed at birth.
- The large septal defect or PDA causes less cyanosis but may have symptoms of congestive heart failure.
- Cyanosis from birth and tachypnea (worsens with cry).
- Gallop rhythm
- Tachycardia
- Hepatomegaly
- Cardiomegaly
- Murmurs of ASD, VSD, or PDA, loud S_2
- Diminished exercise tolerance
- Fatigue
- Clubbing

Investigation

- Chest X-ray
  - Right atrial and ventricular enlargement causes a characteristic oblong appearance to heart.
  - Increased pulmonary vascular marking.
- Electrocardiogram
  - Demonstrates the reversed position of the aorta and pulmonary artery.
  - Detects other cardiac defects.
- Cardiac catheterization
  - Decreased oxygen saturation in left ventricular blood and aortic blood.
  - Increased right atrial, right ventricular, and pulmonary artery oxygen saturation.
  - Right ventricular systolic pressure equal to systemic pressure.
  - Dye injection reveals transposed vessels and the presence of any other cardiac defects.

Complications

- Bacterial endocarditis.
- Congestive heart failure, main hypoxia is the major cause for death.

Management

Medical Management

- Prostaglandin E to maintain potency of the ductus arteriosus.
- Prophylactic antibiotics to prevent bacterial endocarditis.
- Atrial ballon septostomy done during cardiac catheterization to enlarge the patent foramen ovale, which improves oxygenation by allowing greater mixing of the pulmonary and systemic circulations.

Surgical Treatment

- *Arterial switch procedure*: Corrective surgery to redirect blood flow by switching the position of the major blood vessels. Procedure of choice performed in first week of life.
- *Palliative surgery*
  1. Surgical creation of ASD. (Blalock–Halenoperes).
  2. Enlargement of an existing ASD by pulling balloons through the defect (balloon septotomy).
  3. Pulmonary artery banding to decrease blood flow to the lungs.
  4. Creation of a ductus arteriosus if pulmonic stenosis is present.

Complete Repair

- Intra atrial baffle repairs:
  - Intra atrial baffle repairs are rarely performed, although many adolescents and adults survive today with repairs that were done 10 to 25 years ago.
  - An intra atrial baffle is created to divert venous blood to the mitral valve and pulmonary venous blood to the tricuspid valve using the patient's atrial septum (Senning procedure) or a prosthetic material (Mustard procedure). Performed in first year of life. Atrio septopexy or mustard's operation involves removing the entire strient septum and creating a new atrial septum tream existing pericardium or a prosthesis that tunnels or baffles blood for more effective oxygenation (6–18 years of the age).
  - A disadvantage is the continuing role of the right ventricle as the systemic pump and the late development of right ventricular failure and rhythm disturbances.

- Other potential postoperative complications include loss of normal sinus rhythm, baffle leaks, and ventricular dysfunction.

Rastelli Procedure

- Operative choice in infants with TGA, VSD, and severe pulmonic stenosis (PS).
- It involves closure of the VSD with a baffle, directing left ventricular blood through the VSD into the aorta.
- The pulmonic valve is then closed, and a conduit is placed from the right ventricle to the pulmonary artery, creating a physiologically normal circulation. Unfortunately, this procedure requires multiple conduit replacements as the child grows.

Prognosis: Operative mortality is about 5% to 10% with all procedures; with atrial level repairs, there is a later risk of dysrhythmias and ventricular dysfunction.

Nursing Interventions

- Explain the heart defect to the child and parents and answer any questions to prepare the child for cardiac catheterization or surgery.
- Monitor vital signs, pulse oximetry, and intake and output to assess renal function and detect changes.
- Assess cardiovascular and respiratory statuses to detect early signs of decompensation.
- Monitor fluid status, enforcing fluid restrictions as appropriate to prevent fluid overload.
- Weigh the child daily to determine fluid overload or deficit.
- Weigh soiled diapers to monitor fluid output.
- Organize physical care and anticipate the need to reduce the child's oxygen demands.
- Give the child high-calorie foods that are easy to ingest and digest.
- Encourage parents to help their child assume new activity levels and independence.

Truncus Arteriosus

A single large vessel empties both ventricles. The failure of normal septation and division of the embryonic bulbar trunk in the pulmonary artery and aorta, results in a single vessel that overrides both ventricles. It is usually accompanied by a VSD.

Pathophysiology

Blood ejected from the left and right ventricles enters the common artery and flows either to the lungs or to the aortic arch and body. Pressure in the both ventricles is high and blood flow to the lungs is markedly increased.

Clinical Manifestations

- Cyanosis
- Left ventricular hypertrophy
- Dyspnea
- Retraction
- Increased respiratory infection
- Fatigue
- Clubbing
- Increased pulse pressure
- Activity intolerance
- Retarded growth
- Bounding pulse
- Cardiomegaly
- Poor appetite

Investigation

- Chest X-ray shows cardiomegaly and increased pulmonary blood flow.
- Electrocardiogram—indicates right or biventricular hypertrophy.
- Eechocardiography—provides visualization of the defect and a VSD.

Complications

- Congestive heart failure
- Hypoxia
- Infection endocarditis
- Brain abscess
- Cardiomegaly
- Pulmonary hypertension

Management

Medical Management

- Digoxin and diuretics to control heart failure

Surgical Management

Palliative surgery: Banding both pulmonary arteries as they arise from the truncus artieriosus, to the amount of blood flow to the lungs.

Corrective surgery: Closing the VSD and create a passage to pulmonary arteries, inserting a prosthetic valve (Rastelli) operation.

HYPOPLASTIC LEFT HEART SYNDROME

Definition

- Hypoplastic left heart syndrome is the underdevelopment of the left side of the heart defect and includes the following conditions:
  - Aortic valve atresia or stenosis.
  - Mitral valve atresia or stenosis.
  - Diminutive or absent left ventricle.
  - Severe hypoplasia of the ascending aorta and aortic arch.

Pathophysiology

- Blood from the left atrium travels through a patent foramen ovale to the right ventricle and pulmonary artery, entering the systemic circulation via the ductus arteriosus.
- Patency of the ductus arteriosus, which allows blood flow to the systemic circulation, is necessary to sustain life.

Clinical Manifestations

- Signs include tachpnea, retractions, cyanosis
- Peripheral edema
- Decreased peripheral pulses, poor peripheral pulses, poor peripheral perfusion,
- Pulmonary edema, and congestive heart failure eventually leading to shock, acidosis, and death

Complications

- Heart failure
- Death

Investigation

- Echocardiography provides visualization of the defect.

Management

- Medical management
  - Prostaglandin E to maintain patency of the ductus arteriosus.
  - Digoxin and diuretics to control heart failure.
- Surgical repair is done in three stages:
  - Norwood procedure first—anostomosis of the main pulmonary artery to the aorta to create a new aorta, shunting to provide pulmonary blood flow and creation of a large atrial septal defect.
  - Bidirectional Glenn shunt procedure is a two-stage procedure done at 6 to 9 months of age to relieve the cyanosis and reduce the volume load on the right ventricle. It involves final repair and is a modified Fontan procedure restructuring the heart.
  - Without surgery, death occurs in early infancy.
  - Heart transplantation may be performed depending upon the condition of the child.

Nursing Interventions

- Explain the heart defect to the child and parents and answer any questions to prepare the child for surgery.
- Monitor vital signs, pulse oximetry, and intake and output to assess renal function and detect any change from the child.
- Assess cardiovascular and respiratory status to detect early signs of decomposition.
- Monitor fluid status, enforcing fluid restrictions as appropriate to prevent fluid overload to the child.
- Take the child's apical pulse for one minute before giving dioxin, and withhold the drug to prevent toxicity if the child's heart rate is below 100 beats/minute.
- Weigh the child daily to determine fluid overload or deficit.
- Weigh soiled diapers to monitor fluid output accurately.
- Organize physical care and anticipate the need to reduce the child's oxygen demands.

COMMON SIGNS AND SYMPTOMS OF CARDIAC DISEASES IN INFANTS

1. Cry—weak and muffled, loud and breathless
2. Colour
   (*a*) *Cyanotic*—usually generalized, in supine position often unrelieved by oxygen, usually deepens with crying, gray, dusky, mild, moderate, severe.

(*b*) *Acyanotic*—pale with or without mottling on exertion.

3. Activity level
   - Restless
   - Lethargic
   - Unresponsive except to pain
   - Lack of movement of arms and legs when crying
   - Arms become flaccid when eating
4. Posturing
   - Hypotonic – flaccid even when sleeping
   - Hyper extension of neck
   - Dyspnea when supine
   - Powers knee-chest position
5. Persistent bradycardia < 120/minute
6. Respiration
   - Tachypnea respiratory rate 60/minute
   - Retraction of chest with nasal flaring
   - Dyspnea with grunting
   - Grasping followed by 2–3 minutes gaps
   - Chronic cough
7. Feeding behaviour
   - Anorexia
   - Poor suck-due to dyspnea
   - Difficulty in coordinating, sucking, swallowing, breathing slow
   - Unable to feed by nipple

GENERAL NURSING CARE OF THE CHILD WITH CONGENITAL HEART DISEASES

1. Observe for signs or symptoms of congenital heart disease
   - Observe the physical and behavioural characteristics
   - Observe for signs and complications
   - Unconscious, congestive heart failure
   - Convulsion, cerebral vascular accident
2. Assist with diagnosis
   - History collection
   - Physical assessment
   - Investigation
   - Prepare the child for cardiac catheterization
3. Help the parents and child adjust to diagnosis
4. Improve the efficiency of heart
   - Administration of digoxin
     - Check the medicine dose, before giving check pulse rate for 1 full minute. If heart beat is less than 90–110 beat/minute in young infant, and 70–85 beat/minute in older children, nurse should skip the dose and inform to the physician.
   - Assess adequate intake of the child by maintaining intake and output chart.
   - Monitor the potassium level.
5. Reduce cardiac demand
   - Reduce the physical activity
   - Avoid high temperature (Fever).
6. Maintain Nutrition
   - Encourage the child to take a well balanced diet
   - Discourage food with high salt content; don't add extra salt to the child's food.
7. Prevent infection
   - Avoid contact with infected person
   - Provide for adequate rest
8. Prevent potassium depletion
   - Give potassium rich food
   - Maintain with fruit juice
9. Correct anaemia—administration, iron tablets should be given according to the instructions
10. Recognize signs of complicating factors
    - CHF, pneumonia
    - Digitalis toxicity, Hypoxia
11. Reduce parent's fears and anxieties
    - Expose the feeling of the parents
    - Help child understand his defect
    - Explain about palliative or corrective defect
    - Assist in providing financial support

CONGESTIVE HEART FAILURE

Congestive heart failure is a disorder of circulation in which cardiac output is inadequate to support the body's circulatory and metabolic needs. It may result from a congenital heart defect that causes increased pulmonary blood flow or obstruction to the blood outflow tract, from problems with heart contractility, or from pathologic conditions that require high cardiac output, such as severe anaemia, acidosis, or respiratory problem.

Etiology

- Pulmonary venous congestion
- Systemic venous congestion
- Impaired cardiac output
- High metabolic rate
- Congenital heart defect

Pathophysiology

Congenital heart defects are the most common cause of congestive heart failure in children.

- The congestive heart failure develops as a result of congenital defect. Some defects allow blood to flow from the left side of the heart to the right so that extra blood must be pumped to the pulmonary system rather than through the aorta when the left ventricle contracts. This overloads the pulmonary system, and if prolonged can lead to pulmonary artery hypertension, an often irreversible condition leading to life threatening pulmonary vascular resistance.
- Obstructive congenital defects (*i.e.*, abnormally small pulmonary vessels) restrict the flow of blood so the heart hypertrophies to work harder to force blood through these structures. This increases cardiac output initially, but eventually gets hypertrophied.
- Muscle becomes ineffective. Initially the right or left side of the heart may fail, but eventually failure is bilateral.
- When cardiac output remains insufficient, the body's organs and tissues do not receive adequate oxygen. The kidneys respond to the lowered circulating volume by activating the rennin—angiotensin mechanism to retain salt and water.
- A sympathetic response increases the heart rate and heart muscle contractility. Both responses increase cardiac output to the vital organs. Without intervention, the compensatory mechanisms increase their intensity, demanding more effort from the compromised heart. This results in progressive systemic edema and pulmonary congestion.

Clinical Manifestations

Congestive heart failure often develops subtly, and symptoms may not be recognized at first.

- The infant tires easily, especially during feeding.
- Weight loss or lack of normal weight gain
- Diaphoresis
- Irritability and frequent infections may be evident.
- Older children may have exercise intolerance, dyspnea, abdominal pain or distension, and peripheral oedema.

As the disease progresses, symptoms such as

- Tachycardia, pallor or cyanosis
- Nasal flaring, grunting, retractions, cough, or crackles may occur.
- Generalized fluid volume overload is seen more commonly in toddlers and older children. Periorbital and facial edema, jugular vein distension, and hepatomegaly are signs of fluid volume excess.
- Cardiomegaly occurs as the heart attempts to maintain cardiac output.
- Cyanosis, weak peripheral pulses, cool extremities, hypotension, and heart murmur are precursors of cardiogenic shock, which can occur if congestive heart failure is not adequately treated.

Investigation

- X-ray reveals cardiac enlargement and venous congestion or pulmonary oedema.
- Echocardiography too may be performed to diagnose specific cardiac defect or dysfunction.

Medical Management

Goal

1. Increase the cardiac function (To make the heart work more efficiently).
2. Remove excess fluid, (Decreased preload).
3. Decrease cardiac demand.
4. Improve tissue oxygenation and decrease oxygen consumption.

Improve cardiac function: There are two groups of drugs which are used to enhance myocardial performance in CHF.

1. Digitalis glycosides, which improve the contractility.
2. Angiotensin-converting enzyme inhibitors, which reduce the after load on the heart, it makes easier for the heart to pump. (to lessen the workload of the heart and help it to work more efficiently).

Digitalis has three actions:

- Increases the force of contraction (positive inotropic).
- Decreases the heart rate (negative chronotropic) and slows conduction of impulses through the AV node (negative dromotropic).
- Indirectly enhances diuresis by increased renal perfusion.

Digoxin is the drug most commonly used to improve the heart's ability to contract and therefore increase its output. Occasionally a higher than normal dose is given initially, followed by a lower maintenance dose.

This process, called digitalization, speeds the child's response to the drug; B-blockers are used in some cases to reduce the effects of catecholamine on heart rate and contractility.

- Remove accumulated fluid and sodium, diuretics, such as furosemide are the most commonly used medication during hospitalization; thiazides are commonly used to maintain diuresis at home. Because most diuretics (except for spironolactone) cause potassium loss, serum potassium levels are monitored and potassium supplements may be ordered. Avoid salt content of food. Low salt formula are available and should be provided to the child.
- Decrease cardiac demand Vasodilating drugs may be given to reduce pulmonary and systemic vasoconstriction and to decrease the work of the heart.

Surgery or interventional catheterization to correct a congenital heart defect may become the treatment of choice, as occurred with brandy. Cardiac transplantation may be performed for children with end-stage cardiomyopathy or complex congenital heart defects such as hypoplastic left heart syndrome.

Other medical therapy is supportive. Airway management, ventilatory support, rest, and fluid and dietary management are also part of the treatment plan. Oxygen may be ordered. Most children improve rapidly after medication is administered.

Nursing Management

1. Maintain the cardiac output
   - Administer digoxin as ordered.
   - Take apical pulse and listen to heart sounds regularly, especially before each dose of digoxin. Record apical pulse with each recorded dose of digoxin.
   - Use cardiac monitor if ordered.
   - Prevent injury by monitoring for digoxin sideeffects and serum potassium level.
   - Provide for rest periods each hour.
2. Maintain adequate oxygenation
   - Place child in semi-Fowler's position.
   - Evaluate respiratory rate and sounds. Take pulse oximetry readings to determine oxygen saturation.
   - Provide oxygen and humidification if ordered. Observe for diaphoresis, a sign of increased respiratory effort.
3. Maintain fluid balance
   - Nursing care priority intervention: Fluid Management, Promotion of fluid balance and prevention of complications resulting from abnormal or undesired fluid levels.
   - Measure intake and output carefully. Weigh diapers to obtain output of young child.
   - Maintain fluid-restricted diet if ordered.
   - Administer diuretics as ordered.
   - Monitor electrolytes.
   - Weigh daily.
   - Measure abdominal girth daily if present. Observe for peripheral oedema.
4. Maintain the child skin integrity
   - Nursing care priority intervention: pressure management, minimizing pressure to body parts.
   - Provide skin care for edematous body parts and elevate extremities.
   - Change child's position frequently.
   - Inspect skin frequently for redness and skin breakdown over pressure points.
5. Maintain Nutritional Status of the child
   - Nursing care priority intervention involves nutrition management: Assistance with or provision of a balanced dietary intake of food and fluids.
   - Hold the infant at 45° angle for feeding.
   - Record intake carefully.
   - Weigh child daily.
   - Give frequent small meals with rest periods in-between. Give high-calorie snacks.
   - Use soothing approaches such as holding infants for feeding, having parents and eat with older child.

6. Reduce the anxiety of the family
   - Nursing priority intervention: Family Involvement, facilitating family participation in the emotional and physical care of the child.
   - Encourage parents to stay with child, explain procedures and treatment, involve parents in care as much as possible.
   - Involve parents with child during play periods.
   - At discharge, provide clear instructions and information about what to do in an emergency, and whom and where to call with questions.
   - Allow parents to verbalize questions, concerns, and feelings. Refer parents to support groups or other resources as needed.

RHEUMATIC FEVER

Rheumatic fever is a poorly understood autoimmune reaction to group A β–haemolytic, streptococcal pharyngitis. It is a self limited disease that involves the joints, skin, brain, serous surfaces and heart.

Causes

- Streptococcal infections (upper respiratory tract infection).

Pathophysiology

- Hyper sensitivity reaction to a group A beta-haemolytic streptococcal infection in which antibiotics are manufactured to combat streptococci reaction and produce characteristic lesions at specific tissue sites, especially in the heart and joints.
- Results in antigen-antibody complexes that ultimately destroy heart tissue.
- Rheumatic heart diseases refer to cardiac manifestation of rheumatic fever:
  - Pancarditis (myocarditis, pericarditis and endocarditis) during the early acute phase.
  - Chronic valvular disease later.
- The principal manifestation of RF is observed in the heart, joints, skin and central nervous system.
- Inflammatory haemorrhagic bullous lesions called *Aschoff bodies* are formed, which cause swelling, fragmentation and alteration in connective tissue.
- Aschoff bodies are found in virtually all patients with clinical rheumatic activity. These lesions are found in the heart, blood vessels, brain and serous surface of the joints and pleura.

Clinical Manifestations

Guidelines for the diagnosis of initial attach of Rheumatic fever (Jones Criteria, 2009).

Clinical manifestations are classified into two: Major and Minor criteria.

Table 6.1: Major and Minor Clinical Manifestations

Major Manifestations	Minor Manifestations
• Carditis • Polyarthritis • Chorea • Erythema marginatum • Subcutaneous nodules + • Streptococcal infection evidence (ASLO titer)	• Clinical findings • Arthralgia • Fever • Laboratory findings • Elevated acute phase reactions • Erythrocyte sedimentation rate • C-reactive protein • Prolonged PR interval

A firm diagnosis requires that two major or one major and two minor criteria are satisfied in addition to evidence of recent streptococcal infection.

Investigation

- Antistreptolysin –O titer (ASLO) is elevated.
- Throat culture – Positive throat culture or rapid strep antigen test for group A streptococci.
- Erythrocyte sedimentation rate is increased.
- ECG -shows prolonged PR interval.
- Echocardiography helps evaluate valvular damage, chamber size, and ventricular function.
- Cardiac catheterization evaluates valvular damage and left ventricular function in severe cardiac dysfunction.

Medical Management

The goals of medical management are:

- Eradication of haemolytic streptococci.
- Prevention of permanent cardiac damage.
- Palliation of the other symptoms.

- Prevention of recurrences of RF. Penicillin is the drug of choice with erythromycin as a substitute in penicillin-sensitive children.
- Salicylates are used to control the inflammatory process, especially in the joints, and reduce the fever and discomfort.
- Prednisone may be indicated in patients with pancarditis and valvular involvement. Bed rest is recommended during the acute febrile phase but need not be strict.
- Prophylactic treatment against recurrence of RF is started after the acute therapy and involves monthly intramuscular injections of benathine penicillin G (1.2 million U), two daily oral doses of penicillin (200,000 U), or one daily dose of sulfadiazine (1 g).

Nursing Management

The objectives of nursing care for the child with RF are:

1. Encourage compliance with drug regimens.
2. Facilitate recovery from the illness.
3. Provide emotional support.
4. Prevent recurrence of the disease.
   - Monitor vital signs and intake and output to detect fluid volume overload or defect
   - Institute safety measures for chorea; maintain a calm environment, reduce stimulation, avoid the use of forks or glass and assist in walking to prevent injury.
   - Encourage bed rest as ordered; assist in arranging for home schooling and diversified activities as needed.
   - Provide appropriate passive stimulation to maintain growth and development.
   - Provide emotional support for long-term convalescence to help relieve anxiety.
   - Note a history of and monitor for penicillin allergy.
   - Promote good dental hygiene to prevent gingival infection; make sure the child and his family understand the need to comply with prolonged antibiotic therapy and follow-up care and the need for additional antibiotics during dental surgery or procedures.

Chapter 7 ALTERED GASTROINTESTINAL FUNCTIONS

DIAGNOSTIC TESTS

Barium or Meglumine Diatrizoate (Gastrografin) Swallow

- Purpose
  - Primarily used to examine the oesophagus
  - Gastrografin and barium facilitate imaging through X-rays, but gastrografin is less toxic if it escapes from the GI tract
- Nursing interventions
  - Explain the procedure to the child and its parents
  - Maintain the procedure to the child on a nothing–by–mouth status beginning at midnight before the test
  - Tell the child that he must hold still during X-ray
  - After the test
    - Monitor bowel movements for excretion of barium
    - Monitor GI function.

Upper GI Imaging

- Purpose
  - Upper GI series
    - Swallowed barium moves into the oesophagus, stomach and duodenum to reveal abnormalities.
    - Barium outlines stomach walls and delineates ulcer craters and filling defects.
  - Small–bowel series
    - An extension of the upper GI series.
    - Visualizes barium flowing through the small intestine to the ileocecal valve.
- Nursing interventions
  - Explain the procedure to the child and its parents.
  - Tell the child that it must hold still during the X-ray.
  - Make sure the lead apron is properly placed around the genital area.
  - After the test
    - Monitor bowel movement for excretion of barium.
    - Monitor GI function.

Barium Enema (Lower GI Series)

- Purpose
  - Allows X-ray visualization of the colon.
- Nursing interventions
  - Explain the procedure to the child and its parents.
  - Usually, the child will follow a liquid diet for 24 hours before the test.
  - Bowel preparations are administered before the examination.
  - Tell the child that X-rays will be taken on a test table and that it must hold still.
  - Cover the genital area with a lead apron during X-ray.

Stool Specimen

- Purpose
  - Examined for suspected GI bleeding, infection, or malabsorption.
  - Tests include the guaiac test for occult blood and microscopic tests for ova, parasites and fat.
- Nursing interventions
  - Obtain the specimen in the correct container (container may need to be sterile or contain preservative).
  - Be aware that the specimen may need to be transported to the laboratory immediately or placed in the refrigerator.

Fiber-optic Testing

- Purpose
  - Esophagogastroduodenoscopy—a fiber-optic scope is inserted to allow direct visual inspection of the esophagus, stomach and duodenum.
  - Proctosigmoidoscopy—the rectum and distal sigmoid colon are inspected directly.
  - Colonoscopy—the descending, transverse and ascending colon are inspected directly.
- Nursing interventions
  - Explain the procedure to the child and its parents.
  - Obtain written, informed consent.
  - A mild sedative may be administered before the examination.
  - The child may be kept on nothing by mouth status beginning at midnight before the test.
  - The child may be placed on a liquid diet for 24 hours before the examination or require enemas and laxatives until clear.

Endoscopic Retrograde Cholangiopancreatography (ERCP)

- Purpose
  - Contrast media is injected into the duodenal papilla to allow radiographic examination of the pancreatic ducts and hepatobiliary tree.
- Nursing interventions
  - Before the procedure
    - Explain the procedure to the child and its parents.
    - Obtain written, informed consent.
    - Check the child's history for allergies to cholinergic and iodine.
    - Administer a sedative and monitor the child for the drug's effect.
  - After the procedure
    - Monitor the child's gag reflex (the child remains on nothing by mouth status until his gag reflex returns).
    - Protect the child from aspiration of mucus by positioning the child on his side.
    - Monitor the child for urine retention.

GI Intubation

- Purpose
  - To empty the stomach and intestine.
  - To aid diagnosis and treatment.
  - To decompress obstructed areas.
  - To detect and treat GI bleeding.
  - To administer medications or feedings.
- Nursing interventions
  - Maintain accurate intake and output records
    - Record the amount, colour, odour and consistency of gastric drainage every 4 hours.
    - When irrigating the tube, note the amount of normal saline solution instilled and aspirated.
  - Check for fluid and electrolyte imbalances.
  - Provide good oral and nasal care; make sure the tube is secured but that it isn't causing pressure on the nostrils.
  - To support the tube's weight and prevent its accidental removal, anchor the tube to the child's clothing.
  - Check tube placement by checking gastric pH.
  - After removing the tube from a child with GI bleeding, watch for signs and symptoms of recurrent bleeding.
  - Maintain a calm and reassuring manner and provide emotional support because many children panic at the sight of the tube.

NURSING DIAGNOSES

Probable Nursing Diagnoses

- Bowel incontinence
- Constipation
- Delayed growth and development
- Diarrhoea
- Imbalanced nutrition: Less than body requirements
- Imbalanced nutrition: More than body requirements
- Impaired swallowing
- Risk for infection
- Nausea

Possible Nursing Diagnoses

- Feeding self care deficit
- Impaired oral mucous membrane
- Risk for aspiration
- Risk for constipation
- Risk for imbalanced nutrition: More than body requirements.

APPENDICITIS

Definition

- Inflammation and obstruction of the blind sac at the end of the caecum (appendix).
- Most common major surgical disease in children.

Causes

- Results from an obstruction of the appendicial lumen caused by a foecal mass, stricture, or viral infection.
- Common in school age children.

Pathophysiology

- Obstruction starts an inflammatory process that can lead to infection, thrombosis, necrosis and perforation.

Complications

- Ischemic bowel
- Gangrene
- Bowel perforation
- Peritonitis.

Assessment Findings

- Abdominal pain and tenderness that begins as diffused, then localizes in the lower right quadrant at McBurney's point.
- Fever.
- Increased White Blood Cell (WBC) count.
- Rebound tenderness, especially in the right lower quadrant.
- Decreased bowel sounds, nausea, vomiting and anorexia.
- Abdominal distension, rigidity and guarding.
- Symptoms of peritonitis if a rupture occurs: fever, sudden relief of pain followed by a diffused pain.

Diagnostic Test Findings

- Elevated WBC count, with increased immature cells.

Medical Management

- Surgical intervention (appendectomy)
- If peritonitis develops:
  - GI intubation.
  - Parenteral replacement of fluids and electrolytes.
  - Administration of antibiotics.

Nursing Interventions

- Position the child preoperatively in a semi-Fowler's or right side lying position to decrease pain.
- Never apply heat to the right lower abdomen; this may cause the appendix to rupture.
- Be aware that, postoperatively, the child with a ruptured appendix may have a drain and a Nasogastric (NG) tube is attached to low intermittent suction.
- Resume oral nutrition when bowel sounds reappear.
- Administer antibiotics and pain medication.

MECKEL'S DIVERTICULAM

Meckel's Diverticulam, is a pouch or a small bulge at the omphalomesentric duct which connects the mid gut to the yolk sac. During early embryonic development period, ducts to completely obliterate. By the small appendiceal process it grows long and wide at times, it may be connected to the umbilicus by a cord.

Cause

Congenital defect.

Pathophysiology

Ectopic mucosa (gastric acid or pepsin)

↓

Irritates the bowel, erodes the surface

↓

It produces ulceration in the ileum or in the diverticulam

↓

Leads to haemorrhage, perforation and peritonitis

↓

Diverticulam causes intestinal adhesions

↓

Causes Strangulation or Intussusception

↓

Leads to Intestinal Obstruction

Clinical Manifestations

- Rectal bleeding
- Bright red or dark red rectal to bleeding
- Black tarry stools
- Severe anaemia and shock (due to haemorrhage)

Investigation

- History of the child—present and past history
- Rectosigmoidoscopy
- Barium enema
- Blood studies to identify infection and anaemia

Management

- If severe increase, the surgical risk

Medical Intervention

- To correct hypovolemic shock,
  - By administration of blood replacement.
  - Intravenous adminstration of fluid
  - Administration of oxygen.
  - Administration of antibiotics

Surgical Treatment: Recesection of diverticulam by Laporatomy.

INTUSSUSCEPTION

Intussusception is invaginations of a bowel segment or telescoping of one portion of the intestine into another, the most common site being the ileocecal valve.

Causes

- Unknown in most cases
- May result from polyps, hyperactive peristalsis or an abnormal bowel lining
- Viral infections

Pathophysiology

Telescoping of gut

↓

Obstruction of the passage in intestinal contents occurs beyond the defect.

↓

Two walls of the intestine press against each other-causing

↓

Inflammation, edema

↓

Decreased blood flow to affected part

↓

Necrosis results with haemorrhage, perforation and peritonitis.

Clinical Manifestations

- Acute abdominal pain.
- Vomiting and passing of one normal brown stool.
- Screaming of child and drawing his knees up to his chest.

If worse condition:

- Vomiting increases
- Child apathetic
- Intermittent attacks of colicky pain (screaming, drawing knees to chest, sweating, grunting).
- Emesis containing bile or foecal material.
- Child passes red, currant jelly like stool, nonfaecal stool mixed with blood and mucus.
- Abdominal distension.
- Mass felt-in upper Right quadrant region.
- Fever
- peritonitis
- Distended and tender abdomen with a palpable, sausage shaped abdominal mass.

Complications

- Bowel obstruction
- Strangulation of the intestine
- Gangrene
- Shock

- Bowel perforation
- Peritonitis
- Death, especially if treatment is delayed for more than 24 hours.

Investigation

- Barium enema
- Rectal examination
- Abdominal X-ray
- Ultrasound or computerized tomography shows a soft tissue mass and signs of complete or partial obstruction.
- Increased WBC count in blood.

Medical Management

- Insertion of an NG tube to decompress the intestine and minimize vomiting.
- Hydrostatic reduction
  - Air pressure or solution of barium or water – soluble contrast is introduced to the rectum.
  - Force from fluid or air moves invaginated bowel back into its original position.

Surgery

- Indications
  - Failure of hydrostatic reduction
  - Recurrent intussusception
  - Signs of shock or peritonitis.
- Manual reduction performed first by pulling the intussusception back through the bowel.
- Resection of the affected bowel segment if gangrenous or strangulated and anastomosis of the colon.

Nursing Interventions

- Prepare for enema (barium or water-soluble contrast) to confirm the condition and reduce the invagination by hydrostatic pressure.
- Monitor vital sign's; a change in temperature may indicate sepsis.
- Monitor intake and output to prevent dehydration.
- Monitor NG tube output and replace volume lost, as ordered.
- Monitor the child who has undergone hydrostatic reduction for the passage of stools (and barium if used) to determine the need for surgery.

Postoperative Interventions

- Administer antibiotics as ordered to prevent infection.
- Monitor incision site for any signs of infection (inflammation, drainage, or suture separation).
- Monitor for the return of bowel sounds to allow advancement of the diet.
- Offer emotional support and encouragement to the parents who are usually unprepared for their child's emergency surgery and recovery.

GASTROENTERITIS

It is an inflammation of stomach and intestine. It is a common disorder in children passing of motion or stool more than 3 loose stools in a day or 24 hours called diarrhoea.

There are two types—Acute and Chronic. Diarrhoea for less than 14 days is called acute, if diarrhoea persists for 14 days or more it is called chronic.

Causes

- Bacteria: *Shgella, Salmonella, Vibro cholerae, Staphylococcus, Escherichia coli.*
- Virus: Rota virus, adenovirus, astrovirus, calcivirus.
- Parasites: *Entameoba hystolytica, Giardia, Lambin, Trichuris.*
- Socioeconomic factors: Poverty, malnutrition, low standard of living
- Immuno deficiency
- Poor personal hygiene
- Contaminated foods (milk, water food)
- Lactose intolerance
- Anatomical defect
- Neoplasm
- Faulty preparation of infant formula or other food

Pathophysiology

Invading of organism

↓

Inflammation of the epithelial layer of intestine

↓

Destruction of cells in the intestine

↓

It increase in fluid is the cause of diarrhoea

Clinical Manifestations

Clinical manifestations occur depending upon the severity of the illness. If it is severe it causes dehydration.

- Little to extreme loss of subcutaneous fat
- 50% total weight loss
- Decreased urine output
- Poor skin turgor, dry skin and dry mouth and lips
- Sunken fontanels and eyes
- Low blood pressure and high pulse
- Child has irritability
- Restlessness, weakness
- Colour will be pallor
- Hyperpnoea
- Stools have loose fluid having green or yellow green colour
- Fever (low grade)
- Anorexia
- Vomiting.

Investigation

- History collection for duration of illness
- Frequency of stool/day, appearance, consistency, colour, quantity, mucus or blood, etc.
- Vomiting
- Thirst is normal or more, urine output normal or less.
- Clinical evaluation
- Bacteriological culture from the rectal swabs
- Electrolytic studies
- Stool examination

COMPLICATIONS

Dehydration

Classification of Dehydration According to WHO, IMNCI Manual 2008

- Severe dehydration
- Some dehydration
- No dehydration

Some Dehydration or Mild (Clinical Features)

- Irritability and disrupted sleep or restlessness
- Sunken eyes
- Drinks eagerly, thirsty
- Skin pinch goes back slowly and similar other signs
- Low grade fever
- Possibly vomiting

Treatment

- Assess the degree of dehydration
- Oral dehydration therapy upto 2 years 50–100 ml after each loose stool, 2 years or more 100 to 200 ml after each loose stool.
- Encourage the mother to continue the breast feeding.
- Anti-diarrhoeal treatment (Metronitazole) electrolytic studies.
- Intravenous fluid-RL, Normal Saline 5% stool examination.
- Reduction of formula feeding (Low fat and CHO diets).
- Continue breast feeding.
- Oral 5% glucose saline solution every 3–4 hrs.
- Administration of ORS.

Severe Dehydration (Clinical Feature)

- Temperature (104°C–106°C) with vomiting
- Anorexia
- Abdominal cramps
- Greenish stool because of unchanged bile content, containing mucus and possibly tinged with blood
  - Lethargic or unconscious
  - Sunken eyes
  - Not able to drink or drinks poorly and other signs
  - Stools become frequent
  - Infant may be stupor
  - Irritability
  - Convulsion
  - Mouth or lips become dry and the skin loses its turgor (skin pinch goes back very slowly)

- Pulse is rapid and weak
- The fontanels and eyes are sunken
- Decreased output
- Weight loss (25%)
- Acidosis

Treatment

- Correct the acidosis and dehydration first to replace the water loss and restore the electrolyte balance.

1st 48 hrs

- Continuous IV therapy.
- Observe the stool, vomiting. Glucose and electrolyte may be started orally.
- Antibiotics.
- Tepid sponge bath to reduce the fever.
- Anti-diarrhoeal drugs.

Prevention

- Proper methods for storage of food, its preparation and desired proportions of infant formulas are taught to mothers.
- Encourage the mothers to continue the breast feeding.
- Reduce the temperature by tepid sponge or antipyretics.
- Prevent infection by isolation, to prevent spread of infection proper sewage disposal at site is a must.
- Proper boiling and giving drinking water.
- Control insects and protect the food materials.
- Proper hygienic methods to avoid contamination.

INFLAMMATORY BOWEL DISEASES, CROHN'S DISEASE AND ULCERATIVE COLITIS

Inflammatory bowel diseases encompass two distinct chronic disorders—Crohn's Disease (CD) and Ulcerative Colitis (UC). It can occur randomly throughout the gastrointestinal tract with ileum, colon and rectum being the most common sites.

Incidence

- CD is now more common than UC in the paediatric population, 25% and 30% of the patients with CD and 20% of patients with UC are diagnosed in childhood and adolescence.
- The incidence in males and females is similar, with a slightly higher incidence of CD in females.

Etiology

- Environmental factors:
  - Infectious organisms
  - Dietary habits
  - Environmental toxins
  - Elimination disorders
- Genetic factors.

Ulcerative Colitis (UC)

It is also called colitis, distal colitis, pancolitis and ulcerative proctitis. Ulcerative colitis is a disease that causes ulcers in the lining of the rectum and colon. It is one of a group of diseases called inflammatory bowel diseases.

Ulcers form where inflammation has killed the cells that usually line the colon.

It happens at any age but it usually starts between the ages of 15 and 30.

Clinical Manifestations

- Common symptom is pain in the abdomen
- Bloody diarrhoea

Other Symptoms

- Anaemia
- Severe tiredness
- Weight loss
- Loss of appetite
- Bleeding from the rectum
- Sores on the skin and joint pain
- Child with the disease may have problem

Investigation

- Colonoscopy with biopsy
- Barium enema
- Complete blood count
- C – reactive protein (CRP)
- Erythrocyte sedimentation rate (ESR)

Treatment

- 5-aminosalicylates such as mesalamine or sulfasalazine
- Immunomodulator like azathioprine, cyclosporine, methotrexate
- Cortico steroid such as prednisone, methylprednisone, hydrocortisone enema
- Antibacterial such as metronidazole, ciprafloxacil

Crohn's Disease

The Crohn's disease causes inflammation of the digestive system. The disease can affect any area from the mouth to the anus. It often affects the lower part of the small intestine called the ileum.

Cause

- Immune system response.

Clinical Features

- Pain in the abdomen
- Diarrhoea
- Bleeding from the rectum
- Weight loss
- Joint pain
- Skin problems and fever may also occur.
- Growth retardation
- Other problems can include intestinal blockage and malnutrition.
- Fever
- Loss of appetite.

Complications

- Haemorrhage
- Fistula
- Infection (abscesses)
- Stricture

Investigation

- Physical examination reveals abdominal mass or tenderness, skin rash, swollen joints, mouth ulcers.
- Barium enema
- Colonoscopy
- CT Scan of the abdomen
- Endoscopy
- MRI of abdomen
- Sigmoidoscopy
- Blood examination
  - Serum albumin
  - C-reactive protein
  - White blood cell count
- Stool culture.

Management

- Medical treatment
  - Antidiarrhoea drugs
  - Corticosteroids by oral or rectum
  - Antibiotics
  - Immunomodulators such as Azathioprine or 6– mercaptoprine quiet the immune system's reaction.
- Nutritional supplement
  - Administer carbohydrates, protein and vitamins to avoid malnutrition.
  - Provide small amount of food to the child.
  - Encourage the children to take more fluid or water.
  - Avoid high fibre food.
  - Avoid fatty fried food.
- Surgical management or combination of treatment
  - Bowel resection may be needed to remove a damaged or diseased part of the intestine or to drain an abscess.
  - The temporary colostomy to be done to the child.
  - A procedure called anastomosis is done to connect the remaining two ends of the bowel.

TABLE 7.1: Clinical Manifestations of Ulcerative Colitis and Crohn's Disease

	Ulcerative Colitis	Crohn's Disease
Type of lesions	Continuous, superficial involvement	Segmental, transmural (through the wall) involvement
Clinical manifestations		
Anal or perianal lesions	Rare	Common
Anorexia	Mild to moderate	Can be severe
Diarrhoea	Often severe	Moderate
Growth retardation	Mild	Significant
Pain	Present	Common
Rectal bleeding	Present	Absent
Weight loss	Moderate	Severe
Risk of cancer	Slightly increased	Greatly increased

Nursing Management

- Many of the nursing considerations relate directly to the therapeutic management of IBD. However, the scope of nursing responsibilities includes:
  1. Continued guidance of families in terms of dietary management and drug compliance.
  2. Coping with those factors that increase stress and emotional liability
  3. Adjusting to one of chronic illness and
  4. When indicated, preparing the child and parents for the possibility of diversionary bowel surgery.
- Since nutritional support is a very important component of therapy, encouraging the anorectic child to consume sufficient quantities of food is often a challenge.
- An approach that is more likely to meet with success involves including the child in meal planning: encouraging small, frequent meals or snacks rather than three large meals a day; serving meals around medication schedules, when diarrhoea, mouth pain, intestinal spasm are controlled; and encouraging high-protein, high-calorie foods, such as milk shakes, cream soups, puddings and custard.
- Foods that are known to aggravate the condition are avoided. The routine practice of using bran or a high fiber diet for IBD is under question.
- Gentle mouth care before eating, the selection of bland foods and the avoidance of hot liquids or foods usually relieve the discomfort of mouth sores. A nutritionist may also be consulted to provide dietary counselling for the child and the family.
- Nurses have an important role in preparing children and families to administer NG tube feedings or TPN when indicated.
- Attending to the emotional aspects of a chronic condition requires a thorough assessment of disease-related stress factors.
- Complications of IBD, especially growth failure, can negatively affect self-esteem, school performance and social interactions. Nurses can promote positive coping skills by educating the chid regarding the disease and the rationale for all therapies. Many children benefit from peer support provided by other children with IBD.
- If a permanent colostomy/ileostomy is required, the nurse can assist the child and family in accepting and adjusting to the change by teaching them how to care for the ileostomy, emphasizing the positive aspects of surgery. (Particularly, accelerated growth and sexual development, permanent recovery, and eliminated risk of colonic cancer) and stressing the normality of life despite bowel diversion.

NUTRITIONAL DISORDERS

Protein Energy Malnutrition (PEM)

The relationship of a nutrient (macro-micronutrient) to the body at any particular time is expressed by the term of nutritional status. Such nutrition status is the resultant of the opposing forces of supply and demand. Deficiency on the one hand or toxicity on the other represents a spectrum of nutritional status, while balanced nutrient and energy intake promotes optimal biological function. Children with severe malnutrition are at risk of several life-threatening problems like hypoglycaemia, hypothermia, serious infection and severe electrolyte disturbances. Because of this vulnerability, careful assessment, special treatment and management, with regular feeding and monitoring in addition to outpatient care are essential to complete rehabilitation and to prevent relapse.

PEM is also referred to as protein-calorie malnutrition. It develops in children and adults whose consumption of protein and energy (measured by calories) is insufficient to satisfy the body's nutritional needs. While pure protein deficiency can occur when a person's diet provides enough energy but lacks the protein minimum, in most cases the deficiency will be dual. PEM may also occur in persons who are unable to absorb vital nutrients or convert them to energy essential for healthy tissue formation and organ function.

Types of PEM

Primary PEM results from a diet that lacks sufficient sources of protein and/or energy. Secondary PEM usually occurs as a complication of AIDS, cancer, chronic kidney failure, inflammatory bowel disease and other illnesses that impair the body's ability to absorb or use nutrients or to compensate for nutrient losses. PEM can develop gradually in a patient who has a chronic illness or experiences chronic semi-starvation. It may appear suddenly in a patient who has an acute illness.

Causes and Consequences

Protein energy malnutrition (PEM) is a problem in many developing countries, most commonly affecting children between the ages of 6 months and 5 years. The condition may result from lack of food or from infections that cause loss of appetite while increasing the body's nutrient requirements and losses. Children between 12 and 36 months old are especially at risk since they are the most vulnerable to infections such as gastroenteritis and measles. Chronic PEM has many short-term and long-term physical and mental effects, including growth retardation, lowered resistance to infection and increased mortality rates in young children. Death rates are high among children with untreated PEM and the risk of dying increases with the severity of the condition. Even after treatment begins it is not uncommon for deaths to result from electrolyte imbalance or hypothermia.

Main Causes

1. Ignorance about nutrition and its importance.
2. Poverty, poor and unhygienic living conditions.
3. Inadequate protein intake.
4. Inadequate calorie Intake.
5. Faulty practice of feeding.

Classification of Malnutrition

Mild, moderate and severe classifications have not been precisely defined, but patients who lose 10–20% of their body weight without trying are usually said to have moderate PEM. This condition is also characterized by a weakened grip and inability to perform high-energy tasks. Losing 20% of body weight or more is generally classified as severe PEM. People with this condition can't eat normal-sized meals. They have slow heart rates and low blood pressure and body temperatures. Other symptoms of severe secondary PEM include baggy, wrinkled skin, constipation, dry, thin, brittle hair, lethargy, pressure sores and other skin lesions.

Clinical Manifestations

These are the signs and symptoms will be present always or sometimes present in children:

- Nutritional marasmus
- Kwashiorkor
- Marasmic kwashiorkor

Nutritional Marasmus

It results form prolonged starvation. It may also result from chronic or recurring infections with marginal food intake. The main sign is a severe wasting and the child appears very thin and has no fat. The affected child (or adult) is very thin ("skin and bones"), most of the fat and muscle mass having been expended to provide energy. There is severe wasting of the shoulders, arms, buttocks and thighs, with no visible rib outlines.

Associated signs

- A thin "old man" like face.
- "Baggy pants" (the loose skin of the buttocks hanging down).
- Affected children may appear to be alert in spite of their condition.
- There is no oedema (swelling that pits on pressure) of the lower extremities.
- Ribs are very prominent.

Kwashiorkor

It usually affects children aged 1–4 years, although it also occurs in older children and adults. The main sign is oedema, usually starting in the legs and feet and spreading, in more advanced cases, to the hands and face. Oedema may be detected by the production of a definite pit as a result of moderate pressure for 3 seconds with the thumb over the lower end of the tibia and the dorsum of foot. Because of oedema, children with kwashiorkor may look "fat" so that their parents regard them as well fed.

Associated signs

- Hair changes: loss of pigmentation; curly hair become straight, easy pluckable
- Skin lesions and hypo-pigmentation: dark skin may become lighter in some places especially in the skin folds; outer layers of skin may peel off and ulceration may occur; the lesions may resemble burns.
- Children with Kwashiorkor are usually apathetic, miserable and irritable. They show no signs of hunger and it is difficult to persuade them to eat. The associated signs of Kwashiorkor do not always occur. In some cases, oedema may be the only visible sign, while in others all the signs may be present.

Marasmic Kwashiorkor

It is a mixed form of PEM, and manifests as oedema occurring in children who may or may not have other signs of Kwashiorkor. Clinical features of PEM in older children and adults are basically similar to those in young children, but skin and hair signs are less evident.

Initial assessment of the severely malnourished child involves

A history of:

1. Recent intake of food and fluids
2. Usual diet (before the current illness)
3. Breastfeeding
4. Duration and frequency of diarrhoea and vomiting
5. Type of diarrhoea (watery/bloody)
6. Loss of appetite
7. Family circumstances to understand the child's social background
8. Chronic cough
9. Contact with tuberculosis
10. Recent contact with measles
11. Known or suspected HIV infection.

On examination, telling signs include:

1. Sign of dehydration or shock
2. Severe palmar pallor
3. Eyes having signs of vitamin A deficiency: dry conjuctiva or cornea, Bitot's spot, corneal ulceration and keratomalacia
4. Localized signs of infection, including ear and throat infections, skin infection or pneumonia
5. Signs of HIV infection
6. Fever or hypothermia
7. Mouth ulcers
8. Skin changes of kwashiorkor: hypo or hyper-pigmentation, desquamation, ulceration (spreading over limbs, thighs, genitalia, groin and behind the ears); exudative lesions (resembling severe burns) often with secondary infection, including candida.

General Treatment

All severely malnourished children are at risk of hypoglycaemia, hypothermia, dehydration, electrolyte imbalance, micronutrient deficiencies and infection. The general treatment involves two phases: an initial stabilization phase for management of acute medical conditions and a longer rehabilitation phase.

Hypoglycaemia

Hypoglycaemia is present when the blood glucose is <3 mmol/l (<54 mg/dl). 10% of glucose, sucrose solution or a feed is given immediately on admission. If the child is unconscious glucose is given intravenously or by nasogastric tube. Blood glucose is monitored every 30 minutes using a finger or heelprick blood and dextrostix.

Hypothermia

Low body temperature (hypothermia), <35°C (<95°F) axillary or <35.5°C (<95.5°F) rectally, is associated with increased mortality in severely malnourished children. The child should be wrapped (including the head), with a warmed blanket or a heater or lamp can be placed nearby. Transfer of body heat is another option where the child can be cradled in the arms of the mother while being close to the bare chest or abdomen (skin-to-skin) and a warmed blanket and/or warm clothing covers the two. It is advised that the child's rectal temperature be taken 2-hourly or half-hourly if a heater is being used.

Dehydration

Dehydration tends to be over diagnosed and its severity overestimated in malnourished children. Intravenous route is only accessed in case of shock. Standard WHO-ORS solution has high sodium and low potassium content, which is not suitable for severely malnourished children. Thus a special rehydration solution for malnutrition (ReSoMal) is recommended. The progress of rehydration should be monitored half-hourly for 2 hours, then hourly for the next 6–12 hours.

Electrolyte Imbalance

All severely malnourished children have deficiencies of potassium and magnesium, which may take two weeks or more to be corrected. Extra potassium (3–4 mmol/kg daily) and magnesium (0.4–0.6 mmol/kg daily), with low sodium (generally, <125 mEq/L) is recommended along with food preparation having no salt.

Infection

The usual signs of infection are fever and hypothermia. Treatment includes broad-spectrum antibiotics, measles vaccine if the child is >6 months and not immunized, or is >9 months and had been vaccinated before nine months; delay in vaccination is warranted if the child is in shock. The second dose should be given before discharge. If there is evidence of worm infestation, mebendazole (100 mg orally twice a day) is recommended for three days. In countries where infestation is highly prevalent, mebendazole is recommended as a measure even in light of no infestation after duration of 7 days of admission.

Micronutrient Deficiencies

All severely malnourished children have vitamin and mineral deficiencies. Although anaemia is common, iron supplementation is initially withheld (as iron can worsen the infection) until the child has developed a good appetite and has gained substantial amount of weight.

The following regimen is given daily for at least two weeks:

1. A multivitamin supplement
2. Folic acid (5 mg on day 1, then 1 mg/day)
3. Zinc (2 mg Zn/kg/day)
4. Copper (0.3 mg Cu/kg/day)
5. Once gaining weight, ferrous sulfate (3 mg Fe/kg/day)
6. Vitamin A orally (aged <6 months: 50 000 IU; aged 6–12 months: 100 000 IU; older children: 2000000 IU) on day 1.

Initial Feeding

Feeding is initiated immediately on admission, with feeds carefully worked out to provide just enough energy and protein to maintain basic physiological processes.

Essential **features** of **initial** feeding are:

1. Frequent small feeds of low osmolality and low in lactose
2. Oral or nasogastric feeds (never parenteral preparations)
3. Cabohydreate: 100 kcal/kg/day
4. Protein: 1–1.5 g/kg/day
5. Liquid: 130 ml/kg/day (100 ml/kg/day if the child has severe oedema)
6. Breastfeeding should continue, with scheduled amounts of formula starter first. Milk based formulas, such as start F-75 (with 75 kcal/100 ml and 0.9 g of protein per 100 ml), which is known to be compatible with most children can be a choice. A cup, bowl, spoon, dropper or syringe may be necessary. [Provide therapeutic food]

RICKETS

Definition

- Failure of mineralization of growing bones or osteoid tissue

Causes

- Inadequate dietary intake
- Poor exposure to the sun
- Malabsorption of vitamin D from intestine
- Defects in the metabolism of vitamin D

Clinical Manifestations

- Appears towards the end of 1st year and during the 2nd year of life
- In some cases as early as 2 months
- Craniotabes–early clinical sign
- Rachitic rosary
- Thickening of the wrist and ankle
- Pigeon chest deformity of the chest
- Harrison groove and sulcus
- Anterior fontanel is larger than normal-delayed closure beyond 2nd year
- Caput quadratum – box like head
- Eruption of teeth may be delayed or enamel defect
- Deformity of the pelvis
- Bowlegs or knock knees
- Double malleoli
- Greenstick fractures
- Deformity of the spine kyphosis, scoliosis
- Reduced stature or rachitic dwarfism
- Poorly developed muscles
- Tone-developmental delay or regression

Diagnosis

- Wrist X-ray
- Serum Ca level normal or low
- Serum phosphorus level
- Alkaline phosphatase elevated

Treatment

- Natural and artificial light of appropriate wavelength
- Oral administration of vitamin D.
- A single mega dose of vitamin D–healing is rapid within 2–4 weeks
- Calcium supplementation

Prevention

- Exposure of children to ultraviolet light
- Vitamin D supplementation
- Vitamin D should also be administered to pregnant and lactating mothers.

ALTERED GENITOURINARY FUNCTIONS

UNDERSTANDING KIDNEYS AND URINE

The kidneys clear waste materials from the body and maintain a normal balance of fluids and chemicals in the body.

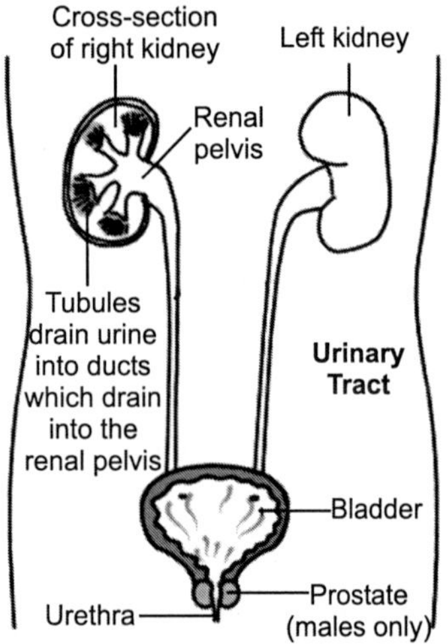

Fig. 8.1: Anatomy of urinary system

The two kidneys lie to the sides of the upper abdomen, behind the intestines, and on either side of the spine. The kidneys are higher up in the body than people imagine—from behind they are actually partially protected by the lowest ribs. The kidneys move slightly with change in your body position and with movement of the diaphragm with breathing. Each kidney is about the size of a large orange, but bean-shaped. 'Renal' is a descriptive medical word, meaning 'related to the kidney'. For example, a renal physician is a doctor who looks after people with kidney (renal) diseases (so-called 'renal medicine').

A large renal artery takes blood to each kidney. The artery divides into many tiny blood vessels (capillaries) throughout the kidney. In the outer part of the kidneys tiny blood vessels cluster together to form structures called glomeruli. Each glomerulus (the singular form of glomeruli) is like a filter. The structure of the glomerulus allows waste products and some water and salt to pass from the blood into a tiny channel called a tubule, while keeping blood cells and protein in the bloodstream. Each glomerulus and tubule is called a nephron. There are about one million nephrons in each kidney.

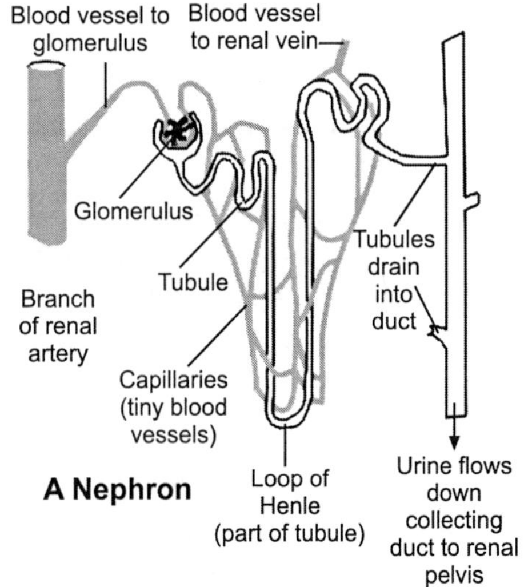

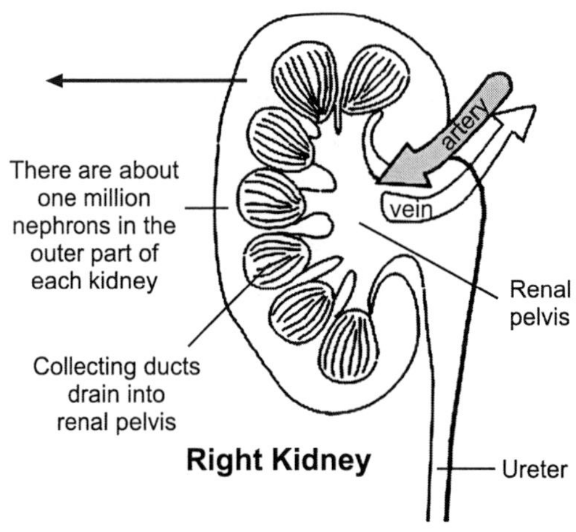

Fig. 8.2: Nephron

As the waste products, water and salts pass along the tubule there is a complex adjustment of the content. For example, some water and salts may be absorbed back into the bloodstream, depending on the current level of water and salt in the blood. Tiny blood vessels next to each tubule enable this 'fine tuning' of the transfer of water and salts between the tubules and the blood. The liquid that remains at the end of each tubule is called urine. This drains into larger channels (collecting ducts) which drain into the renal pelvis (the inner part of the kidney). From the renal pelvis the urine passes down a tube called a ureter which goes from each kidney to the bladder. Urine is stored in the bladder until it is passed out through another tube, called the urethra, when we go to the toilet. The 'cleaned' (filtered) blood from each kidney collects into a large renal vein which takes the blood back towards the heart. The kidneys, ureters, bladder and urethra are, together, called the urinary tract.

URINARY TRACT INFECTION

UTI is a significant childhood problem. It is second infection of children after infection of the respiratory tract.

Incidence

- In the newborn period, UTIs occur most commonly in males, possibly because of the higher incidence of congenital abnormalities.
- 1% to 2% of school age children peak incidence of UTI between 2 and 6 years of age.
- Female children have 10–30 times more UTIs than male children.

Causes

Causative Organisms

- Common gram-negative enteric bacterium
- *Escherichia coli* causes 75% to 90% of all UTIs in females
- Other organisms include *Staphylococcus*, *Klebsiella*, *Proteus*, *Pseudomonas*, *Enterobacter* and *Enterococcus*.

Factors that Predispose to UTI

1. Anatomic and structural factors
   - Incomplete bladder emptying may result from reflux anatomic abnormalities or dysfunction of the voiding mechanism (Vesico Ureteral Reflux).
   - Any congenital abnormal insertion of the ureter into the bladder predisposes to development of infection.
   - Urinary tract obstruction.
2. Physical factors
   - Short, straight urethra
   - Introduction of bacteria during many activities including bath
   - Tight clothing or diapers. Poor hygiene
   - Local inflammation

Renal scarring can result from hydronephrosis or pyelonephritis due to the inflammatory and ischemic effects of the infection. Scars have been associated with hypertension, proteinuria, and kidney failure. The risk of kidney damage increases in the following instances.

- Children less than 1 year of age
- Delay in diagnosis and effective antibacterial treatment for an upper UTI
- Anatomic or neurologic obstruction
- Recurrent episodes of upper UTIs.

Classification

UTI may be present with or without clinical symptoms; it depends on the site of infection and also on the age of the child.

Upper Urinary Tract Infection

Bacteriuria—Growth of bacteria in uncontaminated urine

Urethritis—Inflammation of the urethra

Pyelonephritis—Inflammation of the kidney and upper tract

Lower Urinary Tract Infection

Cystitis—Inflammation of the bladder

Ureteritis—Inflammation of the ureters

- Symptoms in the newborn period tend to be nonspecific—Unexplained fever, failure to thrive, poor feeding, vomiting and diarrhoea, strong smelling urine and irritability. Signs of discomfort before and during in starting urination and stopping the stream intermittently and frequent dripping of small amount of urine.
- In UTIs child has symptoms of
  - High fever

- Chills
- Abdominal pain
- Flank pain
- Persistent vomiting
- Moderate to severe dehydration

- In LUTIs child has symptoms of
  - Frequency, urgency, dysuria
  - Lower abdominal pain
  - Enuresis
  - Strong smelling urine
  - Fever
  - Cloudy urine
  - Haematuria
  - Lethargy and irritability

Complications

- Vesicoureteric reflux
- Bacteremia
- Sepsis
- Septic shock

Investigation

- Urine analysis
- Urine culture
- Blood test
- Intravenous Pyelogram (IVP)
- Voiding Cysto Urethro Gram (VCUG)
- Cystoscopy

Medical Management

- Forced fluid to flush infection from the urinary tract
- Administer Antipyretics
- Antibiotics should be given after identification of the pathogen.
  1. Co-trimoxazole or ampicillin to prevent glomerulonephritis
  2. Antiseptic preparation to maintain urinary stimuli
  3. If anatomical defects surgical correction

Prevention

- Personal hygiene
- Avoid tub bath as it causes ascending infection to the child
- Avoid tight clothing and diaper
- Avoid holding urine for long time
- Encourage to void frequently
- Encourage more fluid intake

Nursing Management

- Prepare for child for the investigation, explain the procedure and purpose of investigation.
- Administer antibiotic as prescribed; instruct parents to complete the entire course of antibiotics even though the child's symptoms may be gone.
- Force fluids to flush the infection from the urinary tract.
- Teach proper toileting hygiene (front-to-back wiping).
- Encourage the child to use the toilet frequently to empty the bladder.
- Discourage the use of bubble baths.
- Instruct the parents measures to prevent future UTIs.

GLOMERULONEPHRITIS

Glomerulonephritis is an inflammation of glomeruli of the kidney.

Types of glomerulonephritis are:

- Acute
- Chronic

Acute Glomerulonephritis

It is an autoimmune immune-complex disorder occurring 1 to 2 weeks after a group *'a'* beta-haemolytic streptococcal infection.

Incidence

It occurs in 2–12 years of children

- More incidence about 6 years of age (peak)
- Less in below 2 years of age.

Etiology

- Caused by group *'a'* beta-haemolytic streptococcal
- Disease secondary to pharyngitis–common in winter or springs season
- Disease associated with pyoderma (impetigo) – skin infection.

Pathophysiology

Streptococcal infection

↓

Inflammatory process occurs due to immunologic reaction

↓

Inflammation of glomeruli + infiltrated with polymorphonuclear leukocytes

↓

Occludes the capillary lumen

↓

Decreases filtration of plasma

↓

It leads to excessive accumulation of water and retention of sodium.

↓

Causes expanded plasma and interstitial fluid volumes

↓

Circulatory congestion and edema

↓

Decreased glomerular filtration rate, Increased Capillary permeability or vascular spasm (It leads to clinical features)

Clinical Manifestations

- Mild fever for 10 days after onset of nephritis
- Initial signs are
  - Puffiness of the face
  - Periorbital edema
  - Anorexia
  - Passage of dark coloured urine
  - Edema more prominent in the face in the morning but spreads during the day to involve the extremities and abdomen.
  - Urine is cloudy, smoky brown (tea or cola colour)
  - Less urine (scanty urination)
  - Child is pale
  - Irritable and lethargic
- Older children complain of
  - Headache
  - Abdominal discomfort
  - Dysuria
- Vomiting not common
- BP elevated mild or moderate (80–120 diastolic, systolic 120–180 mm of Hg.)

Complications

- Chronic renal failure
- Heart failure from hypervolemia leads to pulmonary edema
- Hypertension

Investigation

- Blood exam—Increased erythrocyte sedimentation rate indicates inflammation.
- Increased antistreptolysin-O titer indicates recent streptococcal infection.
- Urine analysis reveals the presence of protein (Proteinuria 3+ or 4+), blood, haematuria, Increased urine specific gravity—more than 1.020.
- Urine microscopic examination reveals RBC, WBCs in the urine, epithelial cells and RBC casts.
- Blood examination shows normal electrolytes, increased blood urea nitrogen, elevated creatinine level.
- Throat culture (pharynx) shows positive for streptococcus
- Renal ultrasound may show a slightly enlarged kidney
- Kidney biopsy may reveal the cause of the inflammation

Medical Management

- No specific treatment for acute glamerulonephritis.
- Supportive measures include bed rest, fluid and dietary sodium restrictions, and correction of electrolyte imbalances,
- Diuretics such as furosemide (Lasix) to reduce fluid overload
- Antihypertensive drug to treat increased blood pressure (Hydralazine),
- Antibiotic (Penicillin) if a staphylococcal infection is documented

Nursing Interventions

- Monitor intake and output and daily weight; watch for signs of acute renal failure, including decreased (less than 1 ml/kg/hours), or no urine output.
- Provide nutritious diet to the child, the diet should contain high carbohydrate, less sodium and protein.
- Teach the parents about possible penicillin therapy to prevent further renal damage in a subsequent streptococcal infection.
- Prevent and control edema by instructing the parent to give moderate sodium restrictions for the child with hypertension or edema.
- Fluid restriction depends upon the child's urine output.
- Administer medications to control hypertension.
- Bed rest is necessary during the acute phase; aid the patient in gradually resuming normal activities.
- Prevent hyperkalemia by restricted diet, monitor laboratory finding and observe the signs of hyperkalemia and treat the child.
- Assess the progress of edema by daily checking of weight, measuring intake and output chart and measuring abdominal girth.
- Observe the signs of complications, by monitoring vital signs, urine output, dyspnea, and vomiting, visual disturbance to the child, severe headache, and abdominal pain.
- Provide comfort to the child.
- Stimulate appetite to the child by providing cheerful, clean, relaxed atmosphere during meals, serve small quantities initially to stimulate appetite, provide special and preferred foods, serve foods in an attractive manner.
- Educate the parents regarding home care to the child.
- Explain about the follow up care.

Chronic Glomerulonephritis

Persistent glomerulonephritis is called as chronic glomerulonephritis (6–12 months); it is a variety of different disease processes that may be distinguished from other by renal biopsy. These include membranoproliferative glomerulonephritis, membranous glomerulonephritis, and focal segmental glomerulosclerosis and IgA nephropathy.

Causes

Variety of disease mentioned as above.

Clinical Manifestations

Clinical manifestation—Laboratory findings reflect to deteriorating renal function.

- Nephrotic syndrome
- Hypertension
- Edema
- Proteinuria
- Cardiac failure
- Dyspnea
- Osteo dystrophy
- Anaemia

Investigation

- Urine analysis shows
  - Proteinuria, with casts
  - Red blood cells and white blood cells
  - Urine specific gravity—shows normal
- Blood analysis evidenced by
  - Renal function test: Elevated blood urea nitrogen, creatinine and uric acid level.
  - Serum electrolytes shows metabolic acidosis, elevated potassium, phosphorus and decreased calcium levels

Medical Management

- Antihypertentive drugs to reduce the hypertension.
- Diuretics to reduce edema.
- Transfusion of fresh packed cells to correct anaemia.
- Salt moderately restricted.

Nursing Management

Prevent and Control Acute Infection

- Avoid contact with an infected person.
- Observe medical aspects
- Administer antibiotics
- Monitor vitals twice a day and also depend upon the child condition, monitor temperature, pulse rate, respiration and blood pressure.
- Keep child dry and warm to prevent infection

Prevent Skin Breakdown

- Provide meticulous skin care
- Cleanse and powder the body
- Support edematous parts
- Change the position frequently to prevent pressure on the skin.

Prevent Further Edema Formation

- Provide salt restricted diet to avoid sodium retention.
- Administer steroids as prescribed to reduce the inflammatory process

Prevent Hypovolemia

- Monitor vital signs to detect hypovolemia
- Take BP – Report any deviations from normal

Conserve Energy

- Bed rest initially
- Balance rest and activity when ambulatory
- Tell the child feels tired ask to take rest

Assess Changes in Edema

- Weight to be checked daily and recorded
- Measure the abdominal girth daily and recorded
- Monitor the intake and output (record) strictly.
- Test the urine for specific gravity and albumin daily and recorded.

Establish Good Nutrition

- Administer high protein, high carbohydrate diet to the child
- Administer supplementary vitamins and iron by oral.

Stimulate Appetite

- Provide cheerful, clean, relaxed atmosphere during meals
- Serve small quantities initially to stimulate appetite
- Provide special and preferred foods
- Serve foods in an attractive manner

Prepare Parents for Home Care of the Child

- Educate the parents how to look after the child at home.
- Educate them regarding administration of medication, personal hygiene, prevention of infection, restricted fluid and salt.
- Instruct them about signs and symptoms of complication, if they identify from the child, should bring the child to the hospital immediately.
- Educate them about the follow up care.

Support Parents

- Ask them to continue the drugs and regular follow up care.
- Psychological support.

NEPHROTIC SYNDROME

Nephrotic syndrome is an autoimmune process that occurs 1 week after an immune assault. Children have signs of hyper albuminuria, hypoalbuminemia, hypovolemia, hyperlipidema. Nephrotic syndrome is a relatively rare but important manifestation of kidney disease. In the US, its annual incidence among children is reported to be 2–7 cases per 100,000. Incidence varies among adults depending on the incidence of underlying causes for the condition, particularly diabetes mellitus. Nephrotic syndrome has an incidence of around three new cases per 100,000 each year in adults.

Causes

It can be caused by a wide range of primary idiopathic (75% of the cases) and secondary glomerular diseases.

Primary Renal Diseases

- Minimal-coliferative glomerulonephritis

Secondary Renal Diseases

- Postinfectious causes, *e.g.*, Group-A beta-haemolytic streptococci, TB, malaria, **syphilis**, viruses such as VZV, HBV, HIV, infectious mononucleosis.
- Collagen vascular diseases, *e.g.*, SLE, rheumatoid arthritis, polyarteritis nodosa, Henoch-Schönlein purpura, vasculitis.
- Metabolic diseases, *e.g.*, diabetes mellitus, amyloidosis.
- Inherited disease, *e.g.*, Alport's syndrome, hereditary nephritis, sickle cell disease.
- Malignant disease, *e.g.*, multiple myeloma, leukaemia, lymphoma, carcinoma of breast/lung/colon/stomach.
- Medications, *e.g.*, NSAIDs, captopril, lithium, gold, diamorphine, interferon-alpha, penicillamine, probenecid and many others.
- Toxins, *e.g.*, bee sting, snake bites, phytotoxins.
- Pregnancy, *e.g.*, pre-eclampsia.
- Transplant rejection.

Pathophysiology

The pathogenesis of the disorder is not understood. There may be a metabolic, biochemical or physiochemical disturbance in the basement membrane of the glomeruli that leads to increased permeability or protein.

The glomerular membrane, which is normally impermeable to albumin and other large protein becomes permeable to protein, especially albumin, which leak through the membrane and are lost in urine (hyperalbuminuria), this reduces the serum albumin level (Hypoalbuminemia). This decreases the colloidal osmotic pressure in the capillaries. As a result the hydrostatic pressure exceeds the pull of the colloidal osmotic pressure and fluid accumulates in the interstitial spaces and body cavities, particularly the abdominal cavity (ascites).

The shift of fluid from the plasma to the interstitial spaces reduces the vascular fluid volume (hypovolemia) which in turn stimulates the rennin—angiotension system and the secretion of anti-diuretic hormone and aldosterone. Tubular reabsorption of sodium and water are increased in an attempt to increase intravascular volume. The elevation of serum cholesterol, phospholipids and triglycerides is unexplained.

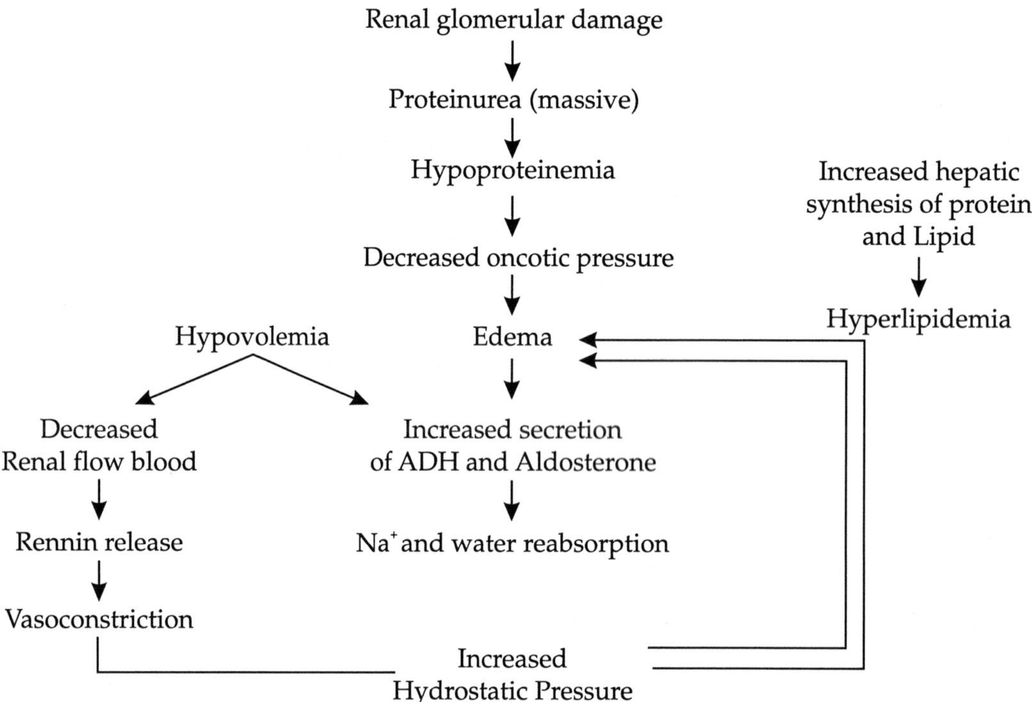

Fig. 8.3: Pathophysiology of nephrotic syndrome

Complications

- Peritonitis
- End-stage renal failure

Clinical Manifestations

- Child begins to gain weight
- Puffiness of the face especially around the eyes is apparent on arising in the morning but subsides during the day.
- Swelling of the abdomen and lower extremities.
- Generalized edema
- Ascites
- Respiratory difficulty—due to pleural effusion.
- Labial or scrotal swelling (edema).
- Edema of the intestinal mucosa may cause diarrhoea, anorexia and poor intestinal absorption.
- Decreased urine output.
- Dark, foamy and frothy urine.
- Poor intestinal absorption.
- Skin pallor.
- Child gets easily fatigue or lethargic.
- Malnutrition from poor appetite and loss of protein.
- Blood pressure is normal or slightly decreased.
- Susceptible to infection like cellulites, pneumonia, peritonitis or septicemia.

Investigation

The aim of investigations is to find the underlying cause, direct future management, establish a baseline of severity and monitor response to treatment. The initial sequence is:

- Confirm proteinuria: urine dipstick positive, Check for concomitant invisible (microscopic) haematuria, Urine specific gravity will be high.
- Exclude urine infection: urine microscopy/ culture and sensitivity.
- Measure amount of proteinuria:
  - Early morning urinary protein : creatinine ratio or albumin : creatinine ratio (mg/mmol).
  - Typically >300–350 mg/mmol in nephrotic syndrome.
- Basic blood testing:
  - Full blood count and coagulation screen.
- Renal function including plasma creatinine and estimated glomerular filtration rate.
- Total serum protein is lowered, concentration (less than 2 g).
  - Alpha 2 globulin and plasma lipids increased, Serum cholesterol shows high (450–1500 mg).
  - Haemoglobin level increased.
- Serum sodium level decreased to 130–135 mg.
- **Liver function tests** to exclude concomitant liver pathology.
- Bone profile—corrected (for albumin) plasma calcium.
- Check for other systemic diseases and causes of nephrotic syndrome:
  - C–reactive protein and erythrocyte sedimentation rate.
  - Glucose.
  - Immunoglobulins, serum and urine electrophoresis.
  - Autoimmune screen if an underlying autoimmune disease is suspected—antinuclear antibody (ANA), anti-double stranded DNA antibody (dsDNA), and complement values (C3 and C4).
  - Hepatitis B and C and HIV (after obtaining informed consent).
- Chest X-ray and abdominal or renal ultrasound scan (especially if renal function is abnormal):
  - To check for pleural effusion or ascites.
  - To check for the presence of two kidneys, their size and shape, and the absence of obstruction.
  - To exclude malignancy and exclude other causes of oedema.
- Be vigilant for complications such as thromboembolism:
  - Doppler ultrasound of leg veins in suspected deep vein thrombosis.
  - Abdominal ultrasound, renal vein Doppler scan, venography of the inferior vena cava, computed tomography and magnetic resonance imaging of the abdomen if renal vein thrombosis is suspected.
  - V/Q nuclear medicine lung scan, computed tomography pulmonary angiography for pulmonary embolism.
- Investigate the underlying renal and systemic cause of nephrotic syndrome:
  - Renal biopsy under ultrasound (to assess size and structural condition of kidneys).
  - Obstructed or small kidneys may contraindicate renal biopsy.
  - Make histological preparations for light microscopy, immunofluoresence or immunoperoxidase, electron microscopy.

Management

- Most cases do not require acute hospitalisation.
- Reduce salt intake in diet (avoid processed foods and adding salt to food).
- Give diet with adequate caloric intake and sufficient protein content (1–2 g/kg daily).
- Hyperlipidaemia does not initially require therapy but may do so if prolonged.
- Fluid restriction is not usually necessary (if severe enough then may need admission).
- Referral to a renal service for urgent outpatient assessment is advisable, to confirm the mode of presentation and direct any future investigations/ therapy.
- Oedema is treated through diuretic therapy with **furosemide** (~1 mg/kg/day) ± **spironolactone** (~2 mg/kg/day).
- Check weight regularly to assess response to **diuretics** and ensure **fluid retention** is not worsening, or that patient is over-diuresed.
- Patients with very low albumin levels may not respond to diuretics and may require admission to receive intravenous albumin therapy.

- Some children with severe oedema may be prescribed **antibiotic prophylaxis** against infection and this should usually be on the advice of a renal specialist.
- Most children will have minimal-change nephrotic syndrome and usually respond to a trial of **steroid therapy** under the direction of a renal specialist.
- Other forms of nephrotic syndrome are less treatment responsive; Angiotension converting enzyme (ACE) inhibitors are used to help reduce protein loss in urine.
- Oral steroid (such as prednisone) therapy to suppress the autoimmune response and to stimulate vascular reabsorption of oedema.
- In children who do not respond to steroids, and in some adults, treatment may be with other immunomodulatory drugs such as **cyclophosphamide, ciclosporin, tacrolimus** and **levamisole**. Cyclophosphamide (cytoxam) 1–2.5 mg/kg/day alternating with prednisone for 2 months then cyclophosphamide is stopped and prednisone is tapered gradually.

Nursing Management

- Provide skin care to oedematous skin; don't use adhesive strip bandage, tape or IM injection.
- Provide warm soaks to decrease periorbital edema.
- Elevate the head of the bed to facilitate to breath well.
- Turn the child frequently to prevent pressure on the skin.
- Provide scrotal support and place padding between body parts to prevent irritation.
- Test the first void of the day for protein.
- Feed small, frequent meals with restricted salt.
- Measure intake and output and daily weight.
- Measure the abdominal girth daily if child has ascitis.
- Prevent contact with persons who have an infection to avoid infection to the child.
- Anticipate diuresis in 1 to 3 weeks
  - Maintain bed rest during rapid diuresis
  - Monitor hydration status and vital signs
  - Corticosteroid (prednisone) single dose (complication growth retardation hypertension, gastrointestinal bleeding, bone demineralization, infection and DM.)
- Provide information to the parents related to the disease condition of their child.
- Educate the parents about home care-restricted fluid intake, salt free diet, skin care, regular medication.
- Inform about follow up care.

WILM'S TUMOR (NEPHROBLASTOMA)

It is a malignant, embryonic adenosarcoma of the kidney. It develops from abnormal tissue in the embryo, beginning to grow before or after the infant is born. The most common intra-abdominal tumour in children; the average age at diagnosis is 2 to 4 years.

- The tumour favours the left kidney and is usually unilateral.
- The tumour remains encapsulated for a long time.
- The prognosis is excellent if metastasis hasn't occurred.

Incidence

It is a most frequent neoplasm that occurs during infancy or toddler age. It is commonly unilateral but may be bilateral.

Causes

- Genetic inheritance
- Associated with several other congenital anomalies including hypospadias, cryptorchidism, Beckwith-Wiederman syndrome, and Denys-Drash syndrome.

Pathophysiology

- Wilms tumour is an embryonal cancer of the kidney originating during foetal life.
- In early stages the tumour is well encapsulated, but it may later spread into the lymph nodes, renal vein, or vena cava; metastasis may occur to the lungs or other sites.
- Staging
  - In stage I, the tumour is limited to one kidney.
  - In stage II, the tumour extends beyond the kidney but can be completely exceed.
  - In stage III, the tumour spreads but is confined to the abdomen and lymph nodes.
  - In stage IV, the tumour metastasis to the lung, liver, bone, and brain.

- In stage V, the tumour involves both kidneys.

Complications

- Metastasis to other organs
- Symptoms of metastasis including shortness of breath, coughing, chest pain, and weight loss.

Clinical Manifestation

- Nontender abdominal mass (most common), usually middling near the liver; commonly identified by the parent while bathing or dressing the child.
- Enlarged abdomen
- High blood pressure
- Vomiting
- Haematuria
- Anaemia
- Constipation

Investigation

- Abdominal ultrasound and CT scan to view tumour size, location, and possible metastasis.
- Excretory urography assesses function of the normal-functioning kidney.
- Blood tests reveal polycythemia if tumour secretes erythropoietin.
- Regional lympnodes (avoid palpation).
- Intravenous pyelography shows the distortion and displacement of the pelvis of the kidney.

Management

- Child with adequate treatment has a rapid rate of cure with early diagnosis.
- If not treated leads to pulmonary metastases via the renal vein and venous circulation to the right side of the lungs and then through the pulmonary artery to the lungs.

Surgical Management

- Treatment is surgical management with possible X-ray irradiation before and after surgery.
- Operation should be done immediately after diagnosis.
- Actinomycin D (dactinomycin) and vincristine are given preoperatively and post operatively.
- Special attention to nutrition for normal infant.
- Avoid abdominal palpation.
- Good skin care keeps the skin clean and dry. If skin has irritation apply bland ointment.
- Nephrectomy surgery to remove the tumour and affected kidney in stages I and II.
- Radiation is indicated with large tumours or those that weren't completely surgically resected.
- Chemotherapy with dactinomycin and vincrestine.

Nursing Interventions

- Preoperative
  - Don't palpate the abdomen, and prevent others from doing so; it may disseminate cancer cells to other sites.
  - Handle and bathe the child carefully.
  - Loosen clothing near the abdomen.
  - Prepare the family for nephrectomy within 24 to 48 hours of diagnosis.
  - Maintain nutritional status of the child.
  - Prevent the child from dehydration.
- Postoperative
  - Provide routine care as for a patient who has had a nephrectomy.
  - Be aware that chemotherapy and radiation will follow.

ALTERED NEUROLOGICAL CONDITIONS

ASSESSMENT OF NEUROLOGICAL CONDITIONS

- History of the child:
  - Birth history
  - Family history
  - Developmental history
- Physical examination
- Altered status of consciousness
  - **Consciousness** is the ability to respond to sensory stimuli and have subjective experiences. There are 2 components of consciousness:
    - Alertness
    - Cognitive power (verbal and motor response)

    An altered status of consciousness usually refers to varying states of unconsciousness that may be momentary or may extend for hours, days or indefinitely.
  - **Unconsciousness** is depressed cerebral function, the inability to respond to sensory stimuli and have subjective experiences.
  - **Coma** is a state of unconsciousness from which the patient cannot be aroused even with powerful stimuli.
- Level of consciousness (LOC)

  It is an assessment of LOC that remains the earliest indicator of improvement or deterioration in neuralgic status.
  - LOC is assessed by child responses to the environment.
  - Other diagnostic tests, like motor activity, reflexes and vital signs.

TABLE 9.1: Levels of Consciousness

Full consciousness	Awake and alert; oriented to time, place and person—behaviour appropriate for age
Confusion	Impaired decision-making
Disorientation	Disorientation to time and place, decreased level of consciousness.
Lethargy	Limited spontaneous movement, sluggish speech.
Obtundation	Arousable with stimulation
Stupor	Remains in a deep sleep, responsive only to vigorous and repeated stimulation.
Coma	No motor or verbal response to noxious (Painful) stimuli.
Persistent Vegetative State (PVS)	The permanently lost function of the cerebral cortex, eyes follow objects only by reflex or when attracted to the direction of loud sounds; all four limbs are spastic but can withdraw from painful stimuli; hands show reflexive grasping and grapping; the face can grimace, some food may be swallowed, and the child may groan or cry but utter no words.

Source: Modified from Hazinski M.F., (ed.), 1992; *Care of the Critically ill Child*, 2nd edn., Mosby St. Louis.

Coma Assessment

This assessment to degree of depressed consciousness.

- The most popular of these is the Glasgow Coma Scale (GCS), which consists of 3 parts of assessment.
- Eye opening
- Verbal response
- Motor response

Numeric values are assigned to the levels of response in each category and they seem of these numeric values give an objective measure of the patients LOC.

- The lower the score the deeper is the coma.
- A person with an unaltered LOC would have score of the highest level, i.e. 15.
- A score of 7 or below is generally accepted as a coma.
- A score of lowest level 3 indicates deep coma.
- In case of irreversible coma, the task force for the determination of brain death in children is involved.

TABLE 9.2: Glasgow Coma Scale for Assessing Neurologic Status

Category	Infant/Younger Children	Numerical Score	Modified Score (Infants)
Eye opening	Spontaneous	4	Spontaneous
	To verbal stimuli	3	To speech
	To pain	2	To pain
	No response	1	No response
Best verbal response	Oriented	5	Coos and babbles
	Confused	4	Irritable cries
	Inappropriate words	3	Cries to pain
	Non-specific sounds	2	Moans to pain
	No response	1	No response
Best motor response	Follows command	6	Normalspontaneous movements
	Localizes pain	5	Withdraws to touch
	Withdraws to pain	4	Withdraws to pain
	Flexes to pain	3	Abnormal flexion
	Extends to pain	2	Abnormal extension
	No response	1	No response

The numerical scores of each of the three categories are added:

- A score of 12–15 (child is alert and awake); it is usually considered unnecessary to obtain a CT scan or to hospitalize such children.
- A score below 12, usually considered an indication to admit the child for careful observation, child should be kept in ICU.
- A score below 8, indicates a severe head injury, usually with considerable cerebral edema, and considerable risk of intracranial hypertension.

Neurological Examination

The neurological examination is to establish an accurate, objective baseline of neurological information.

Vital signs: Normally there are some changes in vital signs in case altered consciousness of the child.

- Body temperature is often elevated
- Pulse: It may vary and may be rapid, slow and bound.
- Blood pressure may be normal
- Respiration is often slow, deep and irregular.

Skin: Skin may offer clues to the cause of unconsciousness.

Eyes: Pupil size and reactivity are assessed

- Pinpoint pupils are seen in poisoning of child.
- Dilated pupils – present in eye trauma
- Widely dilated and fixed pupils paralysis of cranial nerve III due to brain herniation.
- Unilateral fixed pupil—lesion on the same side
- Bilateral fixed pupils—imply brain stem damage.
- Dilated and unreactive pupils—Hypothermia, anoxia, ischemia, poison with atropine.

Motor function: To assess spontaneous activity, posture and response to painful stimuli provides clues to the location and extent of cerebral dysfunction.

Posturing: Posture of the child if affected because, motor function will be altered due to brain dysfunction. There are 2 kinds of posturing.

- **Decorticate posturing:** In this condition of the posturing the motor movement directly related to the area of the brain involved is affected.
- **Decerebrate posturing:** It is a sign of dysfunction at the level of the midbrain.

Special Diagnostic Procedures

- **Lumbar puncture:** To measure spinal fluid pressure, volume, colour, and abnormal compositions.
- **Subdural tap:** Helps to rule out subdural effusions relieve ICP.
- **Ventricular puncture:** Removes CSF to relieve pressure.

Electroencephalography (EEG)

- Measures electric activity of cerebral cortex.
- Detects electric abnormalities in the diagnosis of seizures.
- Used to determine brain death.

Nuclear Brain Scan

- Radioisotope accumulates in areas where blood-brain barrier is defective.
- Identifies focal brain lesions (*e.g.*, tumours, abscesses).
- Positive uptake of material with encephalitis and subdural haematoma.
- Visualizes CSF pathways.

Echoencephalography

- Identifies shifts in midline structures from their normal positions as a result of intracranial lesions.
- May show ventricular dilation.

Real-time Ultrasonography (RTUS)

- Allows high-resolution anatomic visualization in variety of imaging planes.

Radiography

- Shows fractures, dislocations, spreading suture lines, and craniostenosis.
- Shows degenerative changes, bone erosion, calcifications.

Computed Tomography (CT) Scan

- Visualize horizontal and vertical cross section of brain at any axis.
- Distinguishes density of various intracranial tissues and structures, congenital abnormalities, haemorrhage, tumours, demyelingating and inflammatory processes.

Magnetic Resonance Imaging (MRI) or Nuclear Magnetic Resonance

- Permits visualization of morphologic features of target structures.
- Permits tissue discrimination unavailable with many techniques.

Digital Subtraction Angiography (DSA)

- Visualizes vasculature of target tissue.
- Visualizes finite vascular abnormalities.

CONVULSION

It is common in children, a common form of seizures due to febrile convulsion that occurs with fever or acute infection.

Definition

Convulsion is an involuntary muscular contraction and relaxation.

Seizures: It is a spontaneous electrical discharge

Incidence: It occurs in first 2 years.

Causes

Primary causes: idiopathic

Secondary causes:

- Due to infection,
- Genetic factor
- Head trauma: Inadequate oxygen supply to the brain, haemorrhage, tumour, other organic degenerative factors.
- Metabolic disorders such as hypoglycaemia or hypoparathyroidism.
- Ingestion of toxins-mercury, lead or carbon monoxide.

Types

1. Generalized seizures
2. Partial (Focal seizures)

Generalized seizures include:

1. Grand mal (motor)
2. Petitmal seizures

3. Akinetic seizures
4. Myclonic seizures
5. Infantile seizures.

Grand mal seizures: Consist of sudden loss of consciousness with generalized jerking movement. The initial tonic rigidity changes rapidly to generalized jerking movement of the muscles. Children bite the tongue and lose the control of bladder and bowel functions. Jerking movement gradually diminishes, then disappears and the child relaxes. It persists for a minute or lasts 30 minute or more, after seizures child returns to a alert state while others go into a prolonged period of stupor.

Petitmal seizures: Seizures last for only a few seconds, rarely longer than 20 seconds. Child loses consciousness and stares straight ahead but does not fall. They become alert immediately. They will forget what happened during attack.

A kinetic seizure: A momentary loss of consciousness, muscle tone and postural control, it can result in serious facial, head and shoulder injuries.

Myoclonic: Myoclonic seizures are characterized by sudden jerking of a muscle or group of muscles without loss of consciousness.

Infantile spasms: Infantile spasm occurs between 3 months to 12 months of age due to cerebral defect. It occurs followed by a cry. Muscle contractions are sudden, brief, symmetrical, accompanied by rolling of eyes, loss of consciousness does not always occur.

Partial seizures (focal seizures) include:

1. Psychomotor seizures
2. Focal motor seizures
3. Focal sensory seizures

Psychomotor seizures: It's difficult to recognize, they consist of purposeful but inappropriate, repetitive motor acts. Child gradually loses postural tone and falls to the floor.

Focal motor seizures: In this seizure the involuntary unilateral convulsion movement that begins in the extremities such as the fingers, progresses to upper limbs of the body and persists for short time. Child has undisturbed consciousness.

Focal sensory seizures: Produce such sensations as tingling, numbness, pricking pain or parasthesis which originate in one area and spread to the other part of body.

Clinical Manifestations

- Aura just before the seizure's onset (child reports unusual tastes, feelings, or odours)
- Eye deviation to a particular side or blinking
- Usually, unresponsiveness during tonic- clonic muscular contractions; possible incontinence
- Possible disorientation to time and place, drowsiness, and lack of co-ordination immediately after seizure.

Assessment

- Physical and neurological assessment

Investigation

- Electroencephalogram
- CT scan
- MRI
- Brain scan.

Treatment

- Anticonvulsant drugs
- Education and counselling of the child and the parents an important part of treatment
- Early diagnosis and treatment
- Forbidden to drive a motor vehicle, cycling, swimming.

Nursing Care

1. Protect child during seizures
2. Observe seizure
3. Observe postictally
4. Promote rest
5. Reduce parental anxiety.

1. Protect child during seizures

- Protect them from fall,
- Loosen restructure clothing
- Prevent child from hitting sharp objects that might cause injury
- Gently support child
- Apply mouth gag.

2. Observe seizures

- Describe and record characteristics of seizures
- Order of event
- Duration of seizure (child should be observed and recorded)

Observe the onset: Describe and record changes in facial expression such as fear

- Cry or other sound
- Position of head: head should be turned of onset

Movement: Describe and record site of commencement—head thumb, mouth, generalized

Tonic phase: Length, parts of body involved

Clonic phase: Twitching, or jerking movement, part of body involved.

- Lack of movement in any extremities

Face: Colour change – paler, cyanosis, flushing

Mouth: Teeth clenched tongue bitten, frothing at mouth.

Eyes: Reaction to light

Respiratory effort: Presence and length of apnea, presence of stridor

Others: Describe and record

- Involuntary urination
- Involuntary defecation

3. Observe postictally

- State of consciousness
- Orient to time, place, person
- Motor ability of the child
- Speech – Changes
- Complain of discomfort or pain

4. Promote rest and provide comfort

- Allow to take rest
- Reduce sensory stimuli

5. Reduce parental anxiety

- Provide calm, relaxed atmosphere
- Explain purpose of nursing activity
- Provide emotional support.

MENINGITIS

The inflammatory process that can affect the meninges of the brain and spinal cord is called meningitis.

Inflammation of the brain is called as encephalitis.

Inflammation of the spinal cord is called myelitis.

Incidence

Children are affected from 3 months to the 3 years of age group, higher incidence in 6–12 months of infants.

Causes

Organisms

- Bacterial or pyogenic meningitis caused by meningococci
- Tuburculous used by meningitis caused by *Tubercle bacillus*
- Viral or septic meningitis caused by viral agent
- Neonatal meningitis caused by group Beta streptococci and *Escherichicas*

Other Causes

- Skull injury or fracture
- Lumbar puncture
- Surgical procedure for spinabifida shunting procedures
- Sinusitis
- Otitis media
- Encephalitis
- Myelitis
- Brain abscesses.

Pathophysiology

Organism entry by direct implantation by wound (penetration)

↓

Inflammation may involve all meningeal membranes, exudation, white blood cell accumulation, and varying edematous occurences

↓

Infection extends to the ventricles

↓

Thick pus, fibrin may occlude the narrow passages

↓

Obstructing the flow of CSF to cause obstructive hydrocephalus

↓

Subdural effusion and thrombosis may occur.

↓

Destructive changes may take place in cerebral cortex and brain abscesses may form by direct extension of the infection or vascular dissemination

Clinical Manifestations

In Older Children

- Fever,
- Chills,
- Headache and vomiting

- Initial sign is a seizure
- Drowsiness,
- Stupor, and coma
- Child resists flexion of the neck
- Neck stiffness
- Opisthotonos (arching of the back)
- Petechial or purpuric lesions possibly present in bacterial meningitis
- Positive Kernign's sign (the child is unable to extend the leg when the hip and knee are flexed).
- Positive Brudzinski's sign (the child flexes the knees and hips in response to passive neck flexion).

In Infants and Young Children the Age Group of (3 month-2 yrs.)

- Fever,
- Vomiting,
- Marked irritability
- Frequent seizures
- High pitched cry
- Bulging of fontanel
- Poor sucking ability
- Diarrhoea

Neonates

- Hypothermia or fever
- Poor sucking ability
- Vomiting
- Jaundice
- Irritability
- Drowsiness
- Apnea,
- Cyanosis,
- Weight loss
- Bulging of fontanels
- Projectile vomiting causing dehydration; dehydration may prevent a bulging fontanel and thus mask an important sign of increased ICP.

Complications

- Physical injury
- Respiratory compromise or respiratory arrest
- Mental retardation
- Death

Investigation

- Lumbar puncture – CSF shows increased CSF pressure, cloudy colour, increased WBC count and protein level, decreased glucose level if meningitis caused by bacteria.
- Blood culture

TABLE 9.3: Normal Values of Cerebrospinal Fluid in Children

Content	Neonates (<1 mo)	Infants (>1 mo)
White blood cell count	<30	<10
Percent neutrophils	60	0
Protein levels (mg/dl)	<90	<40
Glucose levels (mg/dl)	70-80	50-60

Medical Management

- Isolation of the child
- Analgesics to treat pain of meningeal irritation
- Administration of dexamethasone (decadron)
- Parenteral antibiotics—Ceftazidime (fortaz), ceftriaxone given depending on the age.
- Antimicrobial therapy
- Adequate hydration—IV fluid administration
- Maintain ventilation
- Reduction of ICP—manitol
- Management of bacterial shock
- Control of seizures
- Control of extreme of temperature
- Correct anaemia

Prevention

Vaccination: Administration of HIB

Nursing Management

- Maintain droplet precautions until at least 24 hours of effective antibiotic therapy have elapsed; continued precautions are recommended for meningitis caused by H. influenza or N. meningitides.
- Provide a hypothermia blanket, as indicated.
- Administer oxygen.
- Provide suction to reduce the secretion, to clear the air way.

- Maintain seizure precautions—prevent the child from injury.
- Monitor vital signs and intake and output to assess for excess fluid volume.
- Assess the child's neurological status frequently to monitor for increased ICP.
- Provide a dark and quiet environment to reduce the stimuli.
- Keep the child flat in bed, care should be provided to avoid pressure to take care of bed sore.
- Move the child gently.
- Administer parenteral antibiotics and anticonvulsant drugs to the child on time.

ENCEPHALITIS

Encephalitis is an inflammation of the brain usually caused by a viral infection.

Causes

Common Organisms

- Bacteria
- Spirochetes
- Fungi
- Protozoa
- Virus
  - Entrovirus
  - Adenovirus and herpes virus
  - Arbovirus
  - Hepatitis B virus

Other Causes

- Direct invasion of the CNS
- Post infections involvement of the CNS
- Arbovirus (mosquitoes, arthropod nectar)

Clinical Manifestations

- Malaise and fever
- Headache
- Dizziness
- Apathy
- Stiffness of neck
- Nausea and vomiting
- Ataxia
- Tremor and hyperactivity.
- Speech difficulties
- High fever
- Meningeal irritation signs such as nuchal rigidity, photophobia
- Stupor
- Seizures
- Disorientation
- Spasticity and coma

Investigation

- Lumbar puncture (LP)
- Blood serologic tests–HSV titer
- Urine and stool examination to identify a viral pathogen
- CT scan, MRI may show temporal or frontal lobe haemorrhage
- Electro Encephalogram (EEG)

Complications

- Seizures
- Respiratory failure
- Sensory and motor defects

Medical Management

- Antimicrobial agent
- Antibiotics
- Osmotic diuretics to reduce ICP
- Maintain ventilation

Nursing Management

- Nursing care focuses on monitoring cardio -respiratory function,
- Preventing complications resulting from immobility,
- Maintain the nutritional status of the child.
- Reorienting the child and teaching the parents about the child's condition.

Monitor the Child's Cardiorespiratory Function

- Check the child's airway and ability to handle secretions.
- Monitor respiratory status by observing colour, pulse oximetry readings, and arterial blood gas values.
- Observe cardiopulmonary status by monitoring heart rate, blood pressure, capillary refill time, and urine output.

- Provide seizure precautions, and have appropriate equipment for managing seizures at bedside.

Prevent Complications Resulting from Immobility

- Maintain skin integrity.
- Proper positioning with frequent turning is important.
- When indicated by the physician, perform chest physiotherapy to prevent pneumonia.

Maintain the Nutritional Status of the Child

- Provide small and frequent feeding to the child if child can take orally.
- If child is not taking orally, Ryle's tube feeding to be given or intravenous fluid to be administrated to the child.
- Provide high calorie diet and high protein diet.

Reorienting the Child and Teaching the Parents

- The child whose level of consciousness begins to improve may at first be confused and disoriented and may have residual effects of the disease.
- Orient the child to the hospital environment. Have the family help to reorient the child by bringing favourite stuffed animals or music from home.
- Engage in therapeutic play.
- Give the child age—appropriate toys to encourage a return to normal behaviour.
- Provide the parents with information about their child's condition and prognosis. If the child receives physical, occupational, or speech therapy, explain the treatment regimen to the parents.

CEREBRAL PALSY

Cerebral palsy is a term used to denote a group of disorders arising from a malfunction of motor centers and nerves pathways in the brain. It is a common permanent handicapping condition and is accompanied by seizures, mental retardation, various sensory defects and behavioural disorder.

Causes

Prenatal Causes

- Interference with the O_2 supply to brain such as separation of the placenta, compression of cord or bleeding.
- Maternal infection (rubella)
- Nutritional deficiencies
- Erythroblastosis fetalis or RH incompatibility
- Toxemia
- Radiation during pregnancy

Perinatal Causes

- Anoxia—immediately before, during and after birth
- Intracranial bleeding
- Asphyxia
- Jaundice
- Analgesic (morphine) causes depression of respiratory center
- Birth trauma
- Cerebral haemorrhage

Postnatal Causes

- Head trauma (fall)
- Infection (meningitis, encephalitis)
- Neoplasm
- Cerebral vascular accidents

Clinical Feature

- Difficulty in controlling voluntary muscle movement
- Seizures
- Mental retardation
- Hearing and vision impairment
- Behavioural disorder
- Delays in gross motor development
- Poor sucking and feeding behaviour

Types

Spastic type: This is the most frequent type. They have hyperactive, increased activity of the deep tendon reflexes. Contractures affecting the antigravity, scissoring is present, the child crosses his legs and points his toes when set on his feet.

Athetoid: is marked by involuntary non coordinated motion with varying degrees of muscle tension. These children are likely to have average or above intelligence. Hearing loss is most common.

Ataxia: Lack of coordination caused by disturbances of the kinaesthetic and balance sense. This type is very rare. Their gait is awkward or wide based.

Rigidity: Rigid postures and lack of active movement.

Mixed: Child will have more than one type of cerebral palsy.

Management

Aim of the treatment—To help the child make the most complete use of his residual abilities and achieve maximum possible satisfaction and enrichment.

A team of professionals is needed for this therapy like physician, surgeon, physical therapist, occupational therapist, speech therapist, social worker, and orthopaedic management also needed, dental care, etc.

Medical Management

- Baclofen (Lioresal)
  - Drivers baclofen, a skeletal muscle relaxant, is applied directly to the intrathecal space around the spinal cord
  - Used to treat spasticity
  - Pump lasts for 3 to 5 years; after that time, a new pump must be implanted .
- Muscle relaxants or neurosurgery to decrease spasticity, if appropriate.
- Anticonvulsants, such as phenytoin (Dilantin) and phenobarbital (luminal), to control seizures.
- An artificial urinary sphincter may be indicated for the incontinent child who can use the hands controls.
- Orthopaedic surgery may be indicated to correct contractures.
- Braces or splints and special appliances, such as adapted eating utensils and a low toilet seat arm, to help the child perform activities independently.

Nursing Management

- Institute a high-calorie diet for the child with increased motor function to help him keep up with increased metabolic demands.
- Perform ROM exercises to minimize contractures.
- Assist with locomotion, communication, and educational opportunities to enable the child to attain an optimal developmental level.
- Make food easy to manage to decrease stress during mealtimes.
- Promote age-appropriate mental activities and incentives for motor development to promote growth and development.
- Provide rest periods to promote rest and reduce metabolic needs.
- Provide a safe environment; for example, have the child use protective headgear or bed pads to prevent injury.
- Divide tasks into small steps to promote self-care and activity and increase self-esteem.
- Refer the child for speech, nutrition, and physical therapy to maintain or improve functioning.
- If the child cannot speak, use assistive communication devices to promote a positive self-concept.
- Assist family members in setting realistic goals and managing stress.

MENTAL RETARDATION

Mental retardation is an interference with intelligence that causes a limitation in the way the child is able to adapt to its environment. It is not a disease, but is a complex of symptoms due to variety of causes. The mentally retarded child has adaptive deficits in at least two areas such as communication, self-care, home living, social/interpersonal skills, use of community resources, self-direction, functional academic skills, work, leisure, health or safety. The IQ score and the level of adaptive skills together determine the degree of severity of mental retardation.

Incidence

Mild retardation occurs in 3 to 6 per 1000 people, and mental retardation affects about 3% of the population.

Causes

Hereditary

Other Causes

- Neonatal causes:
  - Intracranial haemorrhage
  - Anoxia or birth injury
- Prenatal causes:
  - Chromosomal defect like
    - Down syndrome
    - Fragile X syndrome
  - Fetal alcohol syndrome
  - Maternal infection
    - Rubella
    - Cytomegalovirus (CMV)

- Metabolic disorder such as phenylketonuria
- Hypothyroidism (cretinism)
- Mongolism—cranial malformation
- Maternal irradiation
- Anoxia
- Isoimmunization (kernicterus)

- Postnatal causes:
  - Intracranial injury
  - Haemorrhage
  - Infections such as meningitis or encephalitis
  - Poisoning such as with lead
  - Cerebrovascular thrombosis—Anoxia/Hypoxia
  - Neoplasm—Recurrent convulsion
  - Environmental deprivation

Clinical Feature

- Epilepsy
- Cerebral palsy
- Severe malnutrition
- Blindness
- Deafness and speech disorder
- MR- severe degree may be recognized as early as birth—failure of the infant to suck the breast or bottle.
- Abnormal development or delayed development.

Investigation

- Intelligence Quotient test (IQ)
- Study the emotional reaction and social adjustment

DSM-IV-TR Diagnostic Criteria for Mental Retardation

A. Significantly sub average intellectual functioning: an IQ approximately 70 or below on an individually administered IQ test (for infants, a clinical judgement of significantly sub average intellectual functioning).

B. Concurrent deficits or impairments in present adaptive functioning (*i.e.*, the person's effectiveness in meeting the standards expected for his or her age by his or her cultural group) in at least two of the following areas: communication, self-care, home living, social/interpersonal skills, use of community resources, self-direction, functional academic skills, work, leisure, health, and safety.

C. The onset is before age 18 years.

Classification

1. *Mildly retardation*: But educable – IQ present between 51–75 can reach a mental age of 8–12 years.
2. *Moderate retardation*: But trainable IQ present between 21–50.
3. *Severe retardation*: Are completely dependent on others for their care—IQ present between 0–20.

Management

- Management shall be done according to the classification
- Every effort should be made to help the child
- Home care
- Institutional care

Nursing Management

Nursing Assessment and Diagnosis

- Nurses can help to identify children with mental retardation through history taking, observation, and developmental screening during early childhood.
- The history should provide information about the mental and adaptive functioning of birth parents and other family members, as mental retardation may cluster in some families and conditions such as fragile X syndrome are genetic in origin.
- The pregnancy and birth history can provide important information relating to alcohol and drug use by the mother during pregnancy. Be alert for a history of difficult pregnancy and problems during delivery.
- When genetic conditions in the family predispose family members to mental retardation, careful assessment of the child is needed
- Children from deprived environments or those at risk because of environmental factors such as lead poisoning are more likely to manifest mental retardation.
- During home visits, clinic appointments, in child care centres, and during hospitalization, be alert for signs of developmental delays, multiple (more than three) physical anomalies associated with a specific condition or neuralgic alterations. Developmental assessment should be part of each healthcare visit.

- Once the diagnosis of mental retardation has been made, assess the adaptive functioning of the child and family.
- A functional assessment of the child should be performed, including toileting, dressing, and feeding skills.
- Assess the home and community for safety hazards.
- Observe how the family is managing with the child.
- Assess the availability of services such as support groups for parents and special education opportunities for children.
- Evaluate the coping skills of family members.

HEAD INJURIES

Traumatic damage to the head (the scalp, skull, meninges, or brain). Head injuries are a common cause of death in children older than age 1. The extent of the brain injury is directly related to the force and location of impact.

Causes

- Motor vehicle-related accidents
- Child abuse
- Vigorous shaking
- Bicycle accidents, especially in those without helmets
- Sports accidents, especially in those without helmets
- Falls
- Blunt trauma
- Penetration of foreign body

Pathophysiology

- The intracranial components are damaged because of a force too great to be absorbed by the skull, muscles, and ligaments that support the head.
- The skulls of infants and children are pliable and can absorb much of the physical impact, providing some level of protection to the intracranial components, but they have a larger head size and less support from muscles and ligaments, making them more prone to acceleration deceleration injuries.

Types of Head Injuries

Scalp laceration—can cause a child to bleed to death because of the vascularity of the surface area:

- Epidural, intracranial haemorrhage—bleeding into the space between the duramater and the skull.
- Subdural haemorrhage—bleeding between the duramater and the arachnoids layer of the meninges.
- Although bleeding may be extensive, hypovolemia or shock is uncommon unless the patient is an infant.

Concussion

- A transient state of neurologic dysfunction caused by a jarring of the brain.
- The most common head injury, it can involve transient impairment of consciousness that usually results from blunt head trauma.
- It is secondary to stretching, compression, or shearing of nerve fibers.
- The child will have an alteration in mental status (*e.g.*, amnesia, dizziness, memory, unsteady gait), but not necessarily loss of consciousness.
- Concussions are categorized by three levels of severity.

TABLE 9.4: Levels of Concussion Severity

Grade	Levels of Concussion
Grade 1	Transient confusion, no loss of consciousness, and duration of mental status abnormalities of less than 15 minutes.
Grade 2	Transient confusion, no loss of consciousness, and a duration of mental status abnormalities of less than 15 minutes and longer.
Grade 3	Loss of consciousness, either brief (seconds) or prolonged (minutes or longer).

Source: Adapted from quality standards subcommittee, American Academy of Neurology (1997) Practice Parameters: The Management of Concussion in Sports, Neurology.

Contusion

- A cerebral contusion, or the bruising of brain tissue, is secondary to blunt trauma and can occur with either coup or countercoup injuries.

- The temporal or frontal sections of the skull are the most common site of this injury, involves damage to the parenchyma with tears in vessels or tissue, pulping and subsequent areas of necrosis or infarction.
- A sign of petechial haemorrhage on the superficial aspects of the brain at the site of the impact.
- A lesion that occurs away from the site of direct trauma.

SKULL FRACTURE

A fracture to any of the eight cranial bones is caused by a considerable force to the head. Any area of the skull with swelling or a haematoma should be evaluated for possible fracture.

- Linear (Simple) fracture
- Depressed (Depression of a bone toward the brain) fracture
- Basilar (at the skull base) fracture
- Compound fracture

Table 9.5: Types of Skull Fractures

Injury	Clinical Therapy
Linear fracture Results from impact to large area of the skull. Usually no symptoms. May have overlying haematoma or soft tissue swelling.	If the fracture is on temporal bone or crosses sagital suture line CT scan to detect the epidural haematoma. consider the possibility of inflicted injury.
Depressed fracture Break in skull itself or an area shattered into many fragments. Pieces of bone may be depressed into brain tissue with haematoma forming on top.	Plain X-ray or CT scan is performed. Surgery to elevate bone fragments when depression is greater than 5 mm. Tetanus Prophylaxis given as needed. Many are associated with intracranial injury and Post traumatic epilepsy.
Compound fracture Combination of a full thickness scalp laceration and depressed skull fracture with the bone exposed. Injuries are considered penetrating fractures if the dura is torn.	Visual diagnosis is performed along with radiographic studies. Surgical debridement, a search for foreign bodies, and copious irrigation are performed. Parenteral antibiotics and tetanus prophylaxis are provided as needed.
Basilar fracture Fracture at the base of the skull that may Involve the frontal, ethmoid, spnenoid, temporal or occipital bones. A dural tear may be present.	Diagnosis is confirmed by signs of blood behind the tympanic membranes, cerebrospinal fluid leakage from the nose or ears, periorbital ecchymosis (raccoon eyes), or bruising of the mastoid (Battle Sign), Radiographic imaging locates the fracture site. Antibiotics may be prescribed. Surgical repair of the site of the cerebrospinal fluid leak is performed. If the leak persists after 7–10 days, transient or permanent cranial nerve injuries occur (e.g., hearing loss).

Source: Rosman, N.P (1999).

Complications

- Haemorrhage
- Infection
- Oedema
- Herniation

Clinical Manifestations

- Change in Level of Consciousness (LOC) or mental status
- Confusion
- Listlessness
- Irritability
- Pale skin
- Vomiting
- Increased head circumference
- Bulging fontanels

- Haemiparesis, quadriplegia
- Headache
- Decreased memory
- Diminished papillary responses

Investigation

- CT and MRI scans show neurologic trauma and injury
- ICP monitoring shows increased ICP
- Skull X-rays show fractures or areas of injury

Emergency Treatment

1. Assess the child
   A - Airway
   B - Breathing
   C - Circulation
2. Stabilize neck and spine.
3. Clean any abrasions with soap and water. Apply clean dressing. If bleeding, apply ice for 1 hour to relieve pain and swelling.
4. Keep NPO or give only clear liquids until no vomiting for at least 6 hours.
5. Give no analgesics or sedatives.
6. Check pupil reaction every 4 hours (including twice during night) for 48 hours.
7. Awaken two times during night to check level of consciousness.
8. Seek medical attention if there is any of the following injury is sustained:
   - At high speed (*e.g.*, auto)
   - Fall from great force (*e.g.*, baseball bat)
   - Under suspicious circumstances
     - Child less than 6 months of age
     - Unconscious more than 5 seconds
     - Discomfort (crying) more than 10 minutes after injury.
     - Headache that is severe, worsening, interferes with sleep.
     - Vomiting three or more times.
     - Swelling in front of or above earlobe or swelling that increases in size.
     - Confused or not behaving normally.
     - Difficult to rouse from sleep.
     - Difficulty with speaking.
     - Blurring of vision or seeing double.
     - Unsteady gait
     - Difficult using upper extremities
     - Neck pain (difficult to touch the neck, baby cries)
     - Pupils dilated or fixed
     - Infant with bulging fontanel.

Management

- Medications, such as diphenhydramine (Benadryl) or chloral hydrate (Aqua chloral Suppurates).
- Surgical management depends upon the child diagnosis and condition.

Nursing Interventions

- Assessing a head injury for the child
- Prepare for surgical evaluation of the injury, if necessary
- Promote bed rest and limit unnecessary body movements; slightly elevate the head of the bed
- Initiate seizure precautions
- Provide a quiet environment
- Awaken the child every 2 hours to check his LOC
- Monitor fluid status carefully; restrict fluids as needed to decrease ICP
- Prevent injury through family and community teaching programs to stress child safety (bicycle helmets, car restraining devices, protective skating equipment)
- Check ear or nose drainage for glucose (CSF tests positive for glucose)
- Note behavioural changes (such as aggression, withdrawal, irritability); watch for alterations in sleep patterns, gait, or school performance.

Altered Musculoskeletal Conditions

DIAGNOSTIC TESTS

Arthroscopy

Purpose

- To perform a visual examination of the interior of a joint with a fiber—optic endoscope.

Nursing Interventions

- Explain the procedure to the parents and the child.
- Obtain written, informed consent.
- Tell the child and its parents that it may need to fast after midnight before the procedure.
- Note allergies because local anaesthesia is used.
- Tell the child that it may feel a thumping sensation as the cannula is inserted in the joint capsule.

Computed Tomography (CT) Scan

Purpose

- Using a strong magnetic field and radio waves, allows cross-sectional imaging of bones and joints and visual assessment of certain muscle and soft-tissue injuries.

Nursing Interventions

- Note if the child has any metal implants, which would be a contraindication for the procedure
- Explain the procedure to the parents and child
- Instruct the child to hold still during the procedure; sedation may be necessary.

Myelography

Purpose

- An invasive procedure that involves injection of a radiopaque contrast medium and serial X-rays used to evaluate abnormalities of the spinal canal and cord.

Nursing Interventions

- Before the procedure
  - Explain the procedure to the parents and the child
  - Obtain written, informed consent
  - Check for allergies to the contrast medium
  - If metrizamide (Amipaque) is used as the contrast medium, discontinue phenothiazines 48 hours before the test.
- During the procedure
  - When the contrast medium is injected, tell the child that he may experience a burning sensation, warmth, headache, salty taste, nausea, and vomiting.
- After the procedure
  - Have the child sit in his room or lie on bed with his head elevated 60 degrees.
  - Make sure he doesn't lie flat for at least 8 hours.
  - Encourage the child to drink extra fluids.
  - Check that the child voids within 8 hours.

X-rays

Purpose

- To help identify joint disruption, calcifications, and bone deformities, fractures, and destruction
- To help measure bone density

Nursing Interventions

- Explain the test to the parents and child
- Tell the child he must hold still during the X-ray
- Cover the genital area with a lead apron

Nursing Diagnoses

Probable Nursing Diagnoses

- Delayed growth and development

- Impaired physical mobility
- Risk for peripheral neurovascular dysfunction
- Impaired walking
- Disturbed body image
- Acute pain
- Activity intolerance
- Risk for injury

Possible Nursing Diagnoses

- Risk for impaired skin integrity
- Impaired gas exchange
- Chronic pain
- Ineffective role performance
- Fatigue
- Compromised family coping
- Powerlessness
- Dressing or grooming self-care deficit
- Ineffective breathing pattern
- Bathing or hygiene self-care deficit
- Anxiety
- Fear.

DEFORMITIES OF SPINE

The spine, consisting of numerous segments, can acquire deformation curves of three types:

1. Kyphosis
2. Lordosis
3. Scoliosis

Kyphosis

Kyphosis is an abnormally increased convex angulation in the curvature of the thoracic spine.

Causes

It can occur secondary to disease processes such as tuberculosis, chronic arthritis, osteodystrophy, or compression fracture of the thoracic spine, most common form of kyphosis is "Postural" children.

Treatment

- Postural exercises to strengthen shoulder and abdominal muscles.
- Bracing for more marked deformity.

Lordosis

Lordosis is an accentuation of the lumbar curvature beyond physiologic limits.

Causes

- Trauma
- Idiopathic
- Associated with flexion contractures of the hip obesity, congenital dislocated hip and slipped femoral capital epiphysis.

Treatment

- Weight reduction and correction of deformities
- Postural exercise.

Scoliosis

Scoliosis is a complex spinal deformity in three planes. It usually involves lateral curvature spinal rotation causing rib asymmetry and thoracic hypokyphosis. Most common is spinal deformity.

Types

- Non-structural, functional or postural scoliosis—a no progressive **C** curvature caused by another condition.
- Structural or progressive scoliosis —a progressive **S** curvature.

Causes

- Idiopathic
- Congenital scoliosis. It may associate with meningomyelocele or failure of segmentation in the vertebrae.
- Neuromuscular scoliosis—due to muscular imbalance, weakness of muscle.
- Lower motor neuron diseases such as poliomyelitis.
- Upper motor neuron diseases such as cerebral palsy.
- Traumatic—thoracotomy or thoracoplasty with rib resection.
- Spinal cord trauma—tumour therapy
  —Fracture
- Miscellaneous—Tumor
  —Inflammation
  —Nutritional deficiencies–rickets
- Mesenchymal diseases—Congenital disorder
  —Dwarfism
- Acquired disorder—rheumatoid arthritis.

Pathophysiology

Non-structural Scoliosis

The pelvic tilt caused by unequal leg lengths, poor posture, para-spinal inflammation, acute disk disease, or head tilt associated with poor vision leads to a spinal deviation.

Structural Scoliosis

- Congenital—usually related to a congenital defect, such as wedge vertebrae, fused ribs or vertebrae, or hemi vertebrae; may result from trauma to zygote or embryo.
- Paralytic or musculoskeletal develops several months after asymmetrical paralysis of the trunk muscles due to polio, cerebral palsy, or muscular dystrophy.
- Idiopathic—the most common form; may be transmitted as an autosomal dominant or multifactorial trait.
  - Appears in previously straight spine during the growing years.
  - Brain stem dysfunction, possibly due to a lesion of the posterior columns or the inner ear, may be the cause.
  - Three classifications.
    - Infantile—affects mostly male infants between birth and age 3 and causes left thoracic and right lumbar curves.
    - Juvenile—affects both sexes between ages 4 and 10 and causes varying types of curvature.
    - Adolescent—generally affects girls between ages 10 to achievement of skeletal maturity and causes varying types of curvature.
- Scoliosis stops progressing when bone growth stops.

Complications

- Impaired growth and development
- Body image disturbances
- Impaired mobility
- Debilitating back pain
- Severe deformity
- With thoracic curve exceeding 60 degrees: possible reduced pulmonary function
- With thoracic curve exceeding 80 degrees: increased risk of corpulmonale in middle age.

Clinical Manifestations

- Preadolescent growth spurt
- Ill fitting of clothes

Non-structural Scoliosis

- C–shaped curvature of the spine
- The curve of the spine disappears when the child bends at the waist to touch the toes.

Structural Scoliosis

- A curve in the thoracic segment of the spine, with convexity to the right, and compensatory curves (S Curves) in the cervical segment above and the lumbar segment below, both with a convexity to the left.
- The spinal curve fails to straighten when the child bends forward with the knees straight and the arms hanging down toward the feet.
- The hips, ribs shoulders, and shoulder blades are asymmetrical
- Backache
- Fatigue
- Dyspnea.

Investigation

- Physical growth—disproposition
- Pain sacral dimpling or hairy patches, absent or abnormal reflexes
- Bowel or bladder incontinence
- X-rays of the spine—reveal curvature
- MRI scan
- Scoliometer—measures the degree of spine curvature.

Management

Medical Management

- **Non-structural Scoliosis**
  - Corrective lenses for the eyes if the problem is associated with poor vision that results in a head tilt
  - Postural exercise
  - Shoe lifts.
- **Structural Scoliosis**
  - Electrical stimulation for mild to moderate curvatures
  - Harrington, Luque, or Cotrel—double set rods for curves greater than 40 degrees (to realign the spine or when curves fail to respond to orthotic treatment)

- Possible prolonged bracing (Milwaukee or Boston brace)
  - Worn over a T-shirt for 23 hours per day
  - Brace adjustments every 3 months
- Skin traction or halo–femoral traction
- Spinal fusion with bone from the iliac crest
- Surgical—realignment and straightening with internal taxation and instrumentation combined with bony fusion of the realigned spine (arthrodesis).

Nursing Intervention

- After spinal fusion and the insertion of rods
  - Monitor vital signs and intake and output to prevent fluid volume deficit.
  - Turn the child only by logrolling to prevent injury.
  - Maintain correct body alignment to promote joint mobility and prevent injury.
  - Keep the bed in a flat position to prevent injury and complication.
  - Help the child adjust to the increase in height and altered self-perception to promote self-esteem and decrease anxiety.
- Teach the child to perform stretching exercises for the spine.
- Help the child to maintain self-esteem
- Teach the child to maintain self-esteem
  - How to apply it and how long to wear it
  - How to prevent skin breakdown
    - Keep the skin beneath the brace clean and dry
    - Wear a tight fitting T-shirt under the brace.

FRACTURES

Definition

Fracture is a discontinuation of the continuity of the tissue of the bones, or a crack, or breakage of bone. When the resistance of bone against the stress being exerted yields to the stress force, it met fracture. Common fracture sites are legs and arms in children.

Causes

Trauma

- Fall
- Sport-related injury
- Child abuse (Suspected in the case of multiple or repeated episodes of fractures)
- Motor vehicle accidents
- Repetitive force on a bone (stress fracture)
- Vigorous play—climbing, falling, running

Pathological Causes

- Bone tumours
- Metabolic disease

Types

- Complete—When fracture fragments are separated.
- Incomplete—When fragments remain attached it is called incomplete.

Fracture line can be

- Transverse
- Oblique
- Bend
- Greenstick fracture
- Buckle fracture—metaphysic, epiphysis
- Complete

Classification

Growth plate fractures are classified depending on the degree of damage to the growth plate itself.

Several classification systems of growth plate fractures have been developed. Perhaps the most widely used is the Salter-Harris system and is described here.

Salter-Harris Classification of Growth Plate Fractures

Type I Fractures: These fractures break through the bone at the growth plate, separating the bone end from the bone shaft and completely disrupting the growth plate.

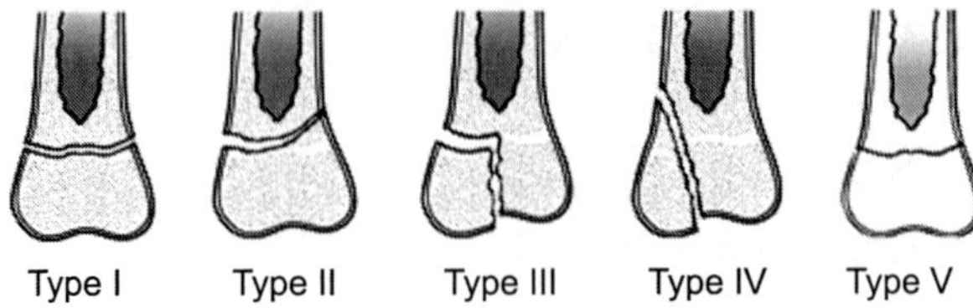

Fig. 10.1: Types of fractures

Type II Fractures: These fractures break through part of the bone at the growth plate and crack through the bone shaft as well.

Type III Fractures: These fractures cross through a portion of the growth plate and break off a piece of the bone end.

Type IV Fractures: These fractures break through the bone shaft, the growth plate, and the end of the bone.

Type V Fractures: These fractures occur due to a crushing injury to the growth plate from a compression force. They are rare fractures.

Complications

- Permanent deformity and dysfunction if bones fail to heal (non-union) or heal improperly (malunion)
- Aseptic necrosis of bone segments from impaired circulation
- Hypovolemic shock as a result of blood vessel damage (this is especially likely to develop in patients with a fractured femur)
- Muscle contractures
- Renal calculi from decalcification (due to prolonged immobility)
- Fat embolism
- Compartment syndrome

Clinical Manifestations

- Pain
- Deformity
- Swelling
- Discoloration
- Crepitus
- Loss of limb function
- If fracture is caused by arterial compromise or nerve damage we can find the symptoms and signs of
  - Numbness and tingling
  - Mottled cyanosis
  - Cool skin at the end of the extremity
  - Loss of pulse distal to the injury.
- Open fractures
  - Skin wound.

Investigation

- History
- X-rays confirm a diagnosis of fracture.

Medical Management

- Simple traction and immobilization until healing takes place
- Position of the bone fragment
- Immobilization
- Restore function to the injured part.

Cast Type

- Short leg cast with walking attachment
- Long leg cast
- Short arm cast
- Long arm cast
- Hip spica casts

Traction

- Manual traction
- Skin traction
- Skeletal traction

Immediate Fracture Management

- Splinting the limb above and below the suspected fracture
- Applying a cold pack
- Elevating the limb to reduce oedema and pain
- Severe fractures that cause blood loss
  - Apply direct pressure to control bleeding
  - Administer fluid replacement as soon as possible to prevent or treat hypovolemic shock
- Reduction
  - Restores displaced bone segments to their normal position.
  - After reduction, the fractured arm or leg must be immobilized by a splint, cast, or with traction.
  - Closed reduction
    - Manual manipulation facilitates the muscle stretching necessary to realign the bone
    - X-rays to determine the outcome of an attempt at closed reduction.
  - Open reduction
    - Used when closed reduction is impossible.
    - Reduces and immobilizes the fracture.
  - Rods
  - Plates
  - Screws

- Casting
  - Traction
    - Uses a series of weights and pulleys.
    - Used when a splint or cast fails to maintain the reduction.
    - Skin traction.
  - Adhesives, moleskin, elastic bandages, and sheepskin coverings are used to attach traction devices to the child's skin.
  - Traction pulls indirectly on the skeleton by pulling on the skin.
- Skeletal traction
  - Pulls directly on the skeleton via pins or wires.
  - A pin or wire inserted through the bone distal to the fracture and attached to a weight allows for prolonged traction.
- Open fractures
  - Tetanus prophylaxis
  - Prophylactic antibiotics
  - Surgery to repair soft-tissue damage
  - Thorough debridement of the wound

Nursing Interventions

- Watch for signs of shock in the child with a severe open fracture of a large bone such as the femur.
- Monitor vital signs, and be especially alert for rapid pulse, decreased blood pressure, pallor, and cool, clammy skin—all of which may indicate that child is in shock.
- Administer I.V. fluids as ordered.
- Offer reassurance to the child, who may be frightened and in pain.
- Ease pain with analgesics as needed.
- Help the child and parents set realistic goals for recovery.
- When a fracture requires long-term immobilization with traction
  - Reposition the child often to increase comfort and prevent pressure ulcers.
  - Assist with active ROM exercises to prevent muscle atrophy.

Nursing Management with Cast

1. Maintain muscle use of an affected area
2. Provide comfort
3. Educate parents
4. Support child during cast removal
   - Encourage deep breathing and coughing to avoid hypostatic pneumonia
     - Urge adequate fluid intake to prevent urinary stasis and constipation
     - Watch for signs of renal calculi (flank pain, nausea, and vomiting)
     - Provide good cast care
   - Support the cast with pillows
   - Observe for skin irritation near cast edges
   - Check for foul odour or discharge
   - Tell the child to report signs and symptoms of impaired circulation

     Skin coldness

     Numbness

     Tingling

     Discoloration
   - Warn the child not to get the cast wet
   - Instruct the child not to insert foreign objects under the cast

- Encourage the child to start moving around as soon as he is able
  - Help him to walk
  - Demonstrate how to use crutches properly
- After cast removal, refer the child to a physical therapist to restore limb mobility.

Teaching about Cast Care

Be sure to include these points in your teaching plan for the parents of a child with a cast:

- Mechanism of bone healing and necessity for casting
- Cast care, including air exposure, elevation, and moving
- Measures to protect the cast
- Measures for skin care
- Methods to relieve itching and irritation
- Measures to keep cast dry
- Ways to test for sensation, movement, and circulation
- Measures to cope with swelling
- Monitoring for wound drainage
- Exercises for the casted extremity.

BURNS

Burns are the second leading cause of injury deaths (after motor vehicle crashes) in children between 5 and 14 years of age (Murphy, 2000). Boys between the ages of 1 and 4 years are twice as likely as girls to be burned; however, the national average age of paediatric burn patients is 32 months. In 1997, 83,000 children were hospitalized for burns. About 4440,000 children are treated for burns each year.

Types

The four main types of burns are thermal, chemical, electrical, and radioactive. Thermal burns, the most common burns in children, may occur through exposure to flames or scalds (such as coffee or grease), or contact with a hot object (such as a wood stove or curling iron). Sherray, described in the opening vignette, sustained a scald burn when a bowl of hot soup fell onto her leg. Chemical burns occur when children touch or ingest caustic agents. Electrical burns occur from exposure to direct or alternating current in electrical wires, appliances, or high-voltage wires. Radiation burns result from exposure to radioactive substances or sunlight. About 10% of all burns in children are due to child abuse.

Etiology

- Residential fires
- Motor vehicle accidents
- Improper use or handling of matches
- Improperly stored kerosene
- Space heater or electric malfunctions
- Contact with faulty electrical wiring
- Child or elder abuse
- Scalding accidents
- Contact ingestion, inhalation, or inunction of acid, alkali
- Contact with high voltage power lines
- Contact with hot liquid or electricity
- Burned by flames

Children at different developmental stages are at risk for different types of burns:

- Infants are most often injured by thermal burns (scalding liquids, house fires).
- Toddlers are at risk for thermal burns (Pulling hot liquids or grease onto themselves), electrical burns (biting electrical cords), contact burns, and chemical burns (ingesting cleaning agents and other substances) associated with exploring the environment.
- Preschool–age children are most often injured by scalding or contact with hot appliances (curling irons, ovens).
- School-age children are at risk for thermal burns (Playing with matches, fireworks), electrical burns (Climbing high-voltage towers wires), and chemical burns (Combustion experiments) associated with their curiosity and interest in experimentation.
- Adolescents also experience thermal, chemical, and electrical burns.

Pathophysiology

Immediately after the burn, intense vasoconstriction occurs in response to substances released by the injured cells; then vasodilatation and capillary permeability allow plasma to seep into the wound. Ischemia due to vasoconstriction may increase the depth of the burn injury. The child experiences increased water and heat loss through the injured epidermis. The child's metabolic rate and need for calories increases as the child tries to maintain body temperature.

Classification explained according to the depth of the injury (layers affected, skin, epidermis, and dermis)

- **Superficial Partial Thickness.** It is called as a first degree burn.
  - Damages only outer layer of the skin
  - Burn is painful and red
  - Heals in a few days
  - Not life threatening *e.g.,* (sunburn)
- **Deep Partial Thickness.** Second degree burn.
  - Involves epidermis and upper layers of the dermis
  - Thin walled and fluid filled blisters
  - May involves sweat gland and sebaceous glands
  - As blisters break, nerve endings are exposed to air
  - Barrier function of the skin is lost
  - Heals in 10–14 days.
- **Full Thickness.** Third degree burn.
  - Involves all of epidermis and dermis
  - Affects every body system and organ
  - May also involve underlying tissue
  - Nerve ending usually destroyed

- **Fourth Degree Burns**
  - Fourth degree burns damage muscles, bones and interstitial tissues
  - Interstitial fluids result in edema
  - Immediate immunolgic response occurs
  - There is wound sepsis threat
  - Painless
  - Scab forms

Complications

- Respiratory complications
- Sepsis
- Hypovolemic shock
- Anaemia
- Malnutrition
- Multiple organ dysfunction syndrome

Clinical Manifestations

Burns are classified by depth. Burn depth may be defined as partial thickness or full thickness.

- Superficial Partial-thickness burn, (first degree burn)
  - Dry, painful, redskin with oedema
  - Look like a sunburn
  - Signs of infection include purulent drainage, focal areas of necrosis, oedema, erythema, discoloration of wound margins, and conversion from partial-thickness to full-thickness injury depth.
- Deep partial thickness (second degree) burn
  - Moist, weeping blisters with oedema
  - Very painful
- Full thickness (third degree) burn
  - Vascular without blanching or pain
  - Dry, pale, leathery skin
  - Diuresis 2 to 5 days after the burns, as fluid shift back
  - Fluid shift from intravascular to interstitial compartments
  - Hypovolemia
  - Symptoms of shock from fluid shift include renal failure
  - Infection due to altered skin integrity.

Assessment of Burn Severity

Table 10.1: Classification of Burns Severity

Minor	Partial thickness <10% BSA Full thickness <2% BSA
Moderate	Partial thickness 10%–20 % BSA Full thickness 3%–10% BSA
Major (severe)	Partial thickness 20% BSA Full thickness >10% BSA Burns involve face, eyes, hands, feet and perineum Electrical burns, Inhalation injury, other injury and pre-existing chronic conditions

Source: Adapted from Stewart, C. (2000). Emergency care of paediatric burns. *Pediatric Emergency Medicine Report*, ***5***(*10*): 101–112.

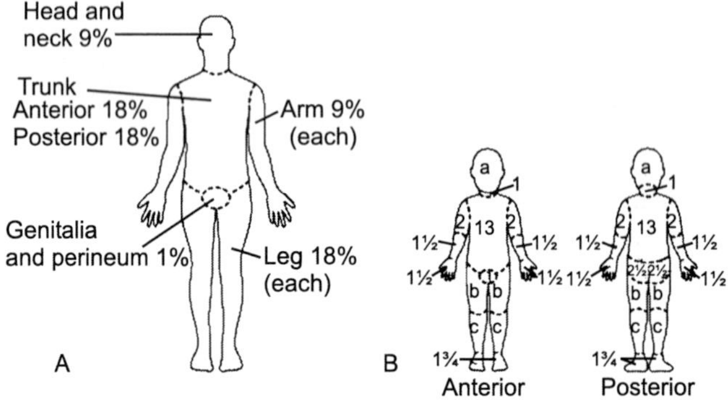

Relative percentage of body surface area (% BSA) affected by growth

Body Part	0 yr	1 yr	5 yr	10 yr	15 yr
	Age				
a = 1/2 of head	9 1/2	8 1/2	6 1/2	5 1/2	4 1/2
b = 1/2 of 1 thigh	2 3/4	3 1/4	4	4 1/4	4 1/2
c = 1/2 of 1 lower leg	2 1/2	2 1/2	2 3/4	3	3 1/4

Fig. 10.2: Percentage of body surface area

Estimation of Burns Distribution in Children, Age from Birth to Older Children

- Burn severity is determined by the depth of the burn injury, Percentage of body surface area (BSA) affected, and involvement of specific body parts (see Table 10.1).
- A Lund and Browder chart with BSA distributions for various body parts at different ages is used to calculate the area affected by the burn injury (see Fig. 10.2).

- Once the affected BSA is calculated, the burn can be classified as minor, moderate, or major. Children with moderate and major burns require hospitalization, and those with major burns will usually be transferred to a burn center.
- The involvement of specific body parts or specific burn distributions increases the burn severity, regardless of the percentage of BSA affected.
- Burns to the face, hands, feet, or perineal area are treated as major injuries because of the potential for functional impairment. Circumferential burns (injury completely surrounding the thorax or an extremity), anterior chest burns, and smoke inhalation are also classified as major burns.

Investigation

- Arterial blood gas
- Complete blood count
- Blood serum electrolytes
- BUN
- Electrocardiogram
- Fiber-optic bronchoscopy (shows oedema of the airway)

Medical Management

Emergency Care

Initial management of the burn patient begins at the scene of injury. The first priority is to stop the burning process. The child should then be transported immediately to the nearest medical facility for definitive treatment.

- *For Minor Burns*
  - The first step is to stop the burning process by removing jewellery and all clothing.
  - Moist soaks or ice (If small surface area is affected) are used to stop the burning process and to relieve pain.
  - Do not apply anything to the wound
  - Cover with a clean cloth if there is risk of damage or contamination.
  - A tetanus vaccine booster is given if more than 5 years have passed since the last vaccine, or when the child has not completed the full vaccine series.
- *For Major Burns*
  - Stop the burning process:
    - Place victim in the horizontal position.
    - Roll victim in a blanket or similar object; avoid covering the head.
  - Assess for an adequate airway and breathing.
  - If not breathing, begin mouth-to-mouth resuscitation.
  - Remove burned clothing and jewellery.
  - Cover wound with a clean cloth.
  - Keep victim warm.
  - Transport to medical aid.
  - Administer intravenous infusion and oxygen therapy.

Management of Minor Burns

Burns classified as a minor can usually be managed adequately on an outpatient department if the caregiver is relied on to carry out the instructions and it requires close follow up.

Wound care includes:

- Clean the wound with soap and water
- Debridement of the wound includes removal of any embedded debris, chemicals and devitalized tissue.
- Removal of intact blisters remains controversial, some authorities argue that blisters provide a barrier against infection; others says that blister fluid is an effective medium for the growth of microorganisms.
- Wound is covered with antimicrobial ointment to reduce the risk of infection, and with light wrap of gauze dressing that avoids interference with movement.
- Instruct the child or parent to keep the wound clean and protect from trauma.
- Instruct them to come for dressing to the hospital.
- The frequency of dressing changes can vary from every other day to twice a day.
- Observe any sign of infection or complication, inform the parent to come for dressing daily.
- Burns of the face are usually treated by an open method, wound must be washed and antimicrobial ointment must be applied twice a day.
- Tetanus prophylaxis is administered if there is no history of immunization or age of the child is more than 5.
- Administration of antibiotics depends upon the hospital policy.

- Administration of mild analgesic like acetaminophen.
- Antipyretic effect of the drug also alleviates the sensation of heat.
- If any complication like function impairment is evaluated, caregiver should be instructed to give exercise and ambulation or physiotherapy.

Management of Major Burns

When a child with extensive burns is admitted to the hospital for treatment, a variety of assessment should be done and treatment must be initiated. The priority concerns include:

- The establishment and maintenance of an adequate airway.
- Initiation of fluid administration.
- Evaluation and treatment of wound and other therapies.
- Nutritional support.
- Positioning and splinting to prevent contractures.
- Treatment of anaemia and hypoproteinemia.
- Psychological support and rehabilitative aspects.

Establishment of an Adequate Airway

The first priority of care is airway maintenance,

- Assessment of the child of oral and nasal membrane that reveals oedema, hyperemia, and blisters or evidence of trauma in upper respiratory passage, administer 100% oxygen.
- Observe the changes in sensorium, air hunger, or other sign of respiratory distress, intubation is performed and ventilatory support is provided.
- Treatment may include bronchodilators to reduce the bronchial spasm.
- Positioning, Provide semi-fowler position, frequently change the position, suctioning is needed to reduce the risk of pneumonia.

Fluid Replacement Therapy

Objectives of the fluid therapy are:

- Compensation for water and sodium losses to the traumatized area and the interstitial spaces, replenishment of sodium deficits.
- Restoration of circulating volume, provision of adequate perfusion, correction of acidosis and improvement of renal function.
- Treatment of fluid replacement is required during the first 24 hours because of fluid shifts that are occurring, Crystalloid solutions are used during this initial phase of therapy. The colloid solutions such as albumin, plasmalytic, a fresh frozen plasma are useful in maintaining plasma volume.
- Ascertain the adequacy of fluid parameters such as vital signs (especially heart rate), urine output volume, adequacy of capillary filling and state of sensorium.
- Ascertain the adequacy of the airway and provide oxygen, insert a large-bore intravenous line, preferably through unburned skin, to deliver fluids at a sufficiently rapid rate to effect resuscitation.
- Insert an indwelling Foley catheter to obtain specimens and monitor hourly output.
- Obtain admission weight.
- Calculate fluid requirements and establish the appropriate regimen.

Nutrition

The enhanced metabolic requirement and catabolism in severe burns make nutritional needs a paramount importance and often difficult to provide.

- Initially the diet must provide sufficient calories to meet the increased metabolic needs and protein to avoid protein breakdown.
- A high protein, high caloric diet is encouraged after resolution of paralytic ileus.
- Child may have poor appetite and may be unable to meet the energy requirement by oral feeding.
- Children with burns in excess of 25% of the TBSA require supplementation with tube feeding.
- Children who have severe burns, if nutritional requirement cannot be met entirely by the central route, parenteral hyperalimentation can be used to supplement intake.
- To facilitate growth and proliferation of epithelial cells, administration of vitamins A and C is begun early in the post burn period.
- Zinc is also supplemented because of its important role in wound healing and epithelialization.

Medication

- Administration of systemic antibiotics to prevent to develop infection.
- Sedation and analgesia is required in the care of burn children *e.g.*, Morphine sulphate is the drug

of choice for severe burn injuries, the dose is 5 to 15 μg/kg.

- Provide IV medication for control of pain and anxiety only after adequate oxygenation is ensured and fluid resuscitation is initiated.
- Administer short acting anaesthetic agent such as propofol and nitrous oxide for eliminating procedural pain.
- Nitrous oxide (50%) and oxygen (50%) a mixture of gases is given for 1 minute (3–5 minutes) to alleviate anxiety and pain.

Burns Wound Care

Initial period is managed with shock management and restoration of fluid balance, and then primary concern is the burn wound. Evaluate the burn wound and determine the extent and depth of injury.

Objective of wound management includes:

- Prevention of infection
- Removal of devitalized tissues and
- Closure of the wound
- Application of dressings and topical antimicrobial therapy reduce pain by minimizing the exposure to air.

Primary excision: Early excision of deep partial-thickness and full-thickness reduces the incidence of infection and the threat of sepsis.

Debridement

Hydrotherapy is employed to cleanse the wound and involves soaking in a tub or showering once or twice a day for not more than 20 minutes.

Hydrotherapy helps to not only clean the wound but also maintenance of range of motion.

Apply topical antimicrobials and dressings to the burn wounds

Method used for managing the burns wound include:

- *Exposure*—Wound is left open to air; crust forms on partial thickness wounds and scar form on full-thickness burns.
- *Open*—Topical antimicrobial agent is applied directly to the wound surface, and the wound is left uncovered.
- *Modified*—Antimicrobial is applied directly or impregnated into thin gauze and applied to the wound; gauze or net secures the area.
- *Occlusive*—Antimicrobial is impregnated in gauze or applied directly to the wound; multiple layers of bulky gauze are placed over the primary layer and secured with gauze or net.
  - Topical agents do not eliminate organism from the wound but can effectively inhibit bacterial growth.
  - To be effective, a topical application must be non-toxic, capable of diffusing through scar, harmless to viable tissue, inexpensive, and easy to apply.
  - It should not encourage the development of resistant strains of bacteria and should produce minimum electrolyte derangement
  - Common topical agents are
    - Silver nitrate 0.5%
    - Silver sulfadiazine 1%
    - Mafenide acetate 10%
    - Bacitracin.
  - Obtain baseline laboratory studies.
  - Administer appropriate tetanus prophylaxis.

Biologic skin coverings: Permanent coverage of extensive burns is a prolonged process that requires repeated operations for debridement and grafting.

- Objectives to early closure shorten the period of metabolic stress and decrease the likelihood of burn wound sepsis.
- In addition, biologic dressings markedly reduce pain and facilitate movement of joints to retain range of motion.

Types of Skin Grafts

Temporary Grafts

Allograft (*homograft*)—Skin is obtained from genetically different members (cadavers) that are screened for communicable diseases.

This graft is useful in the coverage of surgically excised deep partial-thickness and full-thickness wounds in extensive burns when available donor sites are limited.

Xenografts (*heterograft*)—Skin that is obtained from members of a different species, most primarily notably pigskin, is commercially available.

Pig skin dressings are replaced daily or every 2 to 3 days, they are particularly effective in children with partial-thickness scald burns of the hands and face, children relatively have pain free movement, which reduces contracture formation and has the added benefit of improving appetite and morale.

Synthetic skin coverings—are available for the management of partial-thickness burn wounds.

Permanent Grafts

Autograft—Tissue obtained from undamaged areas of the patient's own body.

Isograft—Histocompatible tissue obtained from genetically identical individuals.

Methods of Applying Split Thickness Grafts

Sheet graft—A sheet of skin, removed from the donor site, is placed intact over the recipient site and sutured in place.

Mesh graft—A sheet of skin is removed from the donor site and passed through a mesher, which produces tiny slits in the skin. The meshing allows the expansion of the skin to cover 1½ to 9 times the area of the sheet graft.

Artificial skin—The development of Integra, a product that allows the dermis to regenerate has produced significant improvement in burn wound healing and decreased scar formation.

Perform escharotomy and/or *fasciotomy* to the chest and extremities for constricting circumferential scar or for elevated compartment pressures and for impaired circulation.

Nursing Interventions

- Apply immediate, aggressive burn treatment
- Use sterile technique
- Remove clothing that is still smouldering
- Remove the patient's rings and other constricting items
- Perform appropriate wound care
- Provide adequate hydration
  - By administering lactated Ringer's solution through a large-bore I.V. line.
  - Weigh the patient daily.
  - Monitor urine output; for a child under 30 kg, output should be 1 ml/kg/hour.
  - Important nursing function is to regulate the flow rate of an intravenous infusion, in paediatrics common drops factors is 60 for micro drips.
  - There are two methods of calculating flow rates, the number of millilitres per hour and the number of drops per minute.
  - Millilitres per hour—Hourly rates of infusion can be calculated by dividing the total infusion volume by the total infusion time in hours, *e.g.*, 3000 ml is infused in 24 hrs. The number of millilitre per hour is

$$\frac{\text{3000 ml (total infusion volume)}}{\text{24 hours (total infusion time)}} = \text{125 ml/hr}$$

To calculate the drops per minute

$$= \frac{\text{Total infusion volume} \times \text{drops/minute or (drop factor)}}{\text{Total time of infusion in minute}}$$

For example, 1000 ml in 8 hrs (480 minutes) and the drops factor is 20 drops/ml

The drops per minute

$$= \frac{\text{1000 ml} \times \text{20 drops/ml}}{\text{480 minute}} = \text{41 drops/minute}$$

- Assess for pain and provide medication as needed; medicate before dressing changes.
- Encourage verbalization and provide support.
- Monitor urine specific gravity, which is usually between 1.010 and 1.025; this helps detect dehydration.
- Maintain a patent airway by checking the RR and administer oxygen.
- Assess the signs of complication, infection and the need for and effectiveness of pain management
  - If disorientation in the burned patient is one of the 1st sign of overwhelming sepsis is likely and may indicate inadequate hydration.
  - Assessment of the sensorium is another important indicator of the adequacy of hydration.
  - A spiking fever and diminished bowel sound accompanied by paralytic ileus are noted.
  - Temperature progressively increases over 48 to 72 hours, after which the temperature falls to subnormal limits.
  - At this time the wound deteriorates, the white blood cells count is depressed and septic shock becomes manifest.
- Promote the child comfort
  - Reduce the severe pain of the wound by giving analgesic intravenously.
  - Reduce the anxiety.
  - Promote sleep by giving sedation.
  - Short term anaesthetic propofol.
  - Relaxation techniques and distraction therapy.

- Encourage family participation.
- Care for the burn wound.
- Reducing the stress of burn care procedure.
- Arrange material ready before beginning of the procedure.
- Administer appropriate analgesics.
- Remind the child to test and approve the temperature of the water.
- Allow the child to request a short rest period during the procedure.
- Allow the child to remove the dressing if desired.
- Inform the child when the procedure is near completion.
- Praise the child for cooperation.
- Assist with debridement.
- Elevate the burned part.

- Prevent Complication
  - Maintenance of body temperature (82°F to 91°F).
  - Keep the baby in radiant warmer, warmed solution, warming blanket or heat shields to prevent hypothermia during dressing.
  - Early diagnosis and treatment of infection are essential.
  - Nurses should be aware of the symptoms of sepsis which include a change in the level of consciousness, a rising or falling white blood cells count, hypothermia or hyperthermia, a loss of the progression of wound healing.
  - Increasing fluid requirement, hypoactive or absent bowel sound.
  - A rising or falling blood glucose level, tachycardia, tachypnea and thrombocytopenia.
- Assist with coping skills for disfiguring burns
  - Refer the family to support groups.
  - Address parent's feelings of guilt.
- Reassure the child that the pain isn't punishment; implement measures to decrease fear. Provide psychosocial support to the child and family.

INFECTIOUS DISORDERS

Scabies

Scabies is a transmissible skin infestation with sarcoptes scabei (itcmite). It's characterized by burrows, severe pruritis, and excoriations of the skin.

Causative organism – *Sarcoptes scabei*

Mode of Transmission

- Impregnated female burrows into superficial epidermis, depositing eggs and faecal material, burrows form a minute linear, greyish-brown, thread like lesion transmitted by skin to skin contact.
- Transmissible by direct (Skin to Skin) contact or contact with contaminated articles for up to 48 hours.

Pathophysiology

- Mites burrow into the skin on contact, progressing 2 to 3 mm per day.
- Females live about 4 to 6 weeks and lay about 40 to 50 eggs, which hatch in 3 to 4 days.
- Pruritis occurs only after sensitization to the mite, develops with initial infestation, sensitization requires several weeks with reinfestation, sensitization develops within 24 hours.
- Dead mites, eggs larvae, and their excrement trigger an inflammatory eruption of the skin in infested areas.

Clinical Manifestations

- May be asymptomatic initially.
- Intense pruritis that's more severe at night.
- Characteristic gray-brown threadlike burrows (0.5 to 1 cm long) with tiny papule or vesicle at one end.
- Common sites include flexor surfaces of wrists, elbows, axillary folds, waistline, nipples (in females), and genitalia; in infants, the burrows may appear on the head and neck.
- Maculopapular lesions present in web of the hand, auxiliary region, popliteal fold, inguinal region and scalp.
- Intense pruritis that leads to punctuate discreet excoriation.
- Papules, vesicles, crusting, abscess formation, and cellulites with secondary infection.
- Ova present from skin scrapings.

Complications

- Excoriations
- Secondary bacterial infection
- Abscess formation
- Septicaemia

Investigation

- Wound culture demonstrating secondary bacterial infection.
- Mineral oil burrow-scraping reveals mites, nits, or eggs, and faeces or scybal.
- Punch biopsy may help to confirm the diagnosis.

Medical Management

- Bathing with soap and water before treatment and after medication has been applied for the required time frame.
- After hot bath with soap and water and thorough drying, medicine is applied over entire cutaneous surface from the neck down, it is left on for 24 hrs, is repeated for 3 days clothes should be washed with hot water dry it in sunlight (inner side), family members should be treated at the same time.
- Gamma benzene hexachloride in vanishing cream base.
- Benzyl benzoate emulsion.
- Permethrin, left off for 8 to 12 hours.
- Lindane cream, left on for 8 to 12 hours.
  - Shouldn't be used if the skin is raw or inflamed.
  - Applied from the neck down, covering the entire body.
- Crotamiton (Eurax), left on for 5 days.
- 6% to 10% sulphur solution.
- Systemic antibiotics.
- Antipruritics.
- In infants, include the head in treatment.
- Avoid the use of topical steroids, which may potentiate the infection.

Nursing Interventions

- Prevent secondary infection and the spread of scabies
  - Trim fingernails short.
  - Isolate the child until treatment is completed.
  - Use meticulous hand-washing technique.
  - Have blood pressure cuffs sterilized in gas autoclave before using on others.
  - Decontaminate linens, towels, clothing, and personal articles.
  - Disinfect the room after discharge.
- Administer medications as ordered.
- Notify a child's school of infestation.
- Encourage verbalization of feelings.
- Observe wound and skin precautions for 24 hours after treatment with a scabicide.
- Anticipate treating family members and close contacts because parasite is transmitted by close personal contact and through clothes and linens.

IMPETIGO CONTAGIOSA

Impetigo is a highly contagious, superficial (epidermal) infection caused by streptococci, staphylococci, or both. The most common sites are the face, around the mouth, the hands, the neck, and the extremities. It is the most common bacterial skin condition in children and account for nearly 10% of all skin problems. It is common in toddlers, preschool age group. It's highly contagious until all lesions are healed. Common in children ages 2 to 5.

Causes

- Bacterial infection from group A beta-haemolytic streptococci may also be due to staphylococci
- Spread by autoinoculation through scratching

Predisposing Factors

- Poor hygiene
- Anaemia
- Malnutrition
- Warm climate
  - Most outbreaks occur in the late summer and early fall.

Mode of Transmission

- The infection is spread by direct contact. The incubation period is 2 to 5 days after contact.

Pathophysiology

Two types

- May occur simultaneously and be clinically udistinguishable.

  Nonbullous impetigo
  - Eruption occurs when bacteria inoculate traumatized skin cells.
  - Lesions begin as small vesicles, which rapidly erode.

- ❍ Honey-coloured crusts surrounded by erythema are formed.

Bullous impetigo

- ❍ Eruption occurs in nontraumatized skin via bacterial toxin or exotoxin.
- ❍ Lesions begin as thin-walled bullae and vesicles.
- ❍ Lesions contain clear to turbid yellow fluid; some crusting exists.
- May complicate chickenpox, eczema, and other skin disorders marked by open lesions.

Complications

- Acute glomerulonephritis
  More likely to occur when many members of the same family have impetigo.
- Ecthyma (an infection that occurs usually as a result of untreated impetigo; may be followed by pigmentation and scarring of the skin).
- Exfoliative eruption (Staphylococcal scalded-skin syndrome) in neonates infants, and children younger than age 5.

Clinical Manifestations

- Painless itching
- Nonbullous impetigo
  - ❍ Small, red macule or vesicle that become pustular within a few hours.
  - ❍ Lesions can occur anywhere, but usually occur on the face around the mouth and nose.
  - ❍ Characteristic thick, honey-coloured crust formed from the exudates.
  - ❍ Satellite lesions caused by autoinoculation.
  - ❍ Pruritus ruptures easily, leaving superficial moist erosion.
  - ❍ Tends to spread peripherally in sharply marginated irregular outlines.
  - ❍ Burning sensation of the skin.
  - ❍ Regional lymphadenopathy.
  - ❍ Infants and children develop aural impetigo or otitis, external lesions usually clear without treatment in 2 to 3 weeks, unless there is an underlying disorder such as eczema.
- Bullous impetigo
  - ❍ Thin walled vesicle.
  - ❍ Thin, clear crust formed from exudates.
  - ❍ Lesions that appear as a central clearing circumscribed by an outer rim.
  - ❍ Most commonly appear on the face or other exposed areas.

Investigation

- Gram stain of vesicular fluid-showing infecting organism.
- Culture and sensitivity testing of exudates or denuded crust-showing infecting organism.
- Total blood count, elevated white blood cell count.

Medical Management

- Removal of exudates by washing the lesions 2 to 3 times per day with soap (or antibacterial soap) and water.
- Warm soaks or compresses of normal saline or a diluted soap solution for stubborn crusts.
- Prevention by using benzoyl peroxide soap.
- Medication Topical application of bacterial ointment (Garamycin, Neosporin).
- Systemic administration of oral or parental antibiotics (penicillin) in severe or extensive lesions.
  Antibiotics for 10 days:
  - ❍ Penicillin–resistant penicillin such as dicloxacillin.
  - ❍ Cephalosporins such as Cephalexin (Keftab).
  - ❍ Azithromycin (Zithromax).
  - ❍ Clarithromycin (Biaxin).
  - ❍ Retapamulin (Altabax) a new class of antibiotics called pleuromutilins, inhibit bacteria from making protein and has been approved to treat impetigo. It is prescribed twice per day for 5 days in children age 9 months or older.
- Antihistamines.
- Therapy shouldn't be delayed for laboratory results, which can take up to 3 days.

Nursing Interventions

- Follow standard precautions.
- Prevent secondary infection and the spread of impetigo.
  - ❍ Trim fingernails
  - ❍ Cover the child's hands if necessary
  - ❍ Cover the lesions

- Encourage the patient not to scratch
- Use meticulous hand-washing technique.

- Remove crusts by gently washing with bactericidal soap and water.
- Soften stubborn crusts with warm compresses.
- Administer medications as ordered.
- Remember to check for penicillin allergy.
- Encourage verbalization of feelings about body image.
- Review the importance of not sharing towels, washcloths, or bed linens with other family members.

CONTACT DERMATITIS: DIAPER RASH

It is a local skin reaction in the areas normally covered by a diaper.

Causes

- Body soaps and bubble baths.
- Tight clothes, wool or rough baths.
- Clothing dyes or the soaps used to wash diapers.
- Irritation due to acidic urine and stools or the formation of ammonia in the diaper.
- Moist, warm environment contained by a plastic diaper lining.
- Bacteria.
- Candida.

Pathophysiology

- The skin of a full-term neonate serves as an effective barrier to disease, but the skin barrier may be broken down by a combination of factors:
  - Dampness
  - Lack of air exposure
  - Acidic or irritant exposures
  - Increase in skin friction.
- Prolonged exposure to moisture and diaper contents (urine and stools) causes rash.

Complications

- Pain
- Infection

Clinical Manifestations

- Characteristic bright red, maculopapular rash in the diaper area.
- Irritability because the rash is painful and warm.

Investigation

- Diagnostic testing not necessary.
- Diagnosis is based on inspection or physical examination.

Medical Management

- Cleaning the affected area with mild soap and water.
- Leaving the affected area open to air.
- Medications
  - Zinc oxide ointment or a barrier-type ointment to help the skin heal.
  - Topical antibiotic ointment if secondary infection occurs.
  - Topical antifungal ointment.

Nursing Interventions

- Keep the diaper area clean and dry to maintain skin integrity.
- Change the diaper immediately after the child voids or defecates to prevent skin breakdown.
- Wash the area with mild soap and water to promote healing.
- Completely remove all previous ointments before reapplying.
- Keep the area open to the air without plastic linings, if possible, to promote circulation and comfort.
- Avoid using commercially prepared diaper wipes on broken skin; the chemicals and alcohol in commercially prepared wipes may be irritating.
- Apply medication as ordered.

CONTACT DERMATITIS: POISON IVY

A severe allergic reaction caused by contact with any of several species of climbing vine of the genus **Rhus**.

Causes

- Skin to skin contact with the shiny, three-pointed leaves.

Pathophysiology

- Poisonous oil on the plant leaf causes a delayed hypersensitivity (T cell) response.
- The rash appears 1 to 2 days after contact.
- Oils that remain on the clothes and skin are contagious to others; the eruptions aren't a source of infection and won't spread the disease.
- Animals may carry the oils to human.

Complications

- Infection
- Scarring

Clinical Features

- Pruritus
- Red, localized steaks that precede vesicles

Investigation

- Diagnostic testing not necessary
- Diagnosis is based on inspection

Medical Management

- Wash the oils from the skin with soap and water to prevent absorption through the skin and spread to other areas.
- Don't touch other body parts until the area has been cleaned.
- Carefully wash resin out of the clothes.
- Apply calamine lotion.
- Apply topical steroids to reduce inflammation and itching.
- Oral steroids may be used if dermatitis is severe, especially on the face.

Nursing Interventions

- Follow standard precautions.
- Prevent secondary infection and spreading that may occur as a result of scratching
  - Trim fingernails
  - Cover the child's hands if necessary
  - Cover the lesions
  - Encourage the patient not to scratch
  - Use meticulous hand-washing technique.

Teach the patient and family what the poison ivy plant looks like to prevent future reactions.

Altered Haematological Conditions

DIAGNOSTIC TESTS

Blood Typing

- Purpose
  - To determine the antigens present in a patient's RBCs; reaction with standardized sera indicates the presence of specific antigens.
- Nursing interventions
  - Explain the procedure to the child and its family.
  - Apply pressure to the venipuncture site to prevent haematoma formation and bleeding.

Coagulation Study

- Purpose
  - To analyze platelet function, platelet count, PT, International normalized Ratio, PTT, coagulation time, and bleeding time.
- Nursing interventions
  - Note the child's current drug therapy before the procedure.
  - Check the venipuncture site for bleeding after the procedure.

Nursing Diagnoses

Probable Nursing Diagnoses

- Activity intolerance
- Fatigue
- Imbalanced nutrition less than body requirements
- Impaired gas exchange
- Ineffective thermoregulation
- Ineffective tissue perfusion: peripheral

Possible Nursing Diagnoses

- Acute pain
- Risk for activity intolerance
- Risk for imbalanced body temperature
- Risk for imbalanced fluid volume
- Risk for impaired skin integrity

Table 11.1: Normal Blood Values in Children

	Newborn	2 years	12 years	18 years
Red blood cells (RBC's) (values × 10/μl)	3.4–5.5	4.0–4.9	4.0–5.3	3.8–5.4
Haematocrit (Hct) (%)	37.4–56.1	31.7-37.7	34.0–43.9	33.0–46.2
Haemoglobin (Hgb) (g/dl)	12.7–18.6	10.5–12.7	11.2–14.8	10.7–15.7
White blood cells (WBCs) (values × 10/μl)	6.8–14.3	5.3–11.5	4.5–10.1	4.4–10.2
Platelets (value × 10/μl)	164–351	204–405	165–335	143–326

Source: Modified from Soldin, S.J., Brugnara, C., and Hicks, J.M. 1999, *Paediatric Reference Ranges* (3rd ed.)

BLOOD DISORDERS

The common blood disorders in children are anaemia, haemophilia, leukaemia, etc.

Anaemia

A common blood disorder that occurs when there are fewer red blood cells than normal, or there is a low concentration of haemoglobin in the blood.

Haemophilia

An inherited bleeding, or coagulation, disorder in which the child lacks the ability to stop bleeding because of the low levels, or complete absence, of specific proteins in its blood.

Leukaemia

A cancer affecting the blood-forming cells in the bone marrow.

Hodgkin's Disease

A type of lymphoma, a cancer in the lymphatic system; Hodgkin's disease causes the cells in the lymphatic system to abnormally reproduce, eventually making the body less able to fight infection. Steady enlargement of lymph glands, spleen, and other lymphatic tissue occurs. Also known as Hodgkin's Lymphoma.

Bleeding Disorders in Children

Bleeding disorders involve the blood clotting process. There are many different kinds of bleeding disorders. Normal blood clotting (coagulation) involves as many as 20 different plasma proteins, also called clotting factors. If the clotting system is unbalanced, a patient may either bleed or clot too easily depending on where the problem occurs. Bleeding problems can range from mild to severe. The two most common types of bleeding disorders are Haemophilia and von Willbrand disease. Clotting disorders are at the other end of the spectrum and can result in a variety of problems depending on which blood vessel has clots.

Causes and Treatments

Treatment depends on the type of disorder. It may include factor replacement, transfusion or other therapies.

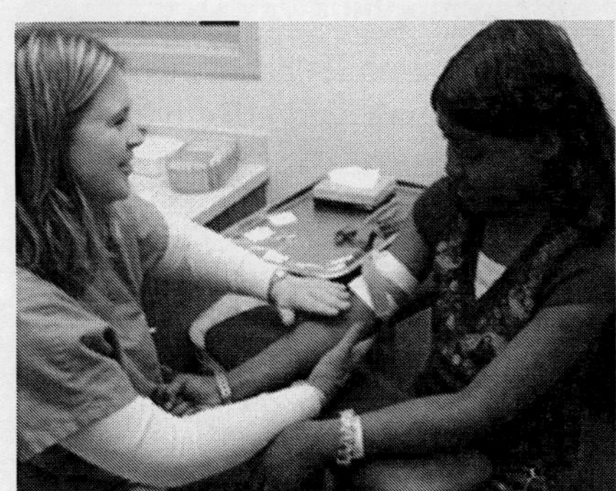

Fig. 11.1: Taking blood sample

Most bleeding disorders can be controlled so a person can have a healthy and full life. It is important to work closely with haematologist and medical support team. Bleeding disorder team includes a haematologist, a nurse coordinator, a social worker, an educational consultant, a physical therapist and a nutritionist.

HAEMOPHILIA

Haemophilia is an inherited bleeding disorder. Children with haemophilia have problems with bleeding because of low levels or complete absence of specific proteins, called "factors" in their blood that are necessary for prevention of excessive bleeding.

Incidence

In the United States, about 20,000 people have haemophilia. People of all races and economic groups are equally affected. Each year, about 400 babies are born with haemophilia.

Causes

- The most common forms of haemophilia result from deficiencies of clotting factor proteins, factor VIII and factor IX. Both factor VIII and factor IX are necessary to form a clot.
- **Haemophilia A,** caused by a missing or reduced amount of the blood clotting protein factor VIII.
- **Haemophilia B,** caused by a missing or reduced amount of the blood clotting protein factor IX (Christmas disease).
- Hereditary bleeding disorder, in about one third of the children with haemophilia, there is no family history of the disorder. A new gene mutation, it is believed may be the cause of the disorder.
- X-linked recessive disorder
  - Haemophilia types A and B are inherited bleeding diseases passed on to children from defective genes located on the X chromosome. Females have two X chromosomes (XX), while males have one X and one Y chromosome (XY). Males (XY) have haemophilia when the gene for clotting factor VIII (Haemophilia A) or clotting factor IX (Haemophilia B) on the single X chromosome is affected.
  - If the father has haemophilia and mother does not, all daughters will be carriers but sons would not have the disease.
  - If the mother is a carrier and the father does not have haemophilia, each son has a 50% chance of getting haemophilia and each daughter has a 50% chance of being a carrier.

Pathophysiology

- Abnormal bleeding occurs because of a specific clotting factor deficiency
  - Factor VIII is a critical cofactor that accelerates the activation of factor X by several thousand fold.
  - Factor IX is an essential factor.
- After a platelet plug forms at a bleeding site, the lack of clotting factors impairs formation of a stable fibrin clot.
- Immediate haemorrhage is not prevalent, delayed bleeding is common.

Complications

- Haemorrhage
- Hepatitis
- Human immunodeficiency virus (HIV) infection secondary to transfusions
- Chronic liver disease

Clinical Manifestations

- The most common symptom of haemophilia is excessive, uncontrollable bleeding.
- Patients with haemophilia do not bleed faster than normal children; they bleed for a longer time.

The severity of symptoms in children with haemophilia depends on the severity of the disease.

Severe haemophilia is when factor VIII or factor IX clotting factor activity is less than 1 per cent.

- Spontaneous bleeding can occur unrelated to injury and is most dangerous when it occurs in the head
- Joint bleeding is common

Moderate haemophilia is when factor VIII or IX clotting factor activity is 1–5 per cent.

- Bleeding episodes are usually related to injury
- Joint bleeding can occur

Mild haemophilia is when factor VIII or IX clotting factor activity is 6–40 per cent.

- Episodes of bleeding are usually related to surgery or dental extractions
- Joint bleeding is uncommon

Other **symptoms** of haemophilia include:

- Bruising
- Soft tissue bleeding
- Bleeding from the nose, gums, or mouth
- Pain, swelling, and limited mobility in the joints and muscles
- Blood found in the urine or stool, or vomiting blood
- Excessive bleeding following circumcision
- Epistaxis
- Fatigue, weakness
- Melena.

Investigation

- A complete medical and family history is taken and a physical examination is performed.
- Blood tests including clotting factor levels, a complete blood count (CBC), and possibly DNA testing.
- PTT test shows prolonged PTT.
- Normal platelet count and function, bleeding time and PT is prolonged.
- Haemophilia B
  - Deficient factor IX assay.
  - Baseline coagulation result similar to those in hemophilia A, with normal factor VIII.
- Haemophilia A and B
  - Degree of factor deficiency defines severity:
    - Mild haemophilia – factor levels 5% to 25% of normal.
    - Moderate haemophilia – factor levels 1% to 5% of normal.
    - Severe haemophilia – factor levels less than 1% of normal.

Treatment for Haemophilia

While a cure for haemophilia is not currently available, the disorder may be managed effectively by doing the following:

- Treat bleeds early and appropriately.
- Avoidance of aspirin, sutures, and cauterization, which may aggravate bleeding.
- Avoid anti-inflammatory agents such as ibuprofen.
- Blood transfusion if necessary.
- Frequent assessment of HIV status (child is at increased risk for acquiring HIV through blood product transfusions).
- Administration of fresh frozen plasma to restore deficient coagulation factors.

- Promotion of vasoconstriction during bleeding episodes by applying ice, pressure, and haemostatic agents.
- Drug therapy:
  - Fibrinolysis inhibitor: aminocaproic acid
  - For haemophilia A
    - Haemostatic: desmopressin (DDAVP) to promote release of factor VIII concentrate
    - Antihaemophilic: cryoprecipitated antihemophilic factor (AHF), lyophilized AHF, or both
  - For haemophilia B
    - Haemostatic: factor IX concentrate
- The goal of factor replacement is to stop or prevent bleeding by increasing the level of the missing or decreased factor VIII or IX. Both factors VIII and IX are available as natural or synthetic (recombinant) powders that can be diluted in sterile fluid and infused directly into a vein.

Nursing Interventions

- Monitor vital signs and intake and output to assess renal status, and monitor for fluid overload or dehydration.
- Assess cardiovascular status and check for signs of bleeding (fever, tachycardia, or hypotension may indicate hypovolemia).
- Measure the affected joint's circumference and compare it with that of an unaffected joint's circumference to assess for bleeding into the joint, which may lead to hypovolemia.
- Note swelling, pain, or limited joint mobility; changes may indicate progressive decline in function.
- Assess for joint degeneration from repeated haemarthroses to detect extent of damage.
- Pad toys and other objects in the child's environment to promote child safety and prevent bleeding; discourage play activities that may result in trauma or injury.
- Recommend using protective head gear, softening as appropriate to prevent bleeding.
- Discourage abnormal weight gain, which increases the load on joints.
- Exercise to maintain healthy joints.
- During bleeding episodes:
  - If the patient has surface cuts or epistaxis, apply pressure; this is commonly the only treatment episode.
  - With deeper cuts, pressure may stop the bleeding temporarily; cut deep enough to require suturing may also require factor infusions to prevent further bleeding.
  - Give the deficient clotting factor or plasma, as ordered.
  - The body uses up AHF in 48 to 72 hours; repeat infusions as ordered, until the bleeding stops.
  - Apply cold compress or ice bags, and elevate the injured part.
  - To prevent recurrence of bleeding, restrict activity for 48 hours after bleeding is under control.
  - Control pain with analgesics as ordered.
  - Avoid I.M. injections because of possible haematoma formation at the injection site.
  - Avoid aspirin and aspirin containing medications, which are contraindicated because they decrease platelet adherence and may increase bleeding.
  - If the patient can't tolerate activities because of blood loss, provide rest periods between activities.
- During bleeding in a joint:
  - Immediately elevate the joint.
  - To restore joint mobility, begin range-of motion (ROM) exercises at least 48 hours after the bleeding is controlled.
  - Restrict weight bearing until bleeding stops and swelling subsides.
  - Administer analgesics for the pain associated with a haemarthrosis.
  - Apply ice packs and elastic bandages to alleviate pain.
- Get an annual comprehensive check up at the haemophilia treatment centre.
- Early treatment of bleeds is important and can be done by intravenous clotting factor replacement. This can even be done at home. Factor replacement prevents serious complications and allows children to live active lives.

ANAEMIA

Anaemia refers to a lower than normal number of red blood cells in the blood. The principal function of red blood cells is to carry oxygen from the lungs and distribute it throughout the entire body.

In general, anaemia is caused by one of the following:

- An inability of the body to make red blood cells.
- Premature destruction of the red blood cells.
- Bleeding, or loss of red blood cells.

Causes

- Blood loss from repeated severe nosebleeds.
- Heavy menstrual periods.
- A bleeding stomach ulcer or certain intestinal disorders.
- Insufficient amounts of important vitamins and other substances that are crucial for the production of new red cells.
- Inherited defects of enzymes, cell membrane structure, or of haemoglobin molecules inside the cell may cause red cells to be more fragile and prone to premature destruction.
- Problems in the bone marrow where red blood cells are produced can also cause anaemia.
- Viral illness or a more severe anaemia because the function of the marrow has been nearly destroyed, such as hepatitis, toxins or, rarely, leukaemia.
- Serious chronic illnesses may give anaemia due to the condition itself or medication used to treat it.

Common Forms or Types of Anaemia

1. Iron deficiency
2. B-Thalassemia
3. Aplastic anaemia
4. Sickle cell anaemia

Iron Deficiency Anaemia

A common form of anaemia in childhood is due to iron deficiency. Iron is an essential component of the molecules inside red blood cells that carry oxygen. Iron is also important for some enzyme systems in the body and for the normal function of certain organs such as the brain.

Causes

- Inadequate iron intake in the diet.
- Chronic diseases
- Iron malabsorption, as in chronic diarrhoea and malabsorption syndromes, such as celiac disease and pernicious anaemia.
- Blood loss secondary to drug induced GI bleeding.
- Whether there are other medical problems.

Pathophysiology

- Insufficient body stores of iron lead to
  - Depleted RBC mass
  - Decreased haemoglobin concentration (hypochromia)
  - Decreased oxygen carrying capacity of blood

Complications

- Infection and pneumonia
- Pica, causing the child to eat lead based paint, which results in poisoning
- Bleeding
- Haemochromatosis

Clinical Manifestations

- When a child has a mild anaemia, he or she may appear almost normal;
- Signs of anaemia may include:
  - Paleness,
  - Headache or dizziness,
  - Fatigue and, in some instances, jaundice (yellowing of the skin and eyes).
  - In cases of sudden very severe anaemia, a child may become restless, extremely pale and may feel like fainted.
  - Dyspnea.
  - Inability to concentrate.
  - Tachycardia.
  - Susceptibility to infection.
- In cases of chronic iron deficiency anaemia, child may have following symptoms:
  - Cracks in corners of the month
  - Dysphagia
  - Neuralgic pain
  - Numbness and tingling in the extremities
  - Smooth tongue
  - Spoon shaped, brittle nails
  - Vasomotor disturbances.

Investigation

- Haematocrit (HCT) and Hb and serum ferritin levels low.
- Mean corpuscular Hb level is decreased.
- RBC count is low, with microcytic and hypochromic cells.
- Serum iron level are low with high binding capacity.

Management

- The treatment of anaemia in general depends on the cause of the anaemia.
- In general, iron deficiency anaemia can be treated successfully with prescription-strength iron by mouth and with changes in diet by increasing iron intake and by adding rich in iron foods to diet.
- Drug therapy
  - Oral preparation of iron or a culmination of iron and ascorbic acid (which enhance iron absorption).
  - Vitamin supplement: cyanocobalamin (vitamin B 12) if intrinsic factor is lacking.
  - Iron supplements: iron dextran.
  - In some cases, blood transfusions must be given.

β-*Thalassemia (Cooley Anaemia)*

Generally Thalassemia is an inherited blood disorder characterized by abnormal synthesis of haemoglobin. Haemoglobin consists of two main protein chains called alpha and beta. There are two subtypes of the disorder (alpha and beta) depending on what portion of the hemoglobin is abnormally synthesized. Each of these subtypes can be further classified depending on the number of thalassemia genes involved. The following conditions have been cited in various sources as potentially causal risk factors related to Thalassemia:

- Italian descent
- Greek descent
- Mediterranean descent
- North African descent
- South-East Asian descent

Types of Thalassemia

Review the cause information for the various types of Thalassemia:

- Alpha thalassemia
- Beta thalassemia
- Delta thalassemia
- Delta-beta thalassemia—a rare type similar to beta thalassemia
- Thalassemia major—homozygous form of beta thalassemia
- Thalassemia minor—a carrier form; heterozygous form of beta thalassemia with variable or mild symptoms.

β-**Thalassemia** is a blood disorder characterized by deficiencies in the rate of production of specific globin chain in Hgb. It is common in those people living near Mediterranean Sea. This disorder has a wide geographic distribution, probably as a result of genetic migration through intermarriage or possibly as a result of spontaneous mutation.

β-Thalassemia is the most common type of thalassemia and occurs in four forms

- Two heterozygous form: Thalassemia minor, an asymptomatic silent carrier and thalassemia trait—which produce microcytic anaemia.
- Thalassemia intermedia—which manifested as splenomegally and moderate to severe anaemia and a homozygous form.
- Thalassemia major(Cooley) which result in a severe anaemia that would lead to cardiac failure and death in early childhood without blood transfusion.

Pathophysiology

Normally in postnatal babies Hgb is composed of 2α-2β polypeptic chains. In β-thalassemia there ia a partial or complete deficiency in the synthesis of the β-chain of the Hgb molecule. Consequently, there is a compensatory increase in the synthesis of α-chains, γ-chain production remains activated, resulting in defective Hbg formation. This unbalanced polypeptide unit is very unstable; when it disintegrates, it damages RBCs, causing severe anemia.

To compensate is formed unless the bone marrow is suppressed by transfusion therapy. Excess iron from hemolysis of supplemental RBCs in transfusion and form the rapid destruction of defective cells is stored in various organs (hemosiderosis).

Investigation

In early condition difficulty to recognise it may identify later half of infant period.

- Thalassemia major—defective synthesis of HbA
- Structurally impaired RBCs
- Shortened life span of erythrocytes

Hematologic studies reveals that:

- RBCs changes are microcytosis, hypochromia, anisocytois, poikilocytosis, target cells and basophilic.
- Hgb, Hct level will be low.
- RBC reduction in the blood
- X-ray bone reveals characteristic findings.

Clinical Manifestation of β-Thalassemia

Child with anaemia manifested by

- Palor
- Unexplained fever
- Poor feeding
- Enlarged spleen /liver

Child with severe anaemia

- Chronic hypoxia
- Headache
- Precordinal and bone pain
- Decreased exercise tolerance
- Listlessness
- Anorexia

Other clinical features like

- Small stature
- Delayed sexual maturation
- Bronzed, freckled complexion

Bone changes in older children

- Enlarged head
- Prominent frontal and partial losses
- Prominent molar eminences
- Flat or depressed bridge of the nose
- Enlarged maxilla
- Protrusion of the lip and upper central incisors and eventual malocclusion
- Generalized skeletal osteoporosis

Treatment

The objective of supportive management is

1. To maintain sufficient Hgb levels to prevent bone marrow expansion and the resulting bony deformities.
2. To provide sufficient RBCs to support normal growth and normal activity.

Medical Management

1. Blood transfusion for the child to maintain Hgb level above 9.5 g/dl. The transfusion must be every 3 to 5 weeks.

Advantages are

- Improve physical and psychological wellbeing because of the ability to participate in normal activities.
- Decreased cardiomegaly and hepatosplenomegaly
- Reduce the bone changes
- Normal or near normal growth and development until puberty.
- Reduce infection

Complication of frequent blood transfusion

- Iron overload
- Development of hemosiderosis

2. Deferoxamine (desferal) an iron chelating agent is given with oral supplement of vitamin C.

   Deferoxamine is given intravenously or subcutaneously, if it is administrated intravenously by infusion pump over 8-24 hours, especially given in night time for 5-7 days a week.

Surgical Management

- Surgical management is splenectomy, in children with severe splenomegaly who demonstrate increased blood transfusion requirements.
- Complication of splenectomy is severe and irresistible infection; therefore these children need prophylactic antibiotics with close medical supervision for many years.
- Children should be vaccinated according to national schedule to prevent infection like pneumococcal and meningococcal.

Nursing Management

- Promote compliance with transfusion and chelation therapy.
- Assist the child in coping with the anxiety about treatment and the side effects of the illness.
- Foster the child's and family's adjustment to a chronic illness.
- Observe the complications of multiple blood transfusion

Based on these nursing objectives, nurses explain to the parents and older children about the disorder, its effect on RBCs and the potential effects of untreated iron overload.

- About prevention of these disorder genetic counselling for the parents and fertile offsprings is mandatory.

- Antenatal care includes prenatal diagnosis using amniocentesis at 20 weeks of gestation or foetal blood sampling at 10 weeks and screening for thalassemia trait.

Aplastic Anaemia

Definition

- Group of disorders characterized by pancytopenia (anaemia, granulocytopenia, and thrombocytopenia) resulting from the decreased functional capacity of a hypoplastic, fatty bone marrow.

Causes

- Congenital
  - Congenital hypoplastic anaemia (Blackfan –Diamond anaemia); develops between ages 2 and 3 months.
  - Fanconisyndrome (characterized by pancytopenia, hypoplasia of bone marrow, and patchy brown discoloration abnormalities usually associated with multiple congenital anomalies).
- Acquired
  - Drug-induced; occurs as an adverse effect from chemotherapy, chloramphenicol (chloromycetin), phenylbutazone (pophenylbutazone), phenytoin (dilantin), some antibiotics, and some recreational drugs.
  - Chemical exposure.
  - Idiopathic (no known cause).
  - Radiation.
  - Viral hepatitis.
  - Human parvovirus.
  - Overwhelming infection.
  - Autoimmune disorders such as lupus.

Pathophysiology

- Aplastic anaemias usually develop when damaged or destroyed stem cells inhibit RBC production.
- Less commonly, they develop when damaged bone marrow microvasculature creates an unfavourable environment for cell growth and maturation.

Complications

- Life-threatening haemorrhage
- Immunosuppression

Clinical Manifestations

- Anorexia
- Dyspnea, tachypnea
- Epistaxis
- Fatigue, weakness
- Gingivitis
- Headache
- Melena
- Multiple infections, fever
- Palpitations, tachycardia
- Purpura, petechiae, ecchymosis, pallor.

Investigation

- Bone marrow biopsy shows fatty marrow with reduction of stem cells.
- Faecal occult blood test is positive.
- Haematology shows decreased granulocytes, thrombocytes, and RBCs.
- Peripheral blood smear shows pancytopenia.
- Urine chemistry reveals haematuria.

Medical Management

- Dietary changes, including establishing a high-protein, high-calorie, high-vitamin diet.
- Transfusion of platelets and packed RBCs.
- Drug therapy.
  - Analgesics: ibuprofen (Motrin), acetaminophen (Tylenol).
  - Androgens: fluoxymensterone (Halotestin), oxymetholone (Anadrol-50).
  - Antibiotics (if infection present): according to the sensitivity of the infecting organism.
  - Antithymocyte globulin and cyclosporine (gengraf).
  - Haematopoietic growth factor: epoetin alfa (procrit).
  - Human granulocyte colony stimulating factor: filgrastim (Neulasta).
- Bone marrow transplantation.
- Peripheral stem-cell transplants.

Nursing Interventions

- Assess respiratory status to detect hypoxemia caused by low Hb levels.
- Assess vital signs for signs of haemorrhage, infection, and activity intolerance.
- Assess cardiovascular status to detect arrhythmias or myocardial ischemia.
- Monitor and record intake and output and urine specific gravity to determine fluid balance.

- Monitor laboratory values to determine effectiveness of therapy.
- Assess stool, urine, and emesis for occult blood loss caused by decreased platelet levels.
- Monitor for infection, bleeding, and bruising caused by decreased levels of WBCs and platelets.
- Encourage fluids and administer intravenous fluids to replace fluids lost by fever and bleeding.
- Administer oxygen to improve tissue oxygen because low Hb levels reduce the blood's oxygen-carrying capacity.
- Administer transfusion therapy, as prescribed, to replace low levels of blood components.
- Maintain the patient's diet to promote RBC production and fight infection.
- Avoid giving I.M. infections to reduce the risk of haemorrhage.
- Avoid taking rectal temperatures to reduce the risk of tissue trauma.
- Prepare for possible bone marrow transplantation, the treatment of choice for anaemia caused by severe aplasia and for the patient who needs constant RBC transfusions.
- Avoid contact sports.
- Avoid excessive exercise.

Sickle Cell Anaemia

It is a congenital haemolytic disease characterized by the partial or complete replacement of normal haemoglobin with abnormal haemoglobin S (Hbs). Sickle cell anaemia occurs primarily in black people.

Causes

- Autosomal recessive inheritance (homozygous inheritance of the Hbs-producing gene).

Pathophysiology

In sickle anaemia,

↓

The haemoglobin in the red blood cells acquires an elongated crescent or sickle shape

↓

The sickle cells are rigid, accumulate in capillaries and smaller vessels, making the blood more viscous and obstruct capillary blood flow

↓

Microscopic obstruction leads to engorgement and tissue ischemia

↓

This local tissue hypoxia causes further sickling and ultimately affects the normal circulation, causing pain, tissue ischemia, infarction and swelling.

↓

Damaged tissues in organs throughout the body become scarred, resulting in impaired function

Complications

- Retinopathy, nephropathy, and cerebral vessel occlusion caused by organ infarction
- Hypovolemic shock and death
- Necrosis
- Infection and gangrene.

Clinical Manifestations

Infants

- Affected children are usually asymptomatic until 4 to 6 months of age because sickling is inhibited by high levels of foetal haemoglobin.
- Colic from pain caused by an abdominal infarction.
- Dactylitis or hand foot syndrome from infarction of the small bones of the hand and feet.
- Splenomegaly from sequestered RBCs.

Toddlers and Preschoolers

- Hypovolemia and shock from sequestration of large amount of blood in spleen.
- Pain at site of vaso-occlusive crisis.
- Possible functional asplenia by age 4, leading to the risk of infection.

School Age Children and Adolescents

- Delayed growth and development, delayed sexual maturity.
- Enuresis.
- Extreme pain at site of crisis.
- History of pneumococcal pneumonia and other infections caused by atrophied spleen.
- Poor healing of leg wounds from inadequate peripheral circulation of oxygenated blood.
- Priapism
  - Suspect any of the following crisis in a patient with sickle cell anemia
    - Who has pale lips, tongue

- Palms or nail beds
- Lethargy
- Restlessness
- Sleepiness
- Irritability
- Severe pain and fever.

Investigation

- Laboratory studies show Hb level is 6 to 9 g/dl (in a toddler).
- More than 50% Hbs indicate sickle cell disease; a lower level of Hbs indicates sickle cell trait.
- RBCs are crescent shaped and prone to agglutination.

Management

- Bed rest.
- Avoidance of stress and extreme temperatures.
- Hydration with I.V. fluid (may be increased to 3 L/day during crisis).
- Short-term oxygen therapy (long-term oxygen decreases bone marrow activity, further aggravating anaemia).
- Transfusion therapy as needed.
- Drug therapy
  - Analgesic: meperidine (Demerol)
  - Antineoplastic: hydroxyurea
  - Vaccine: pneumococcal vaccine.

Nursing Interventions

- Administer sufficient pain medication to promote comfort; concerns regarding addiction are clinically unfounded.
- Assess cardiovascular, respiratory, and neurologic status; tachycardia, dyspnea, or hypotension may indicate fluid volume deficit or electrolyte imbalance; change in level of consciousness may signal neurologic involvement.
- Assess for symptoms of acute chest syndrome from a pulmonary infarction to identify early complications.
- Promote fluid intake to prevent dehydration, which may result from the kidney's inability to concentrate urine.
- Assess vision to monitor for retinal infarction.
- Teach relaxation techniques to decrease the child's stress level.
- Provide proper skin care to prevent skin breakdown.
- Remove tight clothing that impedes circulation.
- Reduce the child's energy expenditure to improve oxygenation.
- Maintain the child's normal body temperature.
- Initiate genetic counselling.
- Suggest family screening for possible carriers of the disease.
- Instruct the child to avoid activities that precipitate a crisis, such as excessive exercise, mountain climbing, and deep sea diving; advise the family to seek early treatment of illness to prevent dehydration.

Common Oncological Conditions in Children

OVERVIEW

Various coping strategies are used by the child with a chronic life-threatening disease. Most of these chronic problems are associated with cancer. Regardless of the problem, supportive, informative nursing care is crucial before, during and after diagnosis. In addition, the nurse must consider the child's stage of development, especially when dealing with the possibility of death.

Definition

- An alteration in cell function resulting from the overproduction of immature and non-functional cells; tissues enlarge for no physiologic function.
- Can be life-threatening.
- Can invade and destroy healthy tissues.
- Paediatric cancers
  - Second to accidents as the leading cause of death in children between ages 1 and 14.
  - Occurs primarily in rapidly differentiating tissues such as bone marrow.
  - Most solid tumours are sarcomas.
  - In order of frequency: leukaemia, neurologic tumours, neuroblastomas, lymphomas, Wilms tumours, bone tumours.
  - Any tumour in a child is considered malignant until histologically identified, even if it is encapsulated.
  - Childhood cancers growth is at high metabolic rate.
  - The incidence of cancer increases with age.

Causes

- Unknown
- Mutations within the genes of cells
- Specific agents that cause mutations
  - Ionizing radiation
  - Asbestos
  - Electromagnetic fields
  - Vinyl chloride
  - Tobacco.
- Some forms of cancer result from genetic predisposition.
- Children who are immunosuppressed, such as those infected with human immuno deficiency virus (HIV) and those with acquired immuno deficiency syndrome (AIDS) or Wiskott-Aldrich syndrome, children on immunosuppressive therapy, and children with chromosomal abnormalities, such as those with Down syndrome, are more prone to developing certain types of cancer.

HOW CANCER METASTASIZES

Cancer usually spreads through the bloodstream to other organs and tissues, as shown here.

Cancer cells secrete enzymes and motility factors
↓
Basement membrane in blood vessels is disrupted
↓
Cancer cells escape into circulation
↓
Undetected cells move out of blood
↓
Enzymes are secreted
↓
Cell wall is cut
↓
New tissue is invaded downstream
↓
Chemical attraction occurs
↓
Malignant cells target specific site
↓
New site is invaded
↓
Cells multiply
↓
Metastatic tumour appears

Pathophysiology

- Rapid, uncontrollable proliferation of cells
- Independent spread from a primary site (site of origin) to other tissues where it establishes secondary foci (metastasis).
- Cancer cells metastasize via circulation through the blood or lymphatics, by unintentional transplantation from one site to another during surgery and by local extension.
- A particular concern with paediatric cancer is the increased risk of development of secondary cancer after successful treatment of the primary cancer.

Complications

- May arise from therapy as well as the disease.
- Anaemia
- Leukopenia
- Thrombocytopenia
- Nausea and vomiting
- Alopecia
- Fluid and electrolyte imbalances
- Death.

Clinical Manifestations

- Signs and symptoms vary with the type and location of cancer.
- Pain, including headache and bone pain.
- Abnormal skin lesions, such as petechiae or bruising.
- Fatigue
- Fever
- Weight loss
- Eye or vision changes.

Investigations

- Biopsy (the removal of a portion of the suspicious tissue) for direct histological study of tumour tissue.
  - The only definitive method to diagnose cancer.
  - Can also provide information about the stage and grade of the cancer
    - The TNM staging system (tumour size, nodal involvement, and metastatic progress) allows comparison of treatments and survival rates among large population groups.
    - Grading compares tumour tissue to normal cells and estimates the tumour's growth rate.
- Imaging studies, such as X-rays, computed tomography (CT) scanning, ultrasonography, and magnetic resonance imaging (MRI), are useful in detecting tumors.
- Bone scans can detect bony lesions, but aren't definitive because they don't distinguish between inflammation and malignancy.

Medical Management

- Goal of treatment is to achieve remission, a 5-year remission is considered a cure.
- Surgery
  - Typically combined with other therapies.
  - May be performed for various reasons.
    - Biopsy to obtain tissue for histological study.
    - Debulking of the tumour.
    - Relieve pain and alleviate pressure.
    - Correct obstruction.
- Radiation therapy
  - Normal cells recover from radiation faster than malignant cells.
  - Approaches
    - External beam radiation
    - Interstitial implants
- Chemotherapy
  - Induces regression of the tumour and its metastasis.
  - Particularly useful in controlling residual disease and relieving pain.
  - Alkylating agents—inhibit cell growth and division by reacting with deoxyribonucleic acid (DNA).
  - Antimetabolites prevent cell growth by competing with metabolites in the production of nucleic acid.
  - Antitumour antibiotics block cell growth by binding with DNA-dependent ribonucleic acid (RNA) synthesis.

- Plant alkaloids prevent cellular reproduction by disrupting cell mitosis.
- Steroid hormones inhibit the growth of hormone–susceptible tumours by changing their chemical environment.

- Biotherapy
  - Interferons have antiviral and antiproliferative effects.
  - Interleukins exert their effects on the T-lymphocytes.
  - Monoclonal antibodies selectively bind to tumour cell surfaces.
  - Haematopoietic growth factors increase the patient's blood counts when chemotherapy or radiation causes a decrease.
- Bone marrow transplant
  - For children for whom other treatments have not been or are unlikely to be successful.
  - Complications may include graft-versus -host disease, veno-occlusive disease, complications from immunosuppressant medications.

Nursing Interventions

- Anticipate the need for pain relief and provide it on a schedule that doesn't allow pain to break through.
- Assist with intravenous and intrathecal chemotherapy
  - Be aware that chemotherapy may include such drugs as Cyclophosphamide (Cytoxan), Methotrexate, Vincrestine (Oncovin), Prednisone (Deltasone) and Asparaginase (Elspar).
  - Monitor for and help the child deal with chemotherapeutic adverse effects.
    - Alopecia.
    - Nausea and vomiting.
    - Infection.
    - Anaemia.
    - Stomatitis.
    - Bleeding.
  - Provide care for the venous access device as necessary.
  - The special protective precautions are essential when administering or disposing of chemotherapeutic drugs because they are easily absorbed through the skin and mucous membranes.
- Assist with radiation and help the child deal with its adverse effects:
  - Vomiting
  - Dry mouth and sore throat
  - Diarrhoea
  - Desquamation (scaling) of the skin
  - May be site specific (dependent upon the site being irradiated).
- Prepare for possible surgery, performed for biopsy, tumour removal, determination of the disease's severity and palliation.
- Anticipate aftereffects years after treatments and counsel parents accordingly
  - Genetic changes
  - Learning disabilities
  - Secondary cancers
  - Altered function of specific organ systems.
- Ensure adequate hydration and nutrition.
- Use coping strategies, such as play therapy, relaxation techniques, and imagery, to deal with the pain and disability.

HODGKIN'S LYMPHOMA

Definition

- A malignant neoplasm of the lymphoid tissue
- Commonly seen in adolescents and young adults
- Prognosis is excellent.

Causes

- Although the cause is unknown, a viral etiology is suspected, with the Epstein-Barr virus as a leading candidate.
- Environmental and immunologic factors may also contribute.

Pathophysiology

- Usually originates in a localized group of lymph nodes.
- Proliferates by way or lymphocytes to other sites including the bone marrow, liver, lungs, mediasternum and spleen.

Complications

- Recurrence of the disease after a period of remission.
- A second malignancy located in another part of the body, such as the bone, breast or blood.
- Hypothyroidism from irradiation of the neck area during the treatment phase.
- Sterility.
- Death.

Clinical Manifestations

- Painless, firm, persistently enlarged lymph nodes
  - Appear insidiously.
  - Most common in the lower cervical region.
- Night sweats and pruritus.
- Recurrent fever
- Weight loss
- Fatigue.

Investigations

- Lymph node and bone marrow biopsies confirm diagnosis by revealing Reed-Sternberg cells (enlarged, abnormal histiocytes).
- Detection of lymph node or organ involvement
  - Chest X-ray
  - CT of abdomen, chest and pelvis
  - Ultrasound
  - Lymphangiogram
    - Dye is injected I.V. into the feet.
    - X-ray tracks the dye as it travels up the body and is absorbed by the lymphatic system (cancerous nodes have a different appearance from normal lymph nodes).
- Blood tests
  - Show mild to severe chromocytic anaemia.
  - Elevated serum alkaline phosphatase indicates liver or bone involvement.
- Position emission tomography scan helps find malignant tumour cells.

Medical Management

- Depends on the number, location and degree of involved lymphnodes.
- Radiation therapy, chemotherapy or a combination may be used for stages I and II.
- Chemotherapy is used for stages III and IV, sometimes inducing a complete remission.
  - MOPP protocol—Mechlorethamine (Mustargen), Vincrestine (Oncovin), Procarbazine (Matulane) and Prednisone.
  - ABVD protocol—Doxorubicin (Adriamycin), Bleomycin (Blenoxane), Vinblastine (Vira-A) and Dacarbazine (DTIC).
  - High dose chemotherapy with autologous bone marrow transplant or autologous peripheral blood stem cell transfusions for a patient who is unresponsive to radiation therapy or chemotherapy.

Nursing Interventions

- Assess for adverse effects of radiation and chemotherapy including anorexia, nausea, vomiting, diarrhoea, fever and bleeding.
- Control pain and bleeding of stomatitis by using a soft toothbrush, applying petroleum jelly to the lips and avoiding astringent mouthwashes.
- Offer appropriate emotional support including information on the Cancer Society.

LEUKAEMIA

Definition

- Leukaemia is the abnormal, uncontrolled proliferation of white blood cells (WBCs).
- Acute lymphocytic leukaemia (ALL) is the most common type of leukaemia and cancer in children.
  - Peak age is 2 to 5 years.
  - 90% to 95% of children with ALL achieve a first remission.
  - Almost 80% live 5 years.
  - The child between ages 3 and 7 with ALL and an initial WBC count of less than 10,000/µl at the time of diagnosis has the best prognosis.
- Acute myeloblastic leukaemia (AML) is more common than ALL in adolescents.
  - 50% to 70 % of adolescents with AML achieve a first remission.
  - 40% live for 5 years.

Causes

- The exact cause of most leukaemias remains unknown.
- Increasing evidence suggests a combination of contributing factors.
- Predisposing factors
  - Familial tendency.
  - Monozygotic twin with leukaemia.
  - Congenital disorders, such as Down syndrome, Bloom syndrome, and ataxia-telangiectasia.
  - Viruses.
  - Ionizing radiation.
  - Exposure to the chemical benzene and cytotoxin such as alkylating agents.

Pathophysiology

- WBCs are produced so rapidly that immature cells (blast cells) are released into the circulation.
- Blast cells are non-functional, can not fight infection and multiply continuously without respect to the body's needs.
- Blast cells appear in the peripheral blood, where they normally do not appear.
- Blast cells may be as high as 95% in the bone marrow (they are normally less than 5%) as measured by marrow aspiration in the posterior or iliac crest (the sternum can not be used in children).
- The increased proliferation of WBCs robs healthy cells of nutrition.
- Bone marrow first undergoes hypertrophy, possibly resulting in pathologic fractures.
- Bone marrow then undergoes atrophy, resulting in a decrease in all blood cells, which leads to anaemia, bleeding disorders and immunosuppression.

Complications

- Organ malfunction, especially the spleen and liver
- Anaemia
- Infection
- Bleeding (petechiae)
- Death.

Clinical Manifestations

- High fever.
- Thrombocytopenia.
- Abdominal or bone pain.
- Pallor, chills and recurrent infections.
- Petechiae and ecchymosis.
- Abnormal bleedings, such as nosebleeds, poor wound healing and oral lesions.
- Confusion, lethargy and headache if the blood-brain barrier has been crossed.
- Fatigue.
- Painless lumps in neck, underarm, stomach and groin.

Investigation

- Bone marrow aspirate showing a proliferation of immature WBCs (greater than 25% blasts).
- Bone marrow biopsy of the posterior superior iliac spine can confirm diagnosis.
- Blood counts show thrombocytopenia, neutropenia and anaemia.
- Differential leukocyte count determines cell type.
- Lumber puncture detects meningeal involvement (if central nervous system (CNS) is involved).
- Cytogenetic analysis shows a "Philadelphia chromosome" in ALL.

Medical Management

- Systemic chemotherapy aims to eradicate leukaemic cells and induce remission.
  - ALL-combination therapy that may include vincristine, prednisone, high-dose cytarabine (Cytosar-U), asparaginase (Elspar), amsacrine (AMSA) and daunorubicin (Cerubidine).
  - AML-combination of I.V. daunorubicin and cytarabine; combination of cyclophosphamide, vincristine, prednisone or methotrxate; high-dose cytarabine alone or with other drugs; amsacrine; etoposide and azacitidine (5-azacytidine) and mitoxantrone (novantrone).
- Intrathecal chemotherapy to prevent or treat CNS infiltration by leukaemic cells.
- Antibiotic, antifungal, and antiviral drugs and granulocyte injections to control infection.

- Transfusions of platelets to prevent bleeding and of red blood cells to prevent anaemia.
- Possible bone marrow transplant (especially in children with the Philadelphia chromosome).

Nursing Interventions

- Prevent infection by placing the patient in a private room, giving special attention to much care and screening staff and visitors for contagious diseases.
- Inspect the skin frequently; avoid taking a rectal temperature or administering rectal medications.
- Use interventions for anaemia and thrombocytopenia.
- Give increased fluids to flush chemotherapy through the kidneys.
- Provide a high-protein, high-calorie, bland diet.
- Provide pain relief.
- Monitor the CNS for involvement (confusion, lethargy and headache).
- Gear nursing measures toward easing the adverse effects of radiation and chemotherapy.
- Help the child and the family verbalize their fears and guilt; allow the family to participate in the child's care, as appropriate.
- Help the child adjust to changes in body image.
- Refer parents and adolescents with cancer to support groups.

RHABDOMYOSARCOMA

It is the fourth most common type of solid tumour that occurs in soft tissues in children. These malignant neoplasms originate from undifferentiated mesenchymal cells in muscles, tendons, bursae and fascia or from such cells in fibrous, connective, lymphatic or vascular tissues.

These disorders derive their name from the specific tissues of origin.

- Myosarcoma originates from muscle (*myo* means muscle).
- Rhabdomyosarcoma originates from rhabdo-striated skeletal muscle.

These may occur at any part of the body, but most common site is head and neck, especially the orbit.

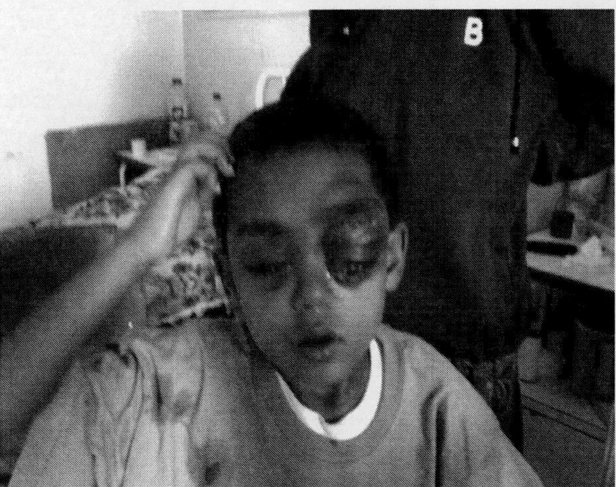

Fig. 12.1: Child with Rhabdomyosarcoma in left eye

Incidence

The disease occurs mostly in the children of age group less than 5 years.

Clinical Manifestations

Clinical features depend on the site the cancer occurs.

- **Orbit**
  - Rapid developing unilateral proptosis.
  - Echymosis of conjunctiva.
  - Loss of extraocular movement (Strabismus).
- **Nasopharynx**
  - Stuffy nose
  - Nasal obstruction
  - Dysphagia
  - Nasal voice
  - Serous otitis media
  - Pain due to sore throat and ear infection
  - Epistaxis
  - Palpable neck nodes
  - Visible mass in oropharynx (late sign)
- **Paranasal sinuses**
  - Nasal obstruction
  - Local pain
  - Discharge
  - Sinusitis and swelling
- **Middle ear**
  - Signs of chronic serous otitis media
  - Pain
  - Sanguinopurulent drainage
  - Facial nerve palsy

- **Retroperitoneal area**
  - Usually a "silent" tumour
  - Abdominal mass
  - Pain
  - Signs of intestinal or genitourinary obstruction
- **Perineum**
  - Visible superficial mass
  - Bowel or bladder dysfunction (from tumour compression)

Investigation

- Physical examination: The common signs and symptoms in children are earache or runny nose.
- Head and neck is very important, careful examination is to be done about palpation of a nontender, firm, hard mass.
- Diagnostic tests include full ocular examination and
- CT or MRI scans of the eye orbit.
- Children with a history or retinoblastoma in the family should be examined by an ophthalmologist after birth.

Treatment

- Treatment for retinoblastoma may include removal of the eye.
- Other surgical treatments involve cryotherapy or photocoagulation (Argon laser therapy).
- Radiation is nearly always used, either as the sole treatment or before surgery to shrink the tumour.
- Chemotherapy is occasionally used but is generally ineffective as the drugs often fail to penetrate sufficiently into the eye.
- Multiple therapies are more commonly used in children with bilateral retinoblastoma.

Nursing Management

- Physiologic assessment of the child with a soft tissue tumour, such as Hodgkin's disease, Non-Hodgkin's Lymphoma, rhabdomyosarcoma, and other Lymphomas, focuses on the children's general condition.
- Accurate height and weight measurements are essential to provide a baseline against which to measure the child's growth during treatment, as well as for calculation of chemotherapeutic drug dosages.
- Observe the area of the tumour, such as the face, neck and abdomen, and describe any changes.
- Monitor the respiratory status if the tumour is on the face or neck; report any changes in respiratory pattern to the physician.
- Avoid palpation of any tumour site or enlarged area; metastasis can be influenced by injudicious palpation and manipulation of a tumour site.
- Observe wounds closely for lack of healing as a result of chemotherapy or radiation. Examine the mouth and extremities for wounds or ulcers.
- Assessment of the family's psychosocial status and coping mechanisms is an essential component of nursing care.
- Children with lymphoma affecting the mediasternum may need respiratory support. Position the child so that the head is elevated.
- Administer chemotherapy drugs as ordered, maintaining adequate fluids to facilitate excretion of the resultant breakdown products.
- Monitor the central line used for chemotherapy administration, and teach parents about care of the central line when the child is home.
- When the child with retinoblastoma undergoes removal of the eye, the parents and child will need detailed instructions on postsurgical care.
- Attention is directed at the body changes of the cancer and its treatment. Children and adolescents may need suggestions to deal with hair loss, disfigurement, and living with serious illness.
- Referral to other children and teens with similar concerns may be helpful.
- Parents of all children need help to encourage normal development in the child with cancer.
- Educate about Retinoblastoma. The family members should be examined by an ophthalmologist after birth and on a regular basis to aid in early diagnosis.
- Teach the family about the chemotherapy drugs and their side effects.
- Teach about the care of venous access devices surgically placed.
- Provide written and illustrated information about the chemotherapy protocol(s).
- Provide radiation and surgery education specific to the tumour treatment.

- Refer the family to nutrition resources such as dieticians to improve the child's nutritional status.

OESTOSARCOMA

Oestosarcoma is the most common bone cancer in children. Peak age is late adolescence but rare in young age. The tumour is usually located at metaphysis of the distal femur, proximal tibia and fibula, or proximal humerus, ileum, vertebra, or mandible. Survival rate is about 60%; increases to 85% if no metastasis.

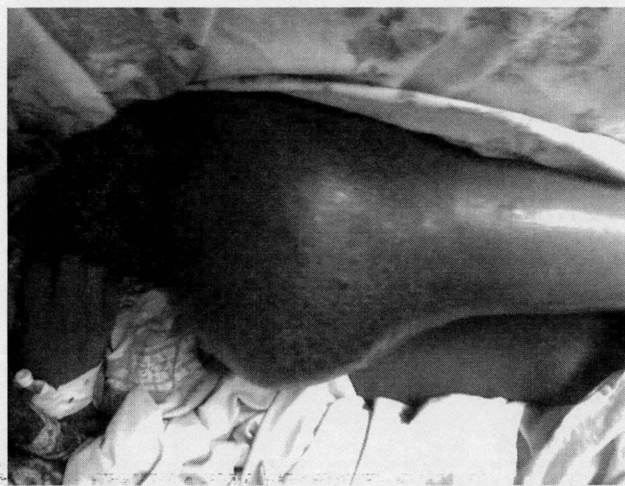

Fig. 12.2: Oestosarcoma in thigh

Causes

- Unknown
- Excessive radiotheraphy radiation exposture
- Heredity

Pathophysiology

Tumour arises from bone-forming osteoblast and bone digesting osteoclast.

Complications

- Metastasis to other organs, especially lungs

Clinical Manifestations

- The initial symptoms of oesteosarcomas are pain and swelling.
  - Pain is more intense at night and is not usually associated with mobility.
- Impaired mobility.
- Absence of infection or trauma at the site preceding the pain.
- Pathologic fractures, which may result from bone marrow involvement.

Investigation

- X-rays studies of the affected area-reveal sunburst appearence.
- Bone scan.
- CT or MRI scan of involved bone.
- Blood test for serum alkaline phosphatase–shows elevated figures.
- Tumour biopsy to confirm the diagnosis.
- Arteriography may be performed if limb-sparing surgery is contemplated.
- Lung tomography reveals lung metastasis.

Management

- Treatment involves surgery and chemotherapy

Surgery

1. Either a limb sparing procedure or
2. Limb amputation
   - Limb sparing procedures: The tumour is removed and internal prosthesis is inserted.
   - The limb sparing procedure is possible if bone growth has taken place and a neurobundle (area where several nerves converge) is not involved in the tumour.
   - If these criterias are not met, limb amputation is necessary. Amputation is done at the joint proximal to the tumour; some institutions remove only the bone and salvage the limb.
   - Chemotherapy may be started before surgery, especially in cases where limb-sparing surgery is performed.
   - Chemotherapy agents are used either alone or in combination with one another.
   - Dactinomycin, doxorubicin, bleomycin, cyclophosphamide and high dose of methotrexate are used.
   - May be infused intra-arterially into the long bones of the legs.
- A thoractomy is performed followed by chemotherapy if lung metastasis is present.

Nursing Management

- Reinforce the fact that the child did not cause the tumour.
- Provide psychological support and reinforce child's strengths.

- Provide support through phantom limb pain.
- Provide stump care and help the child prepare for a prosthesis.
- Assist with chemotherapy.
- Complete bedridden care should be given in early stage, then ambulation of the child after operation.
- Prevent infection.
- Sterile wound care.
- Diversional therapy for the child.

NEUROBLASTOMA

It is the most common extracranial solid tumour diagnosed in the infant years.

Tumours usually arise from the adrenal gland but can also arise at multiple other sites usually within the abdomen. It is responsible for 8 % of childhood cancers and 15 % of cancer deaths in children.

- The cancer usually metastasizes before it is diagnosed
  - Highly malignant
  - Poor prognosis (less than 50% chance of survival) for the child older than age 1; prognosis approaches 75% survival) for children diagnosed younger than age 1.
- If a tumour is in the abdomen, manifestations resemble Wilms tumour.

Causes

- Unknown
- Predisposing factors like an environmental factor such as prenatal drug exposure from the mother.

Pathophysiology

- Tumours start from embryonic cells in the neural crest that give rise to the adrenal medulla, paraganglia and the sympathetic nervous system of the cervical sympathetic chain and the thoracic chain.
- Tumours occur most commonly in the abdomen near the adrenal gland or spinal ganglia.
- Most common sites of metastasis include the bone marrow, lower, and subcutaneous tissue.
- Stages
  - In stage I, the tumour is confined to the organ or structure of origin and is completely removable by surgery.
  - In stage II, continuity extends beyond the primary site but not across the midline; tumour can not be completely removed by surgery.
  - In stage III, the tumour extends beyond the midline.
  - In stage IV, the tumour metastasizes.

Complications

- Neurologic impairment
- Obstruction of the airway
- Spinal paralysis

Clinical Manifestations

- Be aware that the symptoms vary and typically result from compression of the tumour on adjacent structures.
- Firm abdominal mass crossing the midline.
- Altered bowel and bladder function occurs when there is mass in the abdomen, urinary frequency or urine retention.
- Abdominal fullness
- Bone pain
- Fatigue
- Fever
- Dyspnea or infection may occur when the tumour is in mediasternum.
- Weakness and lethargy
- Anorexia and weight loss

Investigation

Tests for Initial Diagnosis

- Tumour tissue diagnosis by microscopy or biopsy of tumour cells plus.
- 24 hour urine collection to measure catecholamines, preceded by a vanillylmandelic acid diet for 3 days (eliminate bananas. nuts, chocolate, vanilla).

Tests for Metastases

- Bone marrow biopsy.
- Skeletal X-ray.
- Ultrasound and CT scan allow for a definite diagnosis.
- MRI allows for the evaluation of the extent of the neuroblastoma.
- Radiolabel scanning with metaiodobenzylguanidine (MIBG).

Medical Management

- Complete surgical removal for stages I and II.
- Radiation for stage III may not improve survival rate but may alleviate pain from metastasis.
- Chemotherapy for treatment of extensive disease, including vincrestine, doxorubicin, cyclophosphamide, and cisplatin (platinol).
- Bone marrow stem cell transplantation, when the marrow is completely destroyed by chemotherapy.

Nursing Interventions

- Explain treatment options to the patient and his family including possible adverse effects from radiation and chemotherapy.
- Prepare the patient and his family for operative procedures.
- Offer emotional support to the family because of the high degree of mortality associated with the disease.

ALTERED ENDOCRINE CONDITIONS

DIABETES MELLITUS

Definition

Diabetes mellitus is a disorder characterized by the relative or absolute lack of insulin production resulting in an impairment of glucose metabolism.

Types

Two major types:

1. Insulin–dependent diabetes mellitus (IDDM- Type I)
2. Non Insulin–dependent mellitus (NIDDM – Type II)

In IDDM, the body is completely or almost completely unable to make insulin in the absence of insulin replacement therapy, fat and protein catabolism results in the development of ketosis.

In NIDDM, the body still makes insulin but either produces an inadequate supply or cannot use the insulin properly.

Incidence

- 150,000 people under 20 years of age have diabetics mellitus.
- About in 600 school age children develop the disease.
- The vast majority of children have the insulin dependent type.

Predisposing Factors (Research Shows)

1. Genetic factors
2. Viral infection
3. An autoimmune attack
4. Tumours of the pancreas
5. Pancreatitis
6. Steroid use may contribute to development of the disease

Pathophysiology

Lack of insulin

Metabolic changes | Physiological changes in all parts of the body

↓

Glucose does not leave the blood to enter the muscles and fat cells

↓

Blood glucose level increases (hyperglycaemia) (S. glucose 200 mg/dl)

↓

Kidneys are unable to reabsorb all the glucose in the glomerular filtrate

↓

Obligatory osmotic diuresis, the glucose appears in the urine (glycosuria)

↓

Large amount of electrolytes (e.g., sodium, potassium, calcium, phosphate and magnesium) are also excreted by the kidneys.

↓

Due to diuretic action there is excessive urination (polyuria) and dehydration

↓

Excess thirst (polydipsia)

Compensatory Mechanism

Glucose is unavailable for cellular metabolism (because insulin is inadequate)

↓

The tissue turns to fat for fuel (large amount of fat breaks down into fatty acids and flows to the liver and other tissues) ⟶ Oxidized for energy.

↓

Liver also converts some fatty acids into ketones

↓

Excessive ketone bodies accumulate and are excreted in the urine (ketonuria)

↓

Additional sodium and potassium are lost as ketone bodies are transported out of the nephron tubules

↓

Metabolic acidosis

↓

In addition, the excess ketones are excreted by the lungs, resulting in an acetone (fruity) odour on the breath.

⟶ Without glucose entering the cells. Protein is also metabolized to provide energy for cell activity.

↓

Body protein breaks down ⟶ Gluconeogenesis increases, and further hyperglycaemia develops

↓

Hunger mechanism ⟶ (Polyphagia) Excessive food intake

↓

Increases, the blood glucose level further

↓

Ketoacidosis ⟶ Dehydration

↓

Electrolyte imbalance ⟶ Coma ⟶ Death

Clinical Manifestations

- Three cardinal signs of diabetes mellitus are polyuria, polydipsia, and polyphagia
- Lethargy
- Weight loss and hunger
- Weakness and fatigue
- Dehydration—dry mucous membranes, poor skin turgor
- Frequent skin and urinary tract infection
- Bed wetting,
- Glucosuria without ketonuria
- Kussmaul respiration and acetone breath
- Numbness or pain in the hands or feet
- Skin change—dry, itchy skin
- Characteristic" breath odour in ketoacidosis
- Vision changes—Retinopathy or cataract formation

Investigation

- Fasting blood sugar test (usually greater than 130 mg/dl).
- Random blood glucose level greater than or equal to 200 mg/dl.
- Glucose tolerance test (elevated blood glucose greater than 200 mg/dl, 2 hours after glucose administration).
- Urine test—glucose, acetone.
- Ophthalmologic examination may show diabetic retinopathy.

Treatment

- Insulin therapy
- Meal plan
- Exercise plan

Insulin Therapy

Action

1. Insulin binds to insulin receptors on cell surface, allowing glucose to enter the cell.

Types

1. Rapid acting
2. Intermediate acting
3. Long acting.

TABLE 13.1: Types of Insulins and their Duration of Action

Product	From	Onset	Peak	Duration
1. Rapid Acting				
• Regular	Pork	30 mt	2.5–3 hours	8 hours
• Semilente	Pork	1–2 hours	5–10 hours	16 hours
• Humulin-R	Human	15–30 mts	2–4 hours	6–8 hours
2. Intermediate				
• Humulin-L	Human	1–3 hours	6–12 hours	18–24 hours
• Purified pork-L	Pork	2–3 hours	7–15 hours	22 hours
• Lente	Beef/pork	1–3 hours	6–12 hours	18–26 hours
3. Long Acting				
• Ultra lente	Beef	4 hours	10–30 hours	36 hours
• Humulin	Human	4–6 hours	8–20 hours	24–28 hours

- The most common insulin regimen for children consists of a combination of rapid– acting (regular) and intermediates–acting (NPH or Lente) insulin mixed in one syringe and administered twice daily, before breakfast and before dinner.
- Oral antidiabetic drug (type 2); insulin may be required.
- Insulin pump; gives insulin on a more regular basis.

Route and Dose of Administration

- Normally subcutaneous route
- If acidosis – Intramuscular/IV route
- Dose adjustment depends on child's activity pattern change and child's blood glucose level.

Site of Injection

- Upper arm, thigh, outer areas of the abdomen are common sites for self Injection.
- Buttocks can be used by family members

Diet (Nutrition Plan)

Meal plan should consider two major goals:

1. Keeping Blood sugar near normal levels by avoiding insulin reaction and hyperglycaemia.
2. Providing the calories for normal growth and weight.
   - American diet association recommends distribution of total calories by food group, for children to take 50–60 % of the calories from carbohydrates, 12–20% from protein and rest from fat.
   - Modest caloric restriction for weight loss or maintenance.
   - Although there is no food that a child with diabetes must avoid, certain foods will need to be balanced by extra insulin.
   - A nutritionist can help the family integrate preferred ethnic foods into the child's diet.
   - About 1 unit of regular insulin per 30 g of carbohydrate.

Exercise

- Regular aerobic exercise.

Safety Rules for Diabetic Children

Nutrition

1. Maintain total calorie intake
2. Develop a daily well balance meal plan
3. Eat extra food for extra activity
4. Plan extra activity for extra food
5. Keep consistent meal time
6. Avoid pure-sugar food
7. Increase intake of fiber
8. Decrease cholesterol and saturated fat.

Exercise

1. Check the blood sugar before exercise
2. Carry some form of sugar at all time

3. Wear identity card
4. Inject the insulin into a non-exercising muscle
5. Drink plenty of fluids (more in hot weather).

Nursing Management

- Administer medications as ordered
- Monitor for hypoglycaemia (insulin shock)
  - Can result from increased insulin use, excessive exercise, or failure to eat
  - Recognize signs and symptoms
  - Behaviour changes (belligerence, confusion, slurred speech)
  - Diaphoresis
  - Palpitations
  - Tachycardia
  - Tremors
  - If hypoglycaemia occurs, give rapidly absorbed carbohydrates such as orange juice or, if the child is unconscious, glucagons or I.V. dextrose as ordered.
- Monitor for hyperglycaemia
  - Recognize signs and symptoms
    - Abdominal cramping
    - Dry, flushed skin
    - Fatigue
    - Fruity breath odour
    - Headache
    - Mental status changes
    - Nausea
    - Thin appearance and possibly malnourishment
    - Vomiting
    - Weakness
  - Administer I.V. fluids and insulin replacement for hyperglycaemic crisis as ordered.
- If it can't be determined whether a stuporous diabetic is suffering from hypoglycaemia or hyperglycaemia, treat for hypoglycaemia.
- Provide meticulous skin care, especially to the feet and legs.
- Treat all injuries, cuts and blisters immediately.
- Avoid constricting hose, slippers, or bed linens.
- Encourage adequate fluid intake.
- Consult a nutritionist.
- Encourage verbalization of feelings.
- Offer emotional support.
- Help to develop effective coping strategies.
- Provide patient teaching
  - The disorder, diagnostic studies, and treatment.
  - Insulin (Insulin-dependent Diabetes Mellitus (IDDM) In IDDM, the body unable to make insulin in the absence of insulin replacement therapy, insulin must be administered to the child.
    - When giving a combination of clear and cloudy insulins, draw up clear insulin first to prevent contamination.
    - To prevent air bubbles, don't shake the vial; intermediate forms are suspensions and should be gently rotated.
    - Administer insulin as ordered (commonly twice daily; however, more injections per day may be ordered), 30 minutes before breakfast and 30 minutes before dinner; know that both injections will include a combination of fast-acting and intermediate-acting insulin.
    - Insulin dosages vary; the dosage for one day is based on blood glucose levels of the previous day, with two-thirds of the daily dose usually given in the morning injection and one-third in the evening injection.
    - Watch for hypoglycaemic reaction during the peak action times for fast-acting and intermediate-acting insulins.
    - Rotate injection sites to prevent lipodystrophy.
    - Teach maintenance of insulin pump.
    - Make sure the child eats when the insulin peaks, such as a mid afternoon and bedtime snack.
    - Keep in mind that insulin requirements may be altered with illness, stress, growth, food intake, and exercise; blood glucose measurements are the best way to determine insulin adjustments.
    - Instruct parents in all aspects of insulin therapy as below.
  - When to notify the physician.
  - Appropriate exercise plan.
  - Self-monitoring of glucose.

- Signs and symptoms of hyperglycaemia, hypoglycaemia, infection, and diabetic neuropathy.
- Foot care.
- Safety precautions.

PITUITARY DYSFUNCTION

Pituitary gland is a master gland because of its role in regulating other endocrine glands under the influence of secretions from the hypothalamus, the anterior lobe of the pituitary (adenohypophysis) releases or withholds seven hormones. These hormones control the secretion of other endocrine glands and influence somatic and sexual development.

Functions of Pituitary Gland

- It secretes growth hormone—It promotes growth of bone and soft tissues.
- Thyroid-Stimulating Hormone (TSH) Thyrotropin-Target tissue: adrenal cortex.
- Gonadotropins: Target tissue gonads.
- Follicle-Stimulating Hormone (FSH) Target tissue: ovaries, testes.
- Luteinizing Hormone (LH): Target tissue ovaries, testes.
- Prolactin (Luteotropic hormone): Target tissue ovaries, breasts.
- Melanocyte-stimulating hormone (MSH): Target tissue skin.

Hypopituitarism (Dwarfism)

It is a growth hormone deficiency disorder caused by decreased activity of the pituitary gland. Because most children with this disorder secrete inadequate amount of growth hormone, the term growth deficiency is often preferred to hypopituitarism.

Causes

- Aplasia or hypoplasia
- Developmental defects
  - Idiopathic pituitary growth failure, hypopituitarism
  - Idiopathic-genetic
- Destructive lesions
- Trauma – Perinatal birth trauma such as breech, birth hypoxia,
  - Child abuse; basal skull fracture
  - Infiltrative lesions tumours, tuberculosis, toxoplasmosis
- Irradiation-CNS; eyes, middle ear
- Surgery
  - Removal of pharyngeal pituitary;
  - Ablations of craniopharyngioma or other tumour
  - Vascular abnormalities,
- Functional disorders such as
  - Anorexia nervous
  - Psychosocial dwarfism

Clinical Manifestations

- At birth baby has normal height and weight.
- After one year retarded growth.
- Sexual development is usually delayed but is normal.
- Facial structure may be normal or short or there may be fine wrinkles about the eyes and mouth.
- Prominent frontal bone.
- The bridge of the nose depressed.
- Eruption of primary teeth appears in expected age but eruption of permanent teeth is delayed.
- Under development of jaw because of that teeth become overcrowded and malpositioned.
- Neck is short and a small larynx produces a high pitched voices.

Investigation

- History collection
  - Family History: It is important in relating short stature to genetic background
  - Child History: It includes a thorough prenatal history to rule out maternal disorders that may have influenced growth.
  - Past medical history: It is investigated for evidence of chronic illness that may influence growth pattern such as congenital heart diseases, malabsorption disorders, severe anaemia.
- Physical Examination
  - Accurate measurement of height and weight and comparison with standard growth chart are essential.
  - Other measurements include crown to pubis and pubis to heel length to compare body proportion.
  - Sexual development should be assessed and compared with age-appropriate development.

  - Funduscopic examination and testing for visual activity should be performed to detect evidence of ocular damage from a tumour.
- Radioimmunoassay (plasma growth hormone levels) study.
- X-ray of the wrist/head for centers of ossification.
- Hormone studies.

Treatment

- Replacement of growth hormone (human pituitary hormone).
- The daily administration of GH to short, prepubertal children has resulted in a growth velocity of 8.7 ± 1.5 cm per year. Many children who respond to therapy have maintained this accelerated rate until achievement of height that is more appropriate to family height.
- The decision to stop GH therapy is made jointly by the child, family, and healthcare team. Radiologic evidence of epiphyseal closure is a criterion for ending therapy. Dosage is increased as the time of epiphyseal closure nears in order to gain the best advantage of the GH. Children with other hormone deficiencies require replacement therapy to correct the specific disorders. This may involve administration of thyroid extract, cortisone, testosterone, or estrogens and progesterone. The sex hormones are usually begun during adolescence to promote normal sexual maturation.

Nursing Management

- The principal nursing consideration is identifying children with growth problems.
- The nurse may be the key person in helping to establish a diagnosis. For example, if serial height and weight records are not available, the nurse can question parents about the child's growth in comparison with that of siblings, peers, or relatives.
- The behavioural or physical changes that suggest a tumour are insidious, they are frequently overlooked. It is important to correlate the onset of any positive findings with the initial evidence of growth retardation.
- Part of a nurse's role in helping to establish a diagnosis is assisting with diagnostic tests.
- If a number of tests are being performed, the child will require particular attention during provocative testing.
- Children also have difficulty overcoming hypoglycaemia generated by tests with insulin, so they must be observed carefully for signs of hypoglycaemia, whereas those receiving glucagons are at risk of nausea and vomiting. The dose of insulin may need to be reduced in infants and small children during this procedure.

Child and Family Support

- Once a diagnosis is made confirming an organic cause of the problem, the parents and child need an opportunity to express their thoughts and feelings.
- Children undergoing hormone replacement require additional support. Therapy for GH deficiency requires daily subcutaneous injections.
- Education for patient self-management during the school-age years should be provided. Nursing functions include family education concerning medication preparation and storage, injection sites, injection technique, and syringe disposal.
- Administration of GH is facilitated by family routines that include a specific time of day for the injection.
- Younger children may enjoy using a calendar and colourful stickers to designate received injections.

Care of Children with HIV/AIDS

COMPREHENSIVE PAEDIATRIC HIV/AIDS CARE AND TREATMENT

The WHO approach to paediatric HIV/AIDS care and treatment is to maximize resources while ensuring provision of equitable care. The Table 14.1 gives outline approach to care and treatment for HIV–exposed and infected children. To provide comprehensive HIV/ AIDS care, especially we need family support as well as coordination of medical, supportive service and health provider are essential. The multidisciplinary team need to provide comprehensive HIV/AIDS care for children, the team may include counsellors, peer educators, community health workers, nutritionists, pharmacists, doctors, nurses. This team should meet periodically to exchange information, develop and monitor patient care plans. This group has a team leader, usually a counsellor or nurse, he plans the weekly patient list and agenda and distributes it to the team in advance of the meeting. A specific team member should be assigned to follow-up on the plan and ensure that interventions discussed are implemented.

Table 14.1: Components of Paediatric HIV Care and Treatment

Components
Family-Centred Care • Improve linkages between paediatric, ANC, PMTCT, TB and adult care and treatment programs • Dedicated paediatric care and treatment team at each site providing adult HIV/AIDS services
Prevention of Paediatric Infection • Primary prevention of HIV infection in women • Provision of ARVs to pregnant women to prevent MTCT • Provision of ARV prophylaxis for infants • Identify and follow HIV-exposed infants
Care of HIV-exposed Infants • Linking ANC, PMTCT, maternity to paediatric care and treatment to facilitate identification of the HIV exposed infant • Growth monitoring and developmental assessment • Counselling on infant feeding, maternal nutrition and support • Early infant HIV diagnosis using age appropriate test (DNA PCR or rapid antibody test) • Early infant HIV diagnosis using age appropriate test (DNA PCR or rapid antibody test) • TB risk assessment • Routine preventive paediatric services including immunizations • Facilitated enrolment of HIV-infected children into care and treatment
Care and Treatment of HIV-infected Children • Promote and support active case detection • Growth monitoring and development assessment • Nutrition counselling and support • Clinical and immunological staging • Laboratory tests • Cotrimoxazole prophylactic therapy • TB risk assessment • Treatment of OIS, HIV-associated TB infection and other common childhood illnesses • Routine preventive paediatric services including immunizations • Provision of ART for eligible infants and children • Management of drug toxicities, treatment failure and provision of second-line regimen • Psychosocial support, adherence and disclosure • Management and appropriate referral for complicated patients

The objective of care is

- The goal of comprehensive approach is to reduce barriers within the healthcare system, improve the health of HIV–affected families, reduce the risk of perinatal transmission, support adherence to treatment and understand the role of families in HIV prevention.

Goal of Early Diagnosis of HIV in Infants and Children

- To identify HIV-infected child early in order to provide them with life saving ART, not to exclude infection.
- To facilitate early access to care and treatment, this reduces morbidity and mortality.

Opportunity and Entry Points for HIV Testing in Children

All healthcare facilities are very important area of entry points for HIV testing in children. Most of the healthcare providers often miss the opportunities for identifying children who need testing. Following health facilities have opportunities and entry points for testing HIV in children.

- PMTCT programs and EPI for HIV-exposed infants
- Paediatric inpatient unit
- Malnutrition units
- TB clinics
- Paediatric outpatients units
- Children of adults attending HIV prevention, care and treatment centres
- Siblings of children enrolled in HIV care.
- Orphanages
- Paediatric inpatient units

Diagnosing HIV Infection in Infants and Children upto 18 Months of Age

All infants born to HIV+ mothers will test HIV antibody positive in the first several months of life. Maternal HIV antibody (IgG) is transferred across the placenta during pregnancy.

A positive HIV antibody test in infants <18 months of age will not distinguish whether or not the infant is HIV-infected; rather it shows that:

- Mother is HIV-infected
- Infant is at risk for HIV infection (exposed to HIV)

If the child is not infected, the HIV antibody fades during first 6–18 months of life. Most uninfected infants test negative by 12 months of age, all uninfected infants test negative by 18 months.

To diagnose the infant the following virologic tests to be done:

- HIV DNA PCR
- HIV RNA PCR
- p24 Antigen
- Viral Culture
- Two positive virologic tests = HIV infection
- One positive virologic test = Presumed HIV infection

HIV DNA PCR is a special laboratory test that detects pieces of the viral gene that are incorporated in the human blood cell.

- By comparison, HIV antibody testing detects the antibody that the body makes in response to the HIV virus.
- Sensitivity of HIV DNA PCR increases with time during the first month of life.
- The infant may have HIV infection but there may not be enough virus in the blood to detect it at birth. It becomes easier to find/detect as the infant gets a little older.

The health professional must know that the child is at risk for HIV infection, if

- Born to an HIV-infected woman
- Tests HIV-antibody positive
- Pay close attention to the child's clinical status and growth pattern.
- Use special virologic tests to identify the infected child, not to exclude infection in the exposed child.
- Interpretation of virologic test results should always be done in the context of the clinical presentation of the infant.

In infants under 18 months, special tests are needed because of the persisting presence of maternal antibodies. The main options are DNA PCR or RNA or p24 antigen tests. Each test has advantages and disadvantages that determine which is most appropriate, depending on resources. However, DNA or RNA PCR test is considered a test for infant diagnosis; in most of the settings, the DNA PCR (a qualitative test) is the preferred methods for infant diagnosis. All infants born to HIV infected women should have DNA PCR at six weeks of age or at the first opportunity thereafter.

If the test is positive, the infant is presumed to be HIV infected, infant should be referred for treatment. Infant 12 months of age, with an initial positive DNA PCR, a confirmatory test should be performed. A negative DNA PCR in a breastfeeding infant does not rule out HIV infection.

In infants with 9 months and older at the time of breastfeeding cessation, if the infant is an asymptomatic child, screen with HIV antibody. If positive, virologic testing is indicated, if it is negative, no virologic testing is necessary. If breastfeeding, repeat antibody testing > 6–12 weeks after cessation of breastfeeding. If the infant has a symptom of HIV screen with virologic testing. If the HIV DNA PCR result is positive, the infant is presumed to be HIV infected, if the HIV DNA PCR is negative, the baby is presumed not to be HIV infected.

Note: Infants who are still breastfeeding are at continued risk for acquiring HIV infection.

HIV testing in HIV exposed infants >12 months is easier where virological testing is available.

STAGING AND CLASSIFICATION OF HIV/AIDS IN CHILDREN

Clinical staging should be performed at every visit. The importance of clinical stages is:

- To assess disease severity.
- To monitor disease progression.
- Criteria for ARV therapy and other HIV-related interventions.
- Criteria to switch a failing regimen especially when CD4 is not available.

Clinical Staging of Paediatric HIV/AIDS

Old WHO clinical stages:

- Three stages.
- Did not capture many disease manifestations.
- Did not include measures of immunologic status.

New WHO clinical stages:

- Four clinical disease categories; asymptomatic, mild, advance and severe.
- Expanded comprehensive list of associated conditions based on prognosis.
- Standardized criteria for presumptive and definitive diagnosis.

WHO Staging for <15 Years Old

Clinical Stage 1 (Asymptomatic)
PGL (Persistant Generalized Lymphadenopathy)
Clinical Stage 2 (Mild)
Hepatosplenomeagly Papular pruritic eruptions, Extensive wart virus infection Extensive molluscum contagious Fungal nail infections, Recurrent oral ulcerations Linear gingival erythema (LGE) Angular cheilitis Parotid enlargement Herpes zoster Recurrent or Chronic URTI (otitis media, otorrhea, sinusitis)
Clinical Stage 3 (Advanced)
Moderate unexplained malnutrition not adequately responding to standard therapy Unexplained persistent diarrhoea (14 days or more) Unexplained persistent fever (intermittent or constant for longer than one month) Oral candidiasis (outside neonatal period), Oral hairy leucoplakia Acute necrotizing ulcerative gingivitis/periodontitis Pulmonary TB Severe recurrent bacterial pneumonia Unexplained anaemia (<8 mg/dl),and/or neutropenia (<500/mm^3) and/or thrombocytopenia, (<50,000/mm^3) for >1 month Chronic HIV associated lung disease including bronchiectasis Symptomatic lymphoid interstitial pneumonitis (LIP)
Clinical Stage 4 (Severe)
Unexplained severe wasting or severe malnutrition not adequately responding to standard therapy Pneumocystis pneumonia Recurrent severe bacterial infections (empyema, pyomyositis, bone or joint infection, meningitis, but excluding pneumonia) Chronic herpes simplex infection (orolabial or cutanoeus > 1 month, visceral of any duration) Kaposi's sarcoma, esophageal candidiasis, CNS toxoplasmosis, HIV encephalopathy CMV infection (retinitis or infection of organs other than liver, spleen or lymph nodes; onset at the age of 1 month or more) Extra pulmonary cryptococcosis including meningitis Any disseminated mycosis (e.g., extra pulmonary

histoplasmmosis, coccidiomycosis, penicillosis)
Cryptosporidiosis, isosporiasis
Disseminated non-tuberculous mycobacteria infection
Candida of the trachea, bronchi or lungs
Acquired HIV associated rectal fistula, cerebral or B-cell lymphoma
Progressive multifocal leucoencephalopathy (PML)
HIV associated cardiomyopathy or HIV associated nephropathy

CARE OF THE HIV-EXPOSED INFANTS

HIV- exposed infants need regular follow-up since they are at risk of morbidity and mortality regardless of infection status. Linking PMTCT to infant follow-up is an important step in ensuring that HIV-exposed infants are enrolled into care. Where PMTCT programmes are non-existent, maternal and child health, immunization and under-5 clinics are excellent venues to identify HIV-exposed infants. Rapid antibody tests performed on mother or infant can confirm HIV exposure, enabling these infants to be enrolled into care. Basic care for HIV-exposed infants can be provided in under-clinics, paediatric outpatient clinics and health centres.

Goals of Care for the HIV-exposed Infants

- To minimize risk of vertical transmission of HIV.
- To recognize HIV infection early using age-appropriate testing.
- To prevent opportunistic infections.
- To enroll HIV-infected children into ART care early.

Comprehensive Care for the HIV-Exposed Infants

HIV-exposed infants must have regular visits for health assessment and promotion. Infants should be seen monthly for the first six months, then every three months. Infants with poor growth, failure to thrive, or recurrent illnesses should have more frequent close follow-up

1. Birth

Mothers should be given appointment for the first postnatal visit at delivery. Mothers who do not deliver at a health facility should be given appointments at first contact with the healthcare system. Refer to National Guidelines on PMTCT for details.

HIV status of the mother should be clearly indicated on the infant's immunization card in a non-stigmatizing way. (Use identification method used for the PMTCT enrolled pregnant women on infant's immunization card.)

- Mother should be counselled on infant prophylaxis (Refer the National Guidelines on PMTCT).
- Immunizations—per National Expanded Program on Immunization.
- Counselling on infant feeding, maternal nutrition and support.

2. Initial Visit at 4–6 Weeks

- History includes use of PMTCT, parental concerns, intercurrent illness.

The following questions should be asked to the caregiver at each visit:

  - Has the child been ill?
  - How is the child eating?
  - Ask about the child's new accomplishments.
  - Has anyone in the household been diagnosed or developed symptoms of tuberculosis.
  - Any new medication taken.
- Parents are often first to recognize problems with the infant.
- Reinforcing the positives, effective communication and family care coordination should be part of the care of the exposed infant.
- Nutrition and growth assessment—Growth can be the most sensitive clinical indication of HIV infection in an infant/young child.
  - HIV-exposed infants are at high risk for poor growth.
  - Failure to thrive affects as many as 50% of HIV-infected infants and children.
  - HIV-infected infants who are failing to thrive have a significantly increased risk of mortality.
  - Easy and systematic way to follow changes in growth over time (growth rates) for an individual child.
  - The decrease in growth rates represents problems in growth.
  - Growth rates should be monitored closely for all exposed infants.
  - Plot weight, height and head circumference on the growth chart.

- Developmental assessment—'Development' represents maturation of the brain and central nervous system.
- Delayed development or loss of milestones may be the first sign of HIV infection in an infant or young child.
  - While we think about growth in terms of rates (change over time), development can be viewed more as snapshots of the child at specified points in time.
  - While other causes are possible, abnormal development should raise concerns of HIV infection.
  - Infants are at high risk for HIV encephalopathy and severe neurologic disease.

Development embraces other aspects of differentiation of form, including those driven by genetic endowment, it also involves changes of function, including those that are shaped mainly by interactions with the environment, whether these produce structural, emotional, or social changes.

"Delayed development or loss of milestones" may be the first signs of HIV infection in a young child. While other causes are certainly likely, abnormal development should raise concerns of HIV infection.

- Early identification of developmental delay and neurologic abnormalities can facilitate intervention and remediation. A developmental assessment that includes the following should be conducted at each visit:
  - Cognitive, motor, language, and social skills.
  - Discuss the infant's milestones.
  - Use a developmental check list or observe the infant during the examination.
  - Verify appropriate development for age.
- Developmental checklist:
  - 1 month: raises head, crawling movement, alerts to sound.
  - 2 months: head midline, lifts chest off table, smiles socially.
  - 4 months: rolls front to back, laughs.
  - 6 months: sits unsupported, babbles.
  - 9 months: pulls to stand, says "mama".
  - 12 months: walks alone, two words.

Table 14.2: Developmental Warning Signs in Infant

Age	Warning Signs
1 month	Does not regard face, no eye contact, no smile, poor suck, floppy
2 months	Does not look at you with both eyes at least for a few moments, and does not follow with eyes if you move your face slowly from side to side
3 months	Does not respond to sound by quieting
4 months	Does not hold head steady for a few moments when you sit him up, does not grasp rattle that you put into his palm
5 months	Does not raise head and support weight on arms when in prone position
6 months	Cannot reach for objects with both hands, Floppy, no response to sound, Poor social response to people
9 months	Unable to sit unsupported, hand preference, fisting, persistence of primitive reflexes
12 months	Unable to bear weight on legs
15 months	Does not walk alone, is not using at least one word meaningfully
18 months	Does not use at least 3 words, and does not point to what he wants

- TB risk assessment—to roll out the infection
- Physical examination—Physical examination at each visit must include:
  - A comprehensive initial examination including all organ systems
  - Focused subsequent examinations based on history and caregiver complaints, targeted to HIV-related stigmata
    - Oral thrush
    - Dermatitis
    - Severe wasting
    - Generalized lymphadenopathy
    - Hepatosplenomegaly
- Signs highly suggestive of HIV infection in infants

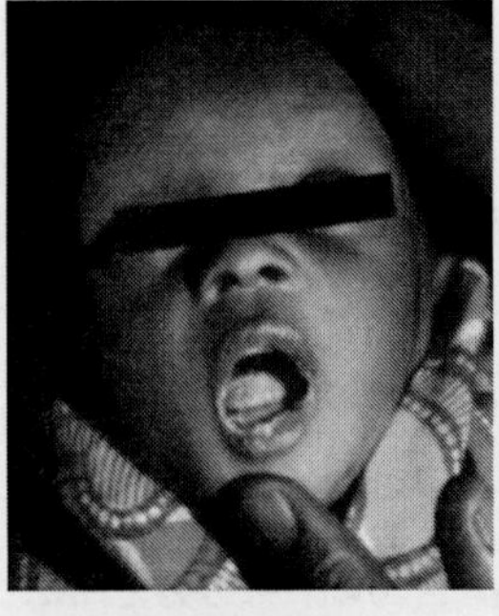
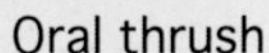
Oral thrush

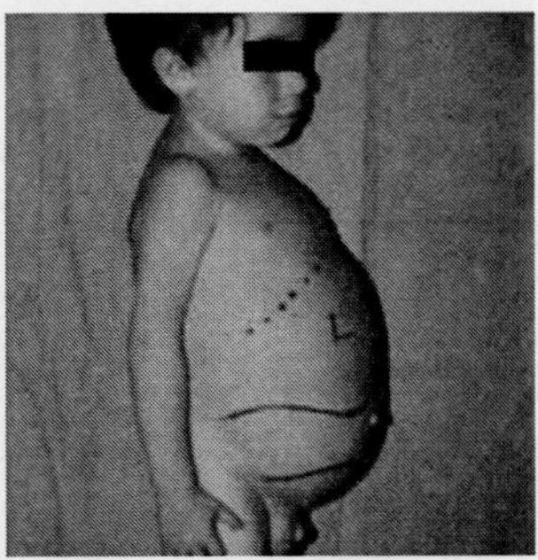
Hepatosplenomegaly

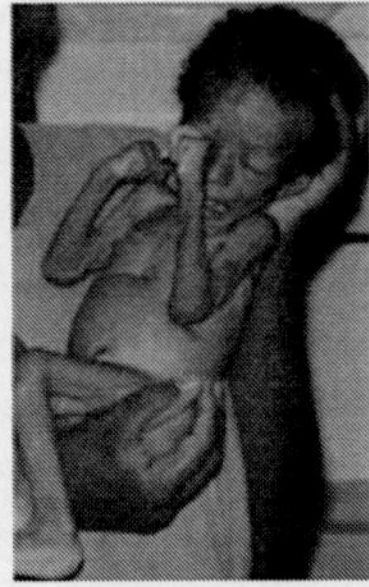
Severe wasting (See Pl. 19)

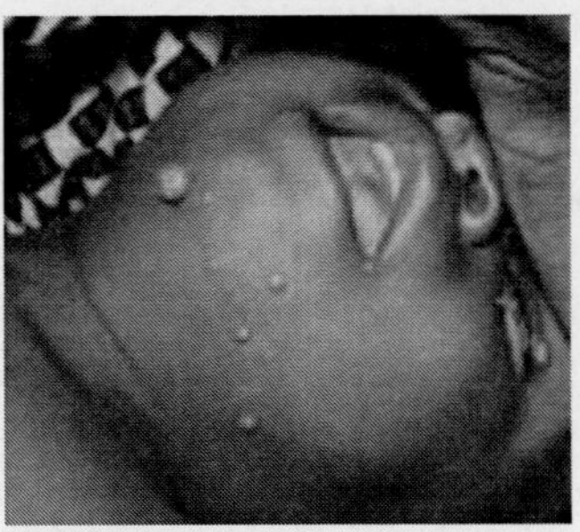
Extensive Molluscum Contagisum

Fig. 14.1: Signs of HIV infection in infant

Source: Ethiopian HIV/AIDS guidelines.

Thrush outside the neonatal period defined as creamy white to yellow soft small plaques on red or normally colored mucosa which cannot easily be scraped off, or red patches on the tongue, palate or lining of the mouth, usually painful.

Hepatosplenomegaly is enlargement of the liver and spleen without apparent course.

Wasting weight for age below the third percentile or crossing two percentiles or low weight-for-age, up to –2 standard deviations (SDs), not explained by poor or inadequate feeding and or other infections, and not adequately responding to standard management.

Severe Molluscum is a relatively common cutaneous infection caused by the DNA pox virus. Lesions are sigle or multiple, white, opalescent, flesh-coloured, or pink papules. They are often dome shaped with a central pinpoint core. It is usually 1–3 mm, they can occasionally be larger than 1 cm and are then refered to as giant molluscum, these are present in face and neck and trunk.

- Determination of HIV status—all exposed infants should have the initial DNA PCR test done at six weeks old. Caregivers should be counselled on the rationale for infant diagnosis; explain the possible test result, and need for additional testing to determine infection status definitely.
- Cotrimoxazole preventive therapy should be provided to all HIV–exposed infants starting at six weeks old, and continued until HIV infection has been excluded and infant is no longer at risk from breastfeeding.

Trimethoprim/sulfamethoxazole CTX/SMZ, Cotrimoxazole, Septrim®, Bactrim®		
Age	**Suspension (40 mg TMP/200 mg SMZ) per 5 ml**	**Single-strength tablet (80 mg TMP/400 mg SMZ)**
<6 months	2.5 ml daily	¼ single strength tab daily
6 months - 5 years	5 ml daily	½ single-strength tab daily

- CTX is generally very well tolerated in children
    - Check for tolerance and adherence at every visit.
- Side effects and toxicities are more common in
    - Adults > children.
    - Advanced disease > early stages of disease.
    - HIV-infected > HIV-exposed children.
- If a child develops severe reaction to CTX dapsone can be used for prophylaxis (2 mg/kg/dose daily, maximum 100 mg daily).
- Immunize according to the National Expanded Programme on Immunization.
- Immunize infants early before there is damage to the immune system.
- HIV-exposed children should receive all recommended vaccines according to the national schedule.
- Children with known or suspected HIV infection should receive all recommended vaccines with the following modifications:
    - An extra dose of measles vaccination at 6 months to improve protection against measles.
    - Children with symptomatic HIV should not receive live attenuated BCG vaccine or Yellow Fever vaccine.
- Counseling on infant feeding, maternal nutrition and support as necessary.
- Make sure to repeat the information at each visit.

- Provide anticipatory guidance (immunizations, healthy habits, nutrition, family support, etc.).
- All family members (infected and non-infected) can benefit from psychosocial support.

3. Follow-up Visit Schedule for HIV–Exposed Infants at Two Months

During the follow-up visit of HIV–exposed infants they should be reviewed same like initial visit.

Basic principles include:

- Early identification of infants who are sick or failing to thrive is critical.
- Careful and frequent clinical monitoring is required.
- Systematic follow up is vital
  - Appointment systems
  - Medical records
  - Family education and support
  - Adherence to care and cotrimoxazole preventive therapy—should be reinforced at each visit.

4. Follow-up Visit Schedule for HIV-Exposed Infants (3 to 18 Months)

HIV-exposed infants who are asymptomatic should be seen monthly until six months of age then every three months until 18 months of age. HIV-exposed infants, who are symptomatic, have poor growth, failure to thrive or recurrent illness should have more frequent follow up. HIV-exposed infants should be discharged from care only after final determination of HIV status. This means the majority of infants will have to be followed until 18 months of age. HIV–infected children determined to be uninfected can be discharged and followed–up in the under-5 clinics.

Review the infant's history, nutrition and growth assessment, developmental assessment, physical examination when looking for symptoms and signs suggestive of HIV infection. For determination of HIV status any symptomatic child should have repeated diagnostic testing during this period and adherence to care and cotrimoxazole therapy should be reinforced at each visit.

CARE OF THE HIV-INFECTED CHILD

Management of the HIV–infected child is best achieved through integrated HIV services and primary health care. A multidisciplinary, family-centred approach to care is effective in engaging children and their families into long-term care.

1. Goals of Care for the HIV-Infected Child

- To promote health and well-being.
- To prevent disease progression.
- To prevent opportunistic infections.

2. Comprehensive Care for the HIV-Infected Child

Comprehensive care and support for the HIV-infected child should be provided in a care and treatment centre, preferably where the parent/caregiver receives treatment. Close regular follow-up is essential since these children are at risk of morbidity and mortality. Mortality estimates in Africa show that without treatment 35.2% of HIV-infected children will die in their first year and 52.5% by age two. This underscores the importance of timely antiretroviral treatment care and support.

3. Initial Intake Visit

Clinical assessment of the HIV-infected child should focus on the following:

- History—with particular emphasis on previous AIDS defining conditions, history of ARV exposure (PMTCT or previous antiretroviral therapy), family members who are aware of the diagnosis, parental concerns, intercurrent illness.
- Nutrition and growth assessment—Check and record the weight, height and head circumference on the growth chart.
- Developmental assessment—Assessment to be done according to the age (refer the care of HIV–exposed content of growth assessment).
- Detailed physical examination should be done to assess for symptoms and signs suggestive of severe HIV infection. Perform careful physical examination at every visit. Initial exam should be comprehensive including examination of all organ systems.
  - Identify any HIV related physical findings; thrush, lymphadenopathy, organomegaly, dermatitis, encephalopathy, etc.
- Subsequent exams can be guided by findings on the symptom/sign checklist:
  - Complete Blood Count
  - CXR if clinically indicated
  - CD4 Count

- ❍ Pregnancy test for sexually active adolescent females
- ❍ CD4 number and percent
  - ■ When infant is determined to be HIV-infected
  - ■ Upon enrolement for older children.

Every six months thereafter laboratory examination.

- CD4 counts and percentages in healthy infants are very high at birth and during the first year of life and then decline.
- The absolute CD4 count varies a lot during the first year of life and is more than 3 times that of adults.
- CD4% is a more stable value than absolute number, so percentage is preferred in children under 5 years of age.
  - ❍ Because of these differences, adult values do not apply in children below the age 5 years.
  - ❍ CD4 count of 500 is considered okay for a 7 year old but is severe suppression for a 6 month old.

Calculating the CD4 Percentage

- Calculate the CD4 percentage for a 13 month old HIV-infected infant.
- CD4 absolute is 640 mm^3.
- WBC is 10,000 mm^3.
- N-38%, L-48%, M-12%, E-2%.
- Calculate the TLC = 10,000 × 0.48 = 4800.
- The CD4 percentage = $\frac{640 \times 100}{4800}$ = 13%.

TABLE 14.3: WHO Classification of Immunodeficiency in Infants and Children

	Age related CD4 values			
Immunological classification	<12 months (CD4%)	12–35 months (CD4%)	36–59 months (CD4%)	≥5 years (CD4 cells/mm^3)
Not significant	>35%	>30%	>25%	>500
Mild	30–35%	25–30%	20–25%	350–499
Advanced	25–30%	20–25%	15–20%	200–349
Severe	<25%	<20%	<15%	<200 or 15%

- Clinical staging should be identified from the infant by using WHO clinical staging criteria (refer to page 210).
- Immunological staging—Using WHO immunological classification.
- TB risk assessment—Collect the history of TB contact, TST for TB screening, and chest radiograph if clinically indicated.
- Cotrimoxazole preventive therapy—Check eligibility based on clinical stage and or CD4 if available.
- Immunization—Immunization should be given according to the national EPI schedule.
- Nutritional Counselling—Nutritional counselling to be given according to the nutritional status of the infant, offer support as necessary.
- ART eligibility—should be reviewed based on clinical stages and immunological criteria.
- Adherence—to care and cotrimoxazole preventive therapy should be reinforced at each visit.
- Disclosure of HIV status—Disclosure of HIV status should be discussed with the caregivers. Disclosure should be introduced early on in a neutral way, and should be tailored to the developmental maturity of the child. It is particularly important that adolescents be informed of their status, so they can become active participants in their own care.

4. Follow-up Visits for the HIV-infected Children

HIV-infected children (both pre-ART and on ART) need close clinical and laboratory monitoring. Follow -up schedule for HIV-infected children on ART is discussed in detail in antiretroviral therapy in children. At each review the following details are to be checked:

- History with particular emphasis on family members who are aware of the diagnosis, parental concerns and illness.
- Nutritional and growth assessment, Developmental assessment—To be checked and recorded.
- Physical examination to assess the symptoms and signs suggestive of HIV disease progression or development of Opportunistic Infection (OI).
- Clinical staging, immunological staging using WHO clinical stage and WHO immunological classification.
- TB risk assessment—Ask about history of household contact with TB, TST annually, and chest radiograph (CXR) if clinically indicated.

- Cotrimoxazole preventive therapy—Check eligibility for cotrimoxazole prophylaxis based on clinical stage and/or CD4 if available.
- ART eligibility—the need for ART should be reviewed based on clinical stage and immunological criteria.
- Adherence to care and medications should be addressed at each visit.
- Disclosure to HIV status to a child should be discussed with the parents or guardians. Disclosure should be introduced early on in a neutral way, and should be tailored to the developmental maturity of the child. It is particularly important that adolescents be informed of their status, so they can become active participants in their own care.

Table 14.4: Follow-up Schedule for HIV-infected Children

Age	Visit Interval
0–12 months	Monthly
12–24 months on ART	Monthly
12–24 months on pre-ART	Every 2–3 months if asymptomatic, monthly if symptomatic
>24 months pre-ART	Every 2–3 months if asymptomatic, monthly if symptomatic
>24 months on ART**	See ART treatment in children

*This is the minimum; children should be seen more frequently if clinically indicated.

** Children >24 months should be seen monthly for the first 6 months after initiation of ART then every 2–3 months if stable.

COMMON ILLNESSES AND TREATMENT IN HIV-INFECTED CHILDREN (OPPORTUNISTIC INFECTIONS)

- Recurrent bacterial infections

  Account for about 20% of AIDS defining illnesses in infants and children. Most are caused by encapsulated organisms such as *S. pnuemoniae* and *Salmonella;* others are *Staphylococcus, Enterococcus,* etc. Most common serious infections are pneumonia, bacteremia, sepsis and meningitis (account for more than 50% of infections in HIV-infected children).
- Clinical features

  Similar as in HIV uninfected children, but may have protracted fulminant course with rapid progression.
- Management
  - Same as in non HIV-infected children
  - Occasionally may require longer duration of treatment.
- Generally occur with severe immune suppression, some occur at higher CD4 counts.
- Young children have primary infection rather than reactivation.
- Lack of immunity leads to more severe course than in adults.
- In children with severe immunodeficiency, the clinical manifestations may vary.

Common OIs, Pneumocystis Pneumonia (PCP)

- Parasitic infection
  - *Pneumocystis jeroveci* (formerly *Pneumocystis carinii*).
- Diffuse and severe pneumonia
- Peak incidence is between the age of 3–6 months
- Characterized by gradual onset of hypoxia, fever, cough and respiratory distress.

Management

- Intravenous/oral 15–20 mg of the trimethoprim and 75–100 mg of the sulfamethoxazole /24 hrs given every 6 hrs for 21 days.
  - If there is severe hypoxia give corticosteroids 2 mg/kg/24 hrs for 7–10 days then gradual tapering over 7–14 days.
- Alternative if intolerant to TMP/SMX: Pentamidine.
- Prophylaxis
  - Secondary-Lifelong after infection
  - Primary-Dependent on clinical stage and/or immunologic suppression.
- In case of allergy to CTX use Dapsone.

Common Oral Manifestations: Candidial Infection

Oral candidiasis is the most common oral condition in HIV infected children. Dysphagia and poor oral intake, irritability indicates involvement of the osophagus

- Three forms
  - Atrophic candidiasis

- ❍ Chronic hyperplasic candidiasis
- ❍ Angular Cheilitis

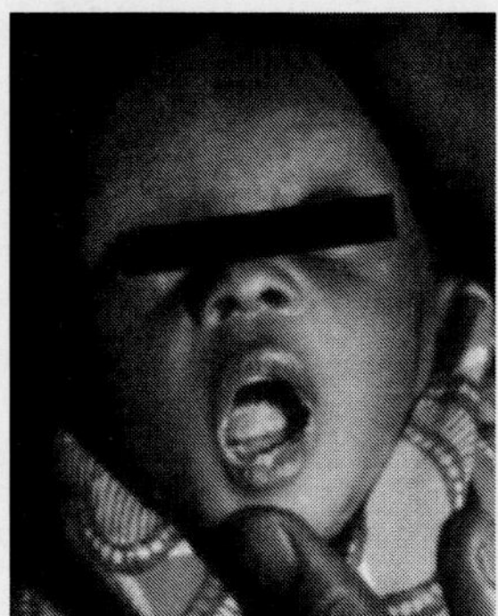

Fig. 14.2: Oral thrush

Management

- Oropharyngeal:
  - ❍ Nystatin 100, units/ml; 1–2 ml four times a day.
  - ❍ Oral miconazole gel 2.5 ml twice a day.
  - ❍ Fluconazole 3–6 mg/kg daily for 7–14 days.
- Esophageal disease: Fluconazole 6 mg/kg on day one then 3–6 mg/kg daily for minimum of 14–21 days.

Common Skin Manifestations

Bacterial Skin Infections

Folliculitis, cellulitis, skin abscesses impetigo, furunculosis and paronychia may occur with increasing frequency. *Staphylococcus aureus* is the cause in most bacterial skin infections. Good hand washing is needed to prevent spread of lesion.

Treatment

Erythromycin or cloxacillin.

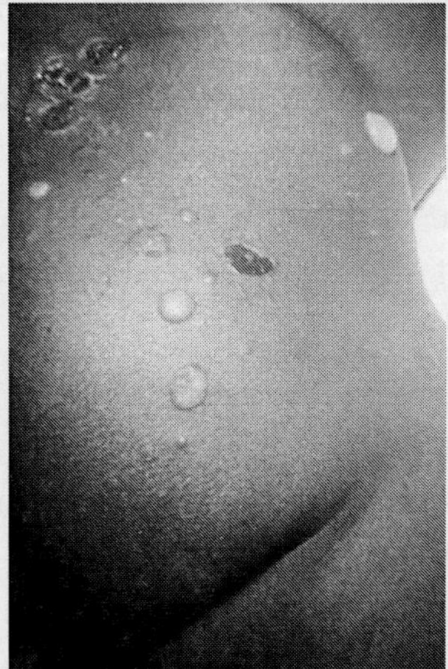

Fig. 14.3: Impetigo

Source: Paediatric HIV/AIDS Ethiopian Guidelines.

Molluscum Contagiosum

Common childhood viral infection is characterized by discrete, dome shaped pearly white papules with central umblication. Transmitted by skin to skin contact, self limited in most cases. In HIV-infected children Mollusum contagiosum tends to be extensive-covering > 5% of the body surface area.

Treatment

Liquid nitrogen, curettage. When patient is put on ART, it tends to resolve.

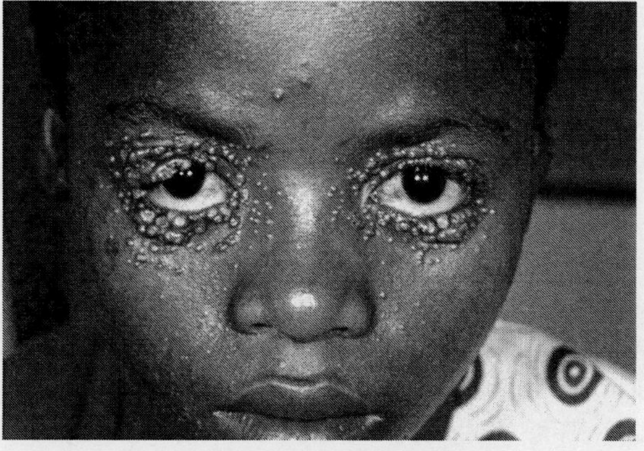

Fig. 14.4: Extensive Molluscum

Source: Paediatric HIV/AIDS Ethiopian Guideline.

Viral Infections

Herpes Zoster

It is recurrent, atypical and chronic, multidermatomes and may need use of acyclovir.

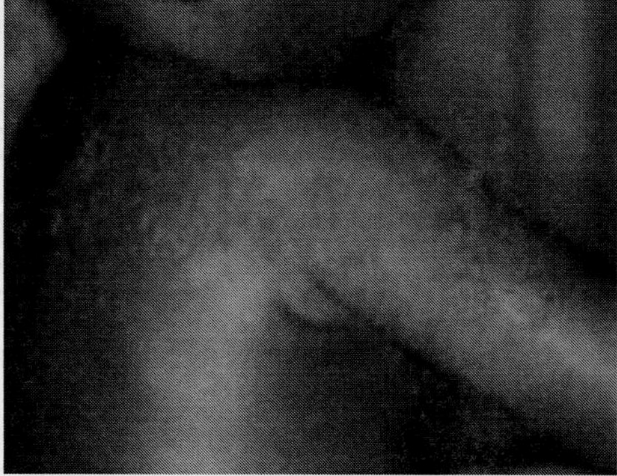

Fig. 14.5: Herpes Zoster

Varicella Zoster

Varicella is a highly contagious disease caused by varicella zoster virus, typically characterized by a generalized pruritic vesicular rash evolving to pustules and crusts which usually heal without scarring. it is treated by acyclovir 20 mg/kg orally four hours/day in patient with minimal decreased CD4 count. Topical antipuritic agents like Calamine lotion can be applied.

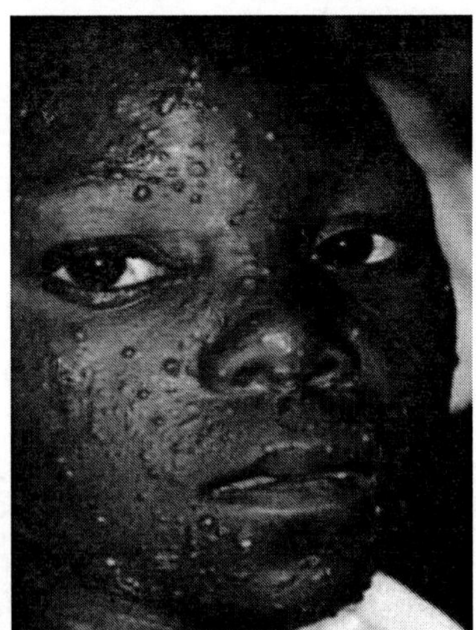

Fig. 14.6: Chicken pox (Varicella Zoster virus)

Scabies

Pruritic papular eruptions. In infants and children tend to involve the sole and the palms, diagnosis is made clinically. Norwegian scabies has generalized scaling and enlarged crusted plaques in the skin.

Treatment

- Benzyl benzoate lotion 25% is drug of choice, 10% sulfur ointment should be applied to the skin.

Seborrheic Dermatitis/Eczema

Seborrheic dermatitis/eczema is extensive and an early non-specific sign of HIV infection in infants.

It is thick yellow scales on the scalp but thin scales over the rest of the body.

Treatment

Topical steroids

Pruritic Papular Eruptions (PPE)

It is a chronic papular lesion of the skin. Etiology is unknown; PPE is evenly distributed over the trunk and extremities. A marker of worsening immunosuppression and may be stigmatizing. It causes secondary bacterial infection.

Treatment

Antihistamines and steroids

Common CNS Manifestations

A CNS manifestation occurs in 50–90% of perinatally infected children in developing countries.

Most common form is progressive encephalopathy; infants have a loss or plateau of developmental milestones, cognitive deterioration, impaired brain growth resulting in acquired microcephaly, apathy, spasticity, hyperreflexia and gait disturbances and loss of language and other motor skills. CT shows cerebral atrophy in 85% of children. Focal neurologic signs and seizure may occur with CNS lymphoma, toxoplasmosis, tuberculoma, and stroke.

Common Cardiovascular Manifestations

Dilated cardiomyopathy, persistent tachycardia and left ventricular hypertrophy are common manifestation in children. In advanced disease high frequency of autonomic instability leads to rhythm abnormality, Gallop rhythm, tachypnea. Hepatosplenomegaly indicates CHF. Treatment is anticongestive therapy. Cardiac complications are associated with poor prognosis.

Common GI Manifestations

Most frequent GI symptoms: Persistent or recurrent diarrhoea with malabsorption, abdominal pain, dysphagia and failure to thrive

- A variety of pathogens cause GI symptoms:
  - Bacteria (*Salmonella*, Campylobacter, MAC)
  - Protozoa (*Giardia, Cryptosporidium, Isosporia, Microsporida*)
  - Viruses (CMV, HSV, Rotavirus)
  - Fungi (Candida).
- MAC and protozoal infections are severe and protracted.
- Other GI manifestations are
  - Chronic liver inflammation with or without jaundice.
  - Pancreatitis with or without abdominal pain.
  - Chronic cholecystitis.
- Management depends on underlying pathology.
- Diarrheal illnesses are managed as per the IMCI guidelines.

Common Malignant Diseases

- Generally less frequent compared to adults and represent less than 2% of AIDS defining illnesses in children.
- Most frequent:
  - Non Hodgkin's lymphoma
  - Primary CNS lymphoma
  - Leiomyosarcoma

- Acute lymphoblastic leukaemia
- Epstein-Barr virus is associated with most cases of lymphomas and all cases of leiomyosarcoma.
- Kaposi sarcoma due to human herpes virus 8 occurs less frequently than in the adults.
- Vascular tumour that is present on the skin and internal organs.
- Treatment
  - Optimize ART
  - Chemotherapy.

ANTIRETROVIRAL THERAPY IN CHILDREN

Antiretroviral therapy is not an emergency intervention. Children need to be properly screened to ensure they meet eligibility criteria and that both children and family are ready for this undertaking.

Goal of ARV Therapy

- To maintain maximal suppression of viral replication.
- Restoration of immune function.
- Reduction of HIV-related morbidity and mortality.
- Improvement of quality of life and to prolong survival.

WHO 2010 Guidelines to Start ART on Children

When to start antiretroviral therapy in infants and children

Infants

1. Initiate ART for all HIV-infected infants diagnosed in the first year of life, irrespective of CD4 count or WHO clinical stage.

Children

2. Initiate ART for all HIV-infected children less than two years of age irrespective of CD4 count or WHO clinical stage.
3. Initiate ART for all HIV-infected children between 24 and 59 months of age with CD4 count of 750 cells/mm^3 or %CD4+ = 25% whichever is lower, irrespective of WHO clinical stage.
4. Initiate ART for all HIV-infected children more than 5 years of age with a CD4 count of 350 cells/mm^3 (as in adults), irrespective of WHO clinical stage.
5. Initiate ART for all HIV-infected children with WHO HIV clinical stages 3 and 4, irrespective of CD4 count.
6. Initiate ART for any child less than 18 months of age who has been given a presumptive clinical diagnosis of HIV infection.

When to start recommended first-line ART regimens for infants and children

Infants

1. For infants not exposed to ARVs, start ART with nevirapine (NVP) + 2 nucleoside reverse transcriptase inhibitors (NRTIs).
2. For infants exposed to maternal or infant NVP or other NNRTIs used for maternal treatment or PMTCT, start ART with lopinavir/ritonavir (LPV/r) + 2 NRTIs.
3. For infants whose exposure to ARVs is unknown, start ART with NVP + 2 NRTIs.

Children

4. For children between 12 and 24 months exposed to maternal or infant NVP or other NNRTIs used for maternal treatment or PMTCT, start ART with lopinavir/ritonavir (LPV/r) + 2 NRTIs.
5. For children more than 24 months and less than 3 years of age, start ART with NVP + 2 NRTIs.
6. For children 3 years of age and above, start ART with NVP or efavirenz (EFV)-containing regimen + 2 NRTIs.
7. For infants and children, the nucleoside backbone for an ART regimen should be one of the following, in preferential order:

   Lamivudine (3TC) + zidovudine (AZT) or 3TC + abacavir (ABC) or 3TC + stavudine (d4T)

Infants and Children with Specific Conditions

8. For children more than 3 years of age with tuberculosis (TB), the preferred regimen is EFV + 2 NRTIs.
9. For infants and children less than 3 years of age with TB, the preferred regimens are NVP + 2 NRTIs or a triple nucleoside regimen.
10. For a child or adolescent with severe anaemia (<7.5 g/dl) or severe neutropenia (<500 cells/mm^3), the preferred regimen is NVP + 2 NRTIs (avoid AZT).

11. For adolescents more than 12 years of age with hepatitis B, the preferred regimen is tenofovir (TDF) + emtricitabine (FTC) + NNRTI.

Table 14.5: WHO 2010 Guidelines when to Start Children on ART

Age	WHO 2010 Guidelines
Less than 24 months	
	All
24–59 months	
Clinical	Stage 3 or 4
Immunological*	<25% or <750
5 years and older	
Clinical	Stage 3 or 4
Immunological	<350

*CD4 percentage/absolute CD4 count mm^3.

Table 14.6: WHO Guidelines 2010 Immunologic Criteria for Starting ART in Children

2010	Immune Marker	Age specific recommendations to initiate ART			Clinical criteria
		<24 months	24–59 months	>5 years	Stage 3 and 4 disease
	CD4 percentage	All	<25%		
	CD4 count mm^3	All	<750 cells	<350 cells	

Source: Adapted from WHO 2010 revision. Essajee S.

Clinical and Laboratory Monitoring

CD4 Monitoring

1. CD4 should be measured at the time of diagnosis of HIV infection, and every 6 months thereafter. Monitor with increasing frequency as CD4 count approaches the threshold for starting ART.
2. CD4 should be measured prior to initiating ART.
3. CD4 should be measured every 6 months after initiating ART.
4. Measure CD4 if new clinical staging events develop, including growth faltering and neurodevelopment delay.
5. Where capacity for CD4 measurement is limited, target the use of CD4 monitoring to assess the significance of clinical events.

Viral Load Monitoring

6. VL determination is desirable, but not essential, prior to initiating ART.
7. VL should be assessed to confirm clinical or immunological failure where possible, prior to switching a treatment regimen.

Routine Clinical and Laboratory Monitoring

8. Baseline haemoglobin level (and white cell count, if available) should be determined at initiation of ART.
9. For infants and children, measure haemoglobin at week 8 after initiation of AZT-containing regimens or more frequently if symptoms indicate.
10. Growth, development and nutrition should be monitored monthly.
11. Laboratory monitoring for toxicity should be symptom directed.

First-line Regimen Treatment Failure; When to Switch Regimens

1. A switch to a second-line regimen is recommended when:
   - Clinical failure is recognized and/or
   - Immunological failure is recognized and/or
   - Virological failure is recognized.
2. Clinical failure is recognized as the appearance or reappearance of WHO clinical stage 3 or stage 4 events after at least 24 weeks on ART in a treatment-adherent child.
3. Immunological failure is recognized as developing or returning to the following age-related immunological thresholds after at least 24 weeks on ART, in a treatment-adherent child:
   - CD4 count of 200 cells/mm^3 or % CD4 + = 10% for a child more than 2 years to less than 5 years of age.
   - CD4 count of 100 cells/mm^3 for a child 5 years of age or more.
4. Virological failure is recognized as a persistent VL above 5,000 RNA copies/ml, after at least 24 weeks on ART, in a treatment-adherent child.

Choice of Second-line Regimens in the Event of Treatment Failure

1. After failure on a first-line NNRTI-based regimen, a boosted PI plus 2 NRTIs are recommended for second-line ART.
2. LPV/r is the preferred boosted PI for a second-line ART regimen after failure on a first-line NNRTI-based regimen.

3. After failure on a first-line regimen of AZT or d4T + 3TC, the ABC + 3TC is the preferred NRTI backbone option for second-line ART; ABC + didanosine (ddI) is an alternative.
4. After failure on a first-line regimen of ABC + 3TC, AZT + 3TC is the preferred NRTI backbone option for second-line ART; AZT + ddI is an alternative.

Considerations for Infants and Children with Tuberculosis and HIV

Isoniazid Preventive Therapy

1. All HIV-infected infants and children exposed to TB through household contacts, but with no evidence of active disease, should begin isoniazid preventive therapy (IPT).
2. Children living with HIV (older than 12 months of age and including those previously treated for TB), who are not likely to have active TB and are not known to be exposed to TB, should receive 6 months of IPT as part of a comprehensive package of HIV care.
3. Infants living with HIV, who are unlikely to have active TB and are not known to have been exposed to TB, should not receive IPT as part of a comprehensive package of HIV care.
4. The recommended dose of isoniazid (INH) for preventive therapy in HIV coinfection is 10 mg/kg/daily for 6 months (maximum 300 mg/day).

Infants and Children Diagnosed with TB and HIV

5. Any child with active TB disease should begin TB treatment immediately, and start ART as soon as tolerated in the first 8 weeks of TB therapy, irrespective of CD4 count and clinical stage.
6. The preferred first-line ARV regimen for infants and children less than 3 years of age, who are taking a rifampicin-containing regimen for TB, is 2 NRTIs + NVP or a triple NRTI regimen.
7. The preferred first-line ARV regimen for children more than 3 years of age, who are taking a rifampicin-containing regimen for TB, is 2 NRTIs + EFV.
8. The preferred first-line ARV regimen for infants and children less than 2 years of age, who have been exposed to NVP and are taking a rifampicin-containing regimen for TB, is a triple NRTI regimen.

HIV-infected Infants and Children Who Develop TB on ART

9. For all HIV-infected children, anti-TB therapy should be started immediately upon the diagnosis of TB; ART should continue.
10. Make adjustments to ART regimens as needed to decrease the potential for toxicities and drug interactions:
    - If on a regimen of 2 NRTIs + NVP, substitute EFV for NVP if the child is 3 years of age or older.
    - If on a regimen of 2 NRTIs + NVP and substitution with EFV is not possible, increase NVP to the maximum dose.
    - If on a regimen of LPV/r, consider adding RTV to a 1 : 1 ratio of LPV : RTV to achieve the full therapeutic dose of LPV.

Consideration for the Nutrition for HIV-Infected Infants and Children

1. HIV-infected children should be assessed routinely for nutritional status, including weight and height at scheduled visits, particularly after the initiation of ART.
2. HIV-infected children on or off ART who are symptomatic, have conditions requiring increased energy (*e.g.* TB, chronic lung disease, chronic opportunistic infections [OIs] or malignancies), have weight loss or have evidence of poor growth, should be provided with 25–30% additional energy.
3. HIV-infected children who are severely malnourished should be managed as per the guidelines for uninfected children and provided with 50–100% additional energy.
4. HIV-infected children should receive one recommended daily allowance (RDA) of micronutrients. If this cannot be assured through the diet, or there is evidence of deficiency, then supplementation should be given.
5. HIV-infected infants and children between 6 and 59 months of age should receive high-dose vitamin A supplementation every 6 months, as per the guidelines for uninfected children.
6. HIV-infected children who have diarrhoea should receive zinc supplementation as a part of management, as per the guidelines for uninfected children.
7. For infants and young children known to be HIV infected, mother are strongly encouraged to exclusively breastfeed for 6 months and to

continue breastfeeding as per recommendations for the general population (i.e., upto two years of age and beyond).

Adherence to ART

1. Pill boxes/calendars/diaries or other practical tools should be used to support adherence.

Table 14.7: Clinical Criteria for Presumptive Diagnosis of Severe HIV Disease in Infants and Children <18 Months of Age

A presumptive diagnosis of severe HIV disease should be made if: • The infant is confirmed HIV antibody positive; and • Diagnosis of any AIDS-indicator conditions can be made; or • The infant is symptomatic with two or more of the following: ❍ Oral thrush ❍ Severe pneumonia ❍ Severe sepsis Other factors that support the diagnosis of severe HIV disease in an HIV seropositive infant include: • Recent HIV-related maternal death, or • Advanced HIV disease in the mother • CD4 < 20% in infant Confirmation of the diagnosis of HIV infection should be sought as soon as possible.

Prior to ART Initiation—Adherence Preparation

- Identify and fully counsel caregivers
- Confirm availability of support services (family, social, inpatients care, etc.)
  - Consistent caregiver for administration, supervision of medication should be available.
- Identify barriers to treatment for the caretaker and address where possible.
- Prepare family and child for adherence
  - Completion of adherence/counseling sessions —may vary at each site.
- Address disclosure where appropriate.

Assessing Adherence Readiness

The Family

- Disclosure, family supports, availability of consistent caregiver for administration/ supervision—will vary with family structure, responsible family member who will be able to keep follow-up appointments, education to caregiver to understand the regimen, dosages, side effects, the caregiver should understand the need for close monitoring and follow-up and understand the need for strict adherence.

Barriers to Address before Starting

ART-health professional should explain about the following:

- Drug taste, volume and burden.
- Poverty and financial variables in general-transportation, employment and work schedule, food availability.
- The caregiver having following traits should not be used
  - Lack of disclosure
  - Lack of emotional support
  - Lack of belief in HIV as the cause of illness and the efficacy of treatment
  - Caregiver is too sick to provide care

Paediatric First-line Therapy

Infants and Children >12 Months of Age

The recommended first–line regimen for children >12 months of age is 2NRTIs + 1 NNRTI. A fixed dose combination of d4T + 3TC and NVP is the preferred first–line drug in children. FDC is available in the right strength and combination and should be used for children.

Infants <12 Months of Age

For HIV-infected infants with no exposure to maternal or infant non-nucleoside reverse transcriptase inhibitors, or whose exposure to maternal or infant antiretroviral is unknown, standard nevirapine-containing triple therapy should be started (2 NRTS + 1 Nevirapine). For infants <12 months of age with a history of exposure to single dose of nevirapine or non–nucleoside reverse transcriptase inhibitors contains maternal antiretroviral therapy or preventive antiretroviral regimens, a protease inhibitor-based triple antiretroviral therapy should be started with close monitoring. These recommendations are based on new WHO guidance released in September 2010.

Zidovudine (AZT)

- Formulation
  - Syrup: 10 mg/ml

- Capsules: 100 mg; 250 mg
- Tablet: 300 mg

- May be crushed and combined with food
- Syrup is light sensitive, needs to be stored in a glass jar
- Should not be used with d4T because of possible antagonism
- Side effects
  - Common-anaemia, granulocytopenia, GI upset
  - Less common-myopathy and mitochondrial disease

Lamivudine (3TC)

- Formulation
  - Oral solution: 10 mg/ml
  - Tablet: 150 mg
- Generally well tolerated
- Store solution at room temperature
- Tablet can be mixed with water or food and taken immediately
- Use within one month of opening the bottle
- Side effects
  - Generally rare, include headache, nausea, rarely pancreatitis and elevated LFTs

Stavudine (d4T)

- Formulation
  - Oral solution: 1 mg/ml
  - Capsules: 15 mg, 20 mg, 30 mg
- Solution must be refrigerated
- Capsules may be opened and mixed with small amount of food
- Should not be used with AZT because of possible antagonism
- Side effects-
  - Common: Headache and GI disturbance, peripheral neuropathy is less common
  - Less common: Metabolic abnormalities, particularly lipoatrophy
  - Life threatening: Lactic acidosis and severe hepatomegaly with steatosis, including fatal cases, have been reported with d4T use

Nevirapine (NVP)

- Formulation
  - Oral solution: 10 mg/ml
  - Tablet: 200 mg
- Can be given with food
- Store suspension at room temperature; must be shaken well
- NVP is initiated at a lower dose and increased in a stepwise fashion
- Side effects
  - Common: Skin rash, do no escalate dose
  - Life threatening: Liver toxicity can occur but is less common than in adults, can be fatal, discontinue for grade 3 toxicity, Steven Johnson Syndrome.

Abacavir (ABC)

- Formulation
  - Oral solution: 20 mg/ml
  - Tablet: 300 mg
- Can be given with food
- Tablet can be crushed and mixed with small amount of water or food and immediately ingested
- Side effects
  - Common: Headache, GI upset
  - Life threatening: Rare (<3%) fatal hypersensitivity reaction, do not rechallenge.

Calculating Doses

- Some drugs are based on weight-mg/kg
- Some drugs are based on Body Surface Area-mg/m^2
- Use standardized weight dosing chart since this is more convenient and reduces chance of errors.

Paediatric Second-Line Therapy

When treatment must be changed because of clinical and/or immunological failure, the entire drug must be changed. Always review adherence and make sure it is adequate. In certain instances Directly Observed Therapy (DOT) may be required. The preferred second line regimen is a boosted PI combined with two new NRTI agents. For children on standard first-line regimen the preferred second-line regimen is ABC + ddI or AZT + ddI. ART sequencing based on resistance patterns associated with specific agents. Goal is to replace failing first-line regimen with a second that has minimal potential for cross resistance. Choices balance potency, toxicity, formulation, and cost, as new data becomes available, these may change.

Table 14.8: Preferred Second-line Regimen for Children

First-line regimen	Preferred second-line regimen
AZT or d4T + 3TC	ABC + 3TC
ABC + 3TC	AZT + 3TC

*NFV can be substituted for LPV/r if no cold chain is available didanosine (ddI) is an alternative.

Abacavir (ABC)

- Formulation
  - Oral solution: 20 mg/ml
  - Tablet: 300 mg
- Can be given with food
- Tablet can be crushed and mixed with small amount of water or food and immediately ingested
- Side effects
  - Common—Headache, GI upset
  - Life threatening—Rare (<3%) fatal hypersensitivity reaction, do not rechallenge

Didanosine (ddI)

- Formulation
  - 25, 50, 100, 200 mg tabs
  - 10 mg/ml liquid
- For proper buffer dose, 2 tabs must be used
- Administer on empty stomach 1 hour before or 2 hours after meal; don't take with acidic drinks but can take with water
- This may make administration of regimen difficult, as drugs may not all be taken together
- Side effects
  - Common: GI intolerance
  - Serious: Peripheral neuropathy, pancreatitis

Lopinavir/Ritonavir (Kaletra)

- Formulation—dose based on lopinavir
  - Solution: 80/20 mg/ml
  - Capsule: 133.3/33.3 mg
- Must take with food
- Can be stored at room temperature once dispensed—stable for 60 days
- Bad taste can be masked with sweets, peanut butter
- A very "forgiving" drug
- Side effects
  - Common: Abdominal pain, nausea, headache, increase in blood lipids
  - Less common: Hyperglycemia, fat redistribution

Note: First line and second line ART treatment regimen varies in different nations.

ADHERENCE IN CHILDREN

ARV treatment requires collaboration between the child, caregiver and medical provider. Adherence in children is challenging, as such efforts to maximize adherence should begin prior to treatment initiation. Continuous assessment and support of adherence is fundamental to successful antiretroviral therapy and to prevent development of drug resistance.

Goals of Adherence

- To ensure patient takes >95% of prescribed doses,
- To prevent development of resistance,

Role of the Healthcare Team in Adherence

Health providers, nurses, pharmacists, counsellors (health professionals, non-health professionals or community counsellors) physicians and social workers (case managers) play an important role in ensuring adherence.

- Health providers should develop a trusting relationship with the patient and family.
- The providers role should be supportive, non-judgemental and honest.
- Feedback from the counsellor to the rest of the team is important.

Factors Associated with Adherence

- Demographic variables: age, sex, caregiver type, caregiver sex, income.
- Disclosure to child, to others.
- Caregiver-child communication.
- Caregiver self-efficacy.
- Caregiver health beliefs.
- Caregiver depression.

- Stress.
- Stigma.

An Approach to Adherence: Giving Medications to Infants and Children

- Promoting Adherence
  - Education
  - Preparation
  - Monitoring
  - Support
- Assessing Adherence
  - Assessment Methods
  - Addressing Barriers

1. Adherence Education
   - Define adherence
     - Never missing a dose
     - Taking >95% of prescribed doses
     - Keeping to specific times of administration
     - Taking it the "right" way
     - Lifelong treatment, even when feeling well
     - Underscore difficulty of task
   - Explain importance of strict adherence
     - Failure of adherence may be temporary, however the effect on treatment choices may be permanent
     - Use simple terms, open–ended questions, visual aids, analogies
   - Emphasize need for communication with health -care team
     - Foster partnership, trust and honesty
     - Negotiate treatment plan that patient and caregiver can understand
     - Encourage disclosure to family who can support treatment plan
2. Adherence Preparation and Practice
   - Assess the family for readiness for therapy
   - Discuss medications Address the WHO, WHAT, WHEN and HOW of medication administration.
   - WHO will administer the medications?

     Every day, weekdays and weekends?
   - WHAT medications will be given?

     Familiarity with medication
   - WHEN will medications be given?

     Establish specific times and routines
   - HOW will medications be given?

     Details of administration: using syringes or measured spoons, cutting and crushing tablets, with or without food, mixed with beverage, mixed together, sequencing.
   - Practice taking medication

     Taste testing, observation of dosing, training for pill swallowing, behavioural reward system, role play.
3. Adherence Monitoring
   - No perfect measures
   - Emphasize the importance of honest reporting
   - Importance of multidisciplinary approach to monitoring
   - Provide all possible support as discussed in adult ART care
4. Adherence Support
   - Psychosocial support in the form of counselling on disclosure
     - Linkages in the community
     - Create links with support groups and encourage discussion on adherence
   - Adherence aids or tools
     - Pill boxes
     - Calendars
     - Pre-labelling syringes
5. Assess the Incomplete Adherence
   - Review current regimen
   - Inquire about problems administering medications—obtain a descriptive assessment
   - Review WHO, WHAT, WHEN, HOW
   - Observe administration

Palliative Care

Children who are terminally ill should be provided with supportive care to:

- Provide emotional support to the dying child and grieving family
- Keep the patient as comfortable as possible and maintain a good quality of life.

Importance of Palliative Care

- Provide relief from pain and other stress from the child
- Treat easily manageable conditions to get the symptomatic benefits of treatment
- Minimizing the hospitalization, encouraging the homecare with available community resources.

Homecare

Palliative care for dying child should be at home if possible. The local primary healthcare service must assist in providing care. It is important to assure the parents/caregivers, that the child has not been abandoned by the healthcare service. Palliative care approach in these children gives relief by providing comfort first then prevents and relieves physical suffering like pain. Pain control is important aspect of palliative care in HIV/AIDS children. Initially it is advisable to use non-opioids such as paracetamol or non-steroidal anti-inflammatory agents even though pain cannot be controlled by these medications. However, we must help the children get freed from pain by providing weak opioids or strong opioids like codine, tramadol, Pethadine, Morphine. Care should be given at the end of the life which includes

- Physical comfort
- Home with loved ones
- Emotional support
- Spiritual support
- Rituals
- Bereavement support

Inpatient Management

Patients should be managed in hospital if they have problem of respiratory distress, dehydration. Due to poor intake of fluids, they need administration of oxygen and adequate hydration by intravenous fluids or nastrogastric tube feeding or if caregivers are unable to cope at home. Pain management is given to relieve the pain and care given to anticipate complications (*e.g.*, constipation) and manage accordingly.

PAEDIATRIC FORMULAS

(1) CALCULATION OF DRUGS

(a) According to body surface area:

$$\text{Child dose} = \frac{\text{Childs body surface area}}{\text{Adults body surface area}} \times \text{Adult dose}$$

(b) Young's Formula:

$$\text{According to age} = \frac{\text{Age of child}}{\text{Age} + 12} \times \text{adult dose}$$

(c) Calculation of flow rate:

$$\text{Drop/min} = \frac{\text{Total volume}}{\text{Time in mnute}} \times \text{drop factor}$$

(2) DEGREE OF MALNUTRITION

$$\text{Malnutrition} = \frac{\text{Actual weight}}{\text{Expected weight}} \times 100$$

(a) Classification by Indian academy of paediatrics:

Grade I – between 71–80% of expected weight for that age

Grade II – between 61–70% of expected weight for that age

Grade III – between 51–60% of expected weight for that age

Grade IV – 50% on less of expected weight for that age

(b) Gomez Classification:

Grade I – between 75–90% of expected weight for that age

Grade II – between 61–75% of expected weight for that age

Grade III – weight less than or equal to 60% of expected weight for that age

(3) CALCULATION OF EXPECTED WEIGHT ACCORDING TO AGE:

(a) For age (1 month to 12 months):

$$\text{Weight} = \frac{\text{age in month} + 9}{2}$$

(b) For age (1 to 6 yrs):

Weight = (age in yrs × 2) + 8

(c) For age (6 to 12 yrs):

$$\text{Weight} = \frac{(\text{age in yrs} \times 7) - 5}{2}$$

(4) CALCULATION OF HEIGHT

(a) At birth–about 50 cms

(b) At 1 yr–about 75 cms

(c) At 2–12 yrs of age: (height = age in yrs × 6) + 77

(5) IDENTIFICATION OF DEHYDRATION

SIGN	WEIGHT CHANGES MILD 2–5%	WEIGHT CHANGES MODERATE 6–10%	WEIGHT CHANGES SEVERE 10–15%	WEIGHT CHANGES DEATH 15 – 20%
Fluid volume loss	< 50 ml/kg	50-90 ml/kg	> 100 ml/kg	
Skin colour	Pale	Gray	Mottled	
Skin elasticity	Decreased	Poor	Very poor	
Mucus membrane	Dry	Very dry	Patched	
Urinary output	Decreased	Oliguria	Marked oliguria	
Blood pressure	Normal	Normal/low	Lowered	
Pulse	Normal or increased	Increased	Rapid and thread	
Capillary refill time	< 2 sec	2–3 sec	> 3 sec	

weight gain 2% mild +ve 5% moderate +ve 8% severe +ve

(6) SIGNS AND SYMPTOMS OF DEHYDRATION:

- Skin colour -- gray
- Temperature -- cold
- Turgor -- poor/fair
- Feel -- dry, cleaning, thickened
- Mucus membrane -- dry, moist, patched
- Tear and salivation -- absent
- Eye ball -- sunken
- Fontanel -- sunken
- Body temperature – subnormal/elevated
- Pulse – rapid
- Respiration -- rapid
- Behaviour -- irritable/lethargic/convulsion/ hyper irritability on stimulation.

(7) NATIONAL IMMUNIZATION SCHEDULE:

At birth	BCG and OPV – 0 dose
At 6 weeks	BCG (if not given at birth) DPT – 1, OPV -- 1, HEP B -- 1
At 10 weeks	DPT – 2, OPV -- 2, HEP B -- 2
At 14 weeks	DPT – 3, OPV -- 3, HEP B -- 3
At 9 months	Measles
At 16–24 months	DPT and OPV
At 5–6 yrs	DT – 2
At 10 and 16 yrs	TT vaccine
Early in pregnancy	TT – 1/booster
One month after TT -	TT – 2

(8) ADVANTAGES OF BREAST FEEDING:

- Safest, cheapest and best protective food
- Essential for brain growth
- Facilitates absorption of calcium, helps in bone growth
- Easily digestable
- Contain Ig A, Ig M, Ig M, Macrophages
- Provides immunity
- Protects the infant from allergy and bronchial asthma
- Promotes physical and emotional bonding
- Economical in terms of saving of money, time and energy

(9) WEANING FOOD AT DIFFERENT AGE

(a) 4–6 months:

- ✓ Fruit juices, suji, biscuit soaked in milk, vegetable soup, mashed banana, mashed and boiled patato.
- ✓ Each food should be given with one/two tea spoon at first 3 to 6 times/day.

(b) 6–9 months:

- ✓ Soft mixture of rice, dal, khichri, pulses, mashed and boiled potato, bread, roti, soaked in milk, dal, mashed fruits like banana, mango, papaya, apple.
- ✓ Egg yolk, curd and khir.
- ✓ The infant can have these foods 5 to 6 times/day and the amount of food to be increased gradually.

(c) 9–12 months:

- ✓ Fish, meat, chicken.
- ✓ Feeds needs not to be mashed but should be soft and well cooked.

(d) 12–18 months:

- ✓ Needs half amount of mothers diet.
- ✓ Number of feeds can be 4 to 5 times or according to the child needs.
- ✓ Breast feeding should be continued especially at night.

(10) CALCULATION OF BODY MASS INDEX:

$$\text{BMI} = \frac{\text{Weight in kg}}{\text{(height in metre) 2}}$$

(11) CALCULATION OF FLUID REPLACEMENT FORMULA

(a) Parkland formula

- 4 ml RL solution x kg of body weight x% total body surface area burned.
- One half of total is given in the first 8 hours post-burn.
- One fourth of total is given in the second 8 hours post-burn
- One fourth of total is given in the third 8 hours post-burn.

(b) Rule of nine for estimation of burns surface area

AREA	AGE (0–5YR)	AGE (5–10YR)	AGE ABOVE 10 YRS
Head and neck	20%	15%	10%
Trunk-front	20%	20%	20%
Trunk-back	20%	20%	20%
Upper limbs	10 × 2 = 20%	10 × 2 = 20%	10 × 2 = 20%
Lower limbs	10 × 2 = 20%	15 × 2 = 30%	15 × 2 = 30%
Total	100% (20 × 5)	105% * (20 × 5) = (105–5) = 100%	100% (20 × 5)

NOTE: *5% to be deducted from trunk

(c) Lund and browder % distribution of burns surface area.

AREA	BIRTH	AGE 1 YEAR	AGE 5 YRS	10 YR	15 YR	ADULT
A = ½ of head	9½	8½	6½	5½	4½	3½
B = ½ of one thigh	2¾	3¼	4	4½	4½	4¾
C = ½ of one leg	2½	2½	2¾	3	3¼	3½

(12) RECOMMENDED CALORIES FOR ALL THE AGE GROUPS:

(a) New born: Calories 120 K Cal/kg

(b) Infant: Calories 120 K Cal/kg

(c) Toddler: Calories 1300 – 1500 K Cal/kg

(d) Pre-scholar: Calories 1300 – 1500 K Cal/kg

(e) School age: Calories 1600 – 2200 K Cal/kg

(f) Adolescence: Calories 2200 – 2800 K Cal/kg.

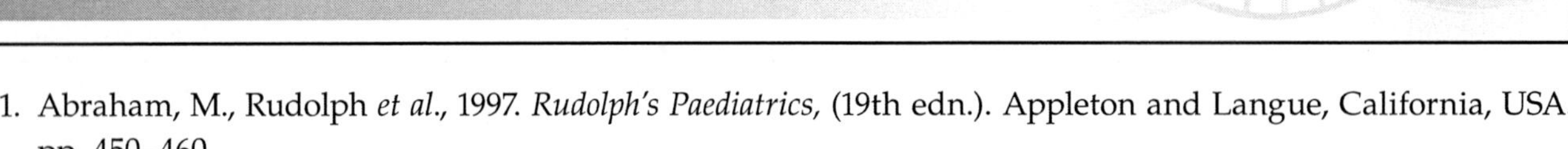

References

1. Abraham, M., Rudolph *et al.*, 1997. *Rudolph's Paediatrics,* (19th edn.). Appleton and Langue, California, USA. pp. 450–460.
2. Abraham M. Rudolph *et al.*, 2002. *Rudolph's Fundamentals of Paediatrics,* (3rd edn.). The McGraw-Hill Companies, Inc., New York, USA. pp. 163–165, 441–422.
3. Achar, 1992. *Textbook of Paediatrics,* (7th edn.). Saunders Publications, New Delhi. pp. 741–765.
4. Addison-Wesley Nursing, 1994. *Essential of Maternal-Newborn Nursing,* (3rd edn.). A division of the Benjamin/ Cummings Publishing Company, Inc.
5. Adele Pillitteri, 1987. *Child Health Nursing Care of Growing Family,* (3rd edn.). Little Brown and Company, Boston. pp. 100–143.
6. African Palliative Care Association, 2009. *Guidelines and a Handbook of Pain Management and Palliative Care in Africa.* Vol. 1. pp. 20–46.
7. Agraharkar M., Gala, G., Gangakhedkar, A. K., 2007. Nephrotic syndrome.emedicine.
8. American Heart Association and American Academy of Paediatrics, 2000. *Neonatal Resuscitation,* (4th edn.).
9. Annaamma Jacob, 2008. *A Comprehensive Textbook of Midwifery,* (2nd edn.). Jaypee Brothers Medical Publication (P) Ltd., New Delhi. pp. 589–595, 562–567.
10. Assaye Kassie Nigussie, 2008. *Manual of Neonatal Basic Life Support,* (2nd edn.) Addis Ababa University Publication, Addis Ababa, Ethiopia. pp. 31–36.
11. Ballard, J. L., Novar, K. K., Driver, M., 1979. A simplified score for assessment of foetal maturation of newly born infants. *J. Pediatrics,* **5:** 769–774.
12. Barbara Aehlert, 2007. *Pals Paediatric Advanced Life Support Study Guide,* (Revised 2nd edn.). Elsevier Mosby Jems, St. Louis. pp. 50–52.
13. Barbara Kozier, Glenora Erb, 1997. *Fundamental of Nursing,* (7th edn.). Addison–Wesley Publishing Company, Health Division. Menlopark, California. pp. 456–520.
14. Behrman Kliegman, 2006. *Nelson Essentials of Paediatrics,* (5th edn.). Saunders Elsevier Company, Philadelphia. pp. 1012–1025.
15. Boggale, W., Assaye, K., 2005. A randomized control trail on effectiveness of early Kangaroo care for the low birth infants. *Journal of Tropical Paediatrics,* **51**(2): 93–97.
16. Carol, Taylor, Carol, Lillis *et al.*, 2005. *Fundamentals of Nursing, The Art and Science of Nursing Care,* (5th edn.). Wolterskluwer Health, Lippincott Williams and Wilkin's, Philadelphia, USA. pp. 782–785.
17. Charpak, N., Ruiz-Pelaz, J., and Figueroa, Z., 2005. Influence of feeding patterns and other factors on early somatic growth of healthy, preterm infants in home-based kangaroo mother care: A cohort study. *Journal of Pediatric Gastroenterol Nutrition,* **41**(4): 430–437.
18. David, N., Herndon, 2007. *Total Burn Care,* (3rd edn.). Saunders Elsevier Inc. Philadelphia. pp. 127, 134, 398–405.

19. Guha, Dipak K., Guha, Rashmi *et al.*, 2006. *Manual of Newborn Critical Care Medicine,* (1st edn.). Jaypee Brothers Medical Publishers (P) Ltd. pp. 95–100, 120–140.

20. Dodd, V., 2005. Implications of kangaroo care for growth and development in preterm infants. *Journal of Obstetrics, Gynecologic, and Neonatal Nursing,* **34**(2): 218–232.

21. Donna, L., Wong Marilyn Hockenberry-Eaton *et al.*, 2001. *Wong's Essentials of Paediatric Nursing,* (6th edn.). Mosby, Inc. St. Louis. pp. 201–216, 290–500, 993–951, 1185–1207.

22. Doroth, R., Barbard, A., Redding, 2002. *Textbook of Paediatric Nursing,* (6th edn.), W.B. Saunders Company, Philadelphia, USA.

23. Federal Ministry of Health, Ethiopia, 2008. *Integrated Management of Newborn and Childhood Illness (IMNCI) Manual,* Family Health Department, Addis Ababa, Ethiopia. pp. 2–74.

24. Federal Ministry of Health, 2008. *Guidelines for Paediatric HIV/AIDS Care and Treatment in Ethiopia.* Federal HIV/AIDS Prevention and Control Office, Addis Ababa, Ethiopia. pp. 40–150.

25. Freed, M. D., 1999. *Moss and Adams' Heart Disease in Infant, Children, and Adolocescents,* (6th edn.). Lippincott-Williams & Wilkins, Philadelphia, USA. pp. 400–600.

26. Leifer Gloria, 2007. *Introduction to Maternity and Paediatric Nursing,* (5th edn.). Saunders Elsevier, St. Louis Missouri, USA. pp. 426–427, 451–468.

27. Guha, D. K., 1997. *Neonatology Principle and Practice,* (2nd edn.). Jaypee Brothers Medical Publication (P) Ltd., New Delhi. pp. 275–289.

28. Hal, B., Jenson, Richard E. Bahrman, 2002. *Essentials of Paediatric,* (17th edn.). Saunders Elsevier, Philadelphia, USA. pp. 537–549.

29. Hazinski, M. F., 1992. *Care of the Critically Ill Children,* (2nd edn.). Mosby, St. Louis, USA. pp. 120–124.

30. Health Concern about Adolescent available at www.who.int/child-adolescent-health/topics/prevention-care/adolescent/dev/en/index.htm/

31. Jane, W., Ball, Ruth, Bindler, C., 2003. *Paediatric Nursing Caring for Children,* (3rd edn.). Pearson Education, Inc. pp. 471–491, 613–615.

32. Keliegman Behrman, Jenson, Stanta, 2007. *Nelson Textbook of Paediatrics,* (18th edn.). Saunders Elsevier, St. Louis, Missouri, USA. pp. 750–900.

33. Lane, J., 2008. Nephrotic syndeome.emedicine.

34. London, M., Ladewig, P., Ball, J. and Bindler, R., 2006. *Maternal and Child Nursing Care,* (2nd edn.). Upper Saddle River, NJ: Pearson Prentice Hall. pp. 573, 791–793.

35. London, Patrica A., Ladewig *et al.*, 2006. *Kangaroo Mother Care for Low Birth Infant.* (2nd edn.).

36. Ludington-Hoe, S., Hosseini, R., and Torowicz, D., 2005. Skin-to-skin contact (Kangaroo Care) analgesia for preterm infant heel stick. *AACN Clinical Issues,* **16**(3): 373–387.

37. Verklan M. Tereses and Marlene Walden, 2000. Neonatal *Intensive Care Nursing,* (3rd edn.). Saunders Elsevier, St. Louis Missouri, USA. pp. 102–113.

38. Duncobe Margaret and Weller Barbara, 1985. *Paediatric Nursing,* (5th edn.). Williams and Wilkins Company, Baltimore. pp. 157–163.

39. Marka, Helfear and David, G., Nichils, 2007. *Manual of Paediatric Critical Care,* (4th edn.). Hazinski, M.F., Saunders Elsevier, St. Louis Missouri, USA. pp. 122–113.

40. May and Mahleister, 1990. *Comprehensive Maternity Nursing,* (2nd edn.). Lippincott Publication, Philadelphia, USA. pp. 535–538.

41. Singh, Meharban, 2004. *Care of the Newborn,* (6th edn.). New Delhi. pp. 47–62.

42. Murphy, S. A., 2000. *The Use of Research Findings Bereavement Programs: Case Studies,* **24:** 584–602.
43. Ghai, O. P., 1993. *Essential Paediatrics,* (3rd edn.). Jaypee Brothers Medical Publications (P) Ltd., New Delhi. pp. 185–200.
44. Castiglia, Partica Thorson Harbin, Richard, E., 1992. *Child Health Care Process and Practice.* J.B. Lippincott Company, New York. pp. 60–73, 218–295. 1240–1290.
45. Revised Jones Criteria for Acute Rheumatic Fever (ARF) (March 2009), available at *http:/www.medical criteria. com/site/Index.*
46. Rheumatic Fever (RF) available at http://www.american heart.org/presenter.jhtml/identifier=4709.
47. Robert, A., Hoekelman *et al.,* 1992. *Primary Paediatric Care,* (2nd edn.). Mosby-Year Book, Inc, St. Louis. pp. 592.
48. Yurt, Roger W., 1999. *Roger's Textbook of Paediatrics,* (2nd edn.). er Wolters Kluwer Health, Lippincott Williams and Wilkin's, Philadelphia, USA. pp. 59–65.
49. Rosan, N. P., 1999. Acute head trauma. *In:* A. Mcmillan, C.D. Deangelis, R.D, Feigin and J.B. Warshawak (eds.), *Oski's Paediatrics: Principles and Practice,* (3rd edn.). Lippincott-Williams and Wilkins, Philadelphia, USA. pp. 603–617.
50. Sheton, T. L., and Steoabejm, I. S., 1994. *Family-Centered Care for Children Needing Specialized Health and Development Services.* Child Life Council, Life Council, 11820 Park Lawn Dr.# 202, MD 20814, pp. 301–881–7090.
51. Stewart, 2000, Emergency Care of Paediatric Burns, *Paediatric Emergency Medicine Report,* **5**(10): 102–112.
52. Thalassemia in Infants available at http://www.wrong diagnosis.com/t/thalassemia/cause.htm/ktract = Kcplink.
53. UNICEF, 2007. *Status of Young Child Survival and Development in Eastern and Southern Africa.* pp. 16–25.
54. Whaly and Wong, 1982. *Essential of Paediatric Nursing,* (6th edn.). Mosby Company, London. pp. 700–1500.
55. When to start antiretroviral therapy in infants and children available at http://www.searo.who/linkfiles/ publication 10, recommendation. pdf.
56. William, W., Hay, J. R. *et al.,* 2007. *Current Diagnosis and Treatment,* (19th edn.). The McGraw Hill Company Inc. New York. pp. 568–700.
57. Wolters Kluwer, 2008. *Straight A's in Paediatric Nursing,* (2nd edn.). Wolters Kluwer/Lippincott Williams and Wilkins. Philadelphia. pp. 268–271, 321–331, 414–418.
58. World Health Organization, 1996. Essential Newborn Care. *Report of a Technical Working Group Trieste,* 25–29 April 1996. WHO Geneva. Division of Reproductive Health. pp. 22–28.

INDEX

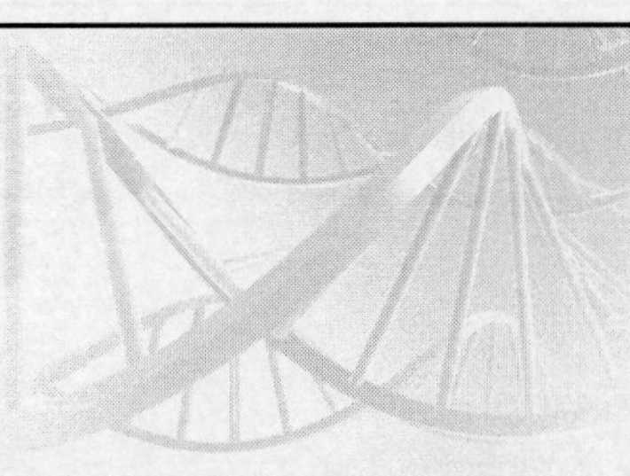